PSRO:

The Promise, Perspective, and Potential

PSRO:
The Promise, Perspective, and Potential

Editors:

John W. Bussman, M.D.

Sharon V. Davidson, R.N., B.S.N., M.Ed.

▲▼ **Addison-Wesley Publishing Company**
Medical/Nursing Division, Menlo Park, California
Reading, Massachusetts • London • Amsterdam
Don Mills, Ontario • Sydney

Sponsoring Editor: Pat Franklin
Production Coordinator: Madeleine Dreyfack
Production Editor: Nancy Sjoberg
Designer: Wendy C. Calmenson

Library of Congress Cataloging in Publication Data
Main entry under title:

PSRO.

  Bibliography: p.
  Includes index.
  1. Professional standards review organizations
(Medicine)—United States. 2. Medical care—
Evaluation. I. Bussman, John W., 1924–
II. Davidson, Sharon Van Sell, 1944–
RA399.A3P17   362.1'068   80-21668
ISBN 0-201-00790-8
ABCDEFGHIJ-HA-8987654321

The authors and publishers have exerted every effort to ensure
that drug selection and dosage set forth in this text are in
accord with current recommendations and practice at the time of
publication. However, in view of ongoing research, changes in
government regulations and the constant flow of information
relating to drug therapy and drug reactions, the reader is urged
to check the package insert for each drug for any change in
indications of dosage and for added warnings and precautions.
This is particularly important where the recommended agent is a
new and/or infrequently employed drug.

⋀ Addison-Wesley Publishing Company
Medical/Nursing Division
2725 Sand Hill Road
Menlo Park, California 94025

Preface

Since the passage of legislation in 1972 that established the Professional Standards Review Organizations (PSROs), these groups have been subjected to scrutiny from many sources, both in and outside of the government. The unique partnership between the bureaucracy and the medical profession has stimulated interest on the part of physicians dedicated to the assessment and assurance of the quality of health care; skepticism in Congress, which is searching for a means of slowing the spiraling rise in the cost of health care; resistance among members of the profession who resent the scrutiny of their practices; and resentment on the part of some health professionals who were excluded from active participation in the program.

Recent developments have demonstrated that PSROs are capable of assuring that health care services provided to federal beneficiaries are medically necessary and are delivered in appropriate settings; they also meet professionally acceptable standards of quality. The rapid expansion of the techniques used to evaluate the quality of health care and determine appropriate utilization has created an exciting movement in which PSROs are playing a leading role. The recent inclusion of PSRO provisions in all the major proposals for national health insurance is reassuring to those who feared for the long-term prospects of PSROs. Additionally, requests for extension of professional review for the privately insured population, either through federal mandate or by private contract with insurance carriers, give further evidence of recognition of the value of this approach.

Although much has been published on the PSRO program, usually by those outside the organizations, it seemed time to publish a comprehensive volume written by those involved in day-to-day operations. In organizing this text, we have first provided a historical perspective on the precursors of PSROs and the early implementation of the program. This section is followed by a description of the functions of the numerous components of PSROs. In the last section, we have attempted to predict the future development of the professional's involvement in utilization, review, and quality assessment. Our efforts should prove useful to students in medical and peer review fields, physicians, and PSRO staffs. Additionally, other professionals who are involved in evaluating the contributions of health care teams will also find this book valuable.

No one individual could attempt to write all the chapters on the many aspects of this complex program. The senior author (J.W.B.) has been involved since the early demonstration projects with the Experimental Medical Care Review Organizations, which predated the legislation. In working in many areas of professional review, he has been fortunate to be able to meet most of the leaders and innovators in the field of quality assurance, and many of them have kindly responded to his request to contribute to the creation of this volume.

ACKNOWLEDGMENTS

We wish to acknowledge our indebtedness to our many contributors, who despite pressing schedules, consented to share their knowledge and experience with others involved in this program. The valuable comments and suggestions of those who received the early drafts of chapters have helped to shape the final manuscript. Lastly, the staff of Addison-Wesley is to be thanked for the patience with which they accepted the frustrating delays in bringing the contributions of many authors together.

John W. Bussman
Sharon V. Davidson
January 1981

Foreword

Throughout history, society has accorded the learned professions a special status. Some might argue that this status is self-proclaimed and expresses private interests, but such reasoning overlooks the fact that more often than not it has been justly earned by commitment and contribution. And society, after all, is greatly benefited by the existence of strong and independent professions.

The feature that most distinguishes the learned professions is self-determination. Nowhere is this trait more evident than in the profession of medicine. Consider, for instance, that physicians select, instruct, examine, license, and determine credentials for their successors; oversee their own ethics; and accept responsibility for the discipline and censure of their own members. They add to, subtract from, and administer the body of knowledge that constitutes their reason for existence. They not only determine the modalities by which they will render their services but also determine their worth.

That society has chosen not to intrude on professional self-determination does not mean, however, that the professions are not held to account, for indeed they are. But such accountability has generally focused on process accountability rather than on technologic justification. Again, using medicine as an example, society asks that educational institutions be subject to accreditation, that licensing be accomplished by public rather than private agencies, that codes of ethics be published, that research be subjected to peer review, that the application of knowledge meet community standards and expectations, and that channels exist for hearing legitimate grievances.

This unwritten contract, wherein technologic and uniquely professional matters are left to the profession while process accountability resides with the public, has made it possible for the professions to grow in strength while society reaps its harvest from their contributions.

The challenge to our value systems and to the integrity of long-established institutions that characterized the movement of the 1960s and early 1970s has, however, resulted in an erosion of this contract. All professions appear to be subject to this erosion, but for three reasons medicine is the most vulnerable. First, for much the same reason that Disraeli concluded that health was power, the American public has declaimed that access to medical services should be accorded the status of a right for all citizens. Second, the unparalleled explosion of new knowledge so changed the profile of American medicine that it produced a gap between the perceived needs of the public and medicine's capacity to accommodate those needs. Third, the cost of medical care began to outstrip our ability (and perhaps even our willingness) to pay for it.

There is an irony here. One of the earliest public pronouncements that "health care is a right" came from a White House conference on aging and was subsequently reiterated in the preamble to myriad pieces of federal legislation. Similarly, advances in medical technology, new knowledge that came from research (and which led to specialism and subspecialism), and the marked increase in the number of independent, decision-making health professionals—all of which contributed enormously to the escalation of health care costs—were, themselves, articulated by government. Then, as if to reconcile this paradox, public funds in huge amounts were forcibly pumped into the health care system to bring modern medicine to large segments of the population.

Whether because of or in spite of this federal investment, the costs of medical care continued to rise while access was not thought to have improved. Blame, to the extent it could be assigned, was principally directed at medicine and served as both an impetus to and a justification for eroding the preexisting contract. No longer was process accountability accepted as a sufficient public role. Instead, a progressive intrusion into medicine's preserve of self-determination began. Educational institutions were enticed to sacrifice their autonomy in exchange for sustenance; recent graduates were persuaded to accept indentured service and geographic assignments in exchange for financial support as students; the responsibility for health facility planning and capital investment strategies were vested by law in consumers; hospital rates were subjected to public review; reimbursement levels for medical services rendered to large segments of our population were set by government; professional dominance of licensing bodies was increasingly diluted with public representation; and codes of professional ethics were openly attacked as inimical to the public interest because they were thought to restrain trade.

The most vigorous challenge to medicine came, however, with public intervention into the uniquely professional area of quality control. Thus, when the Professional Standards Review Organizations amendment to the Social Security Amendments of 1972 was enacted into law, the reaction from American medicine was less than congenial. When one recognizes that no national government has ever before entered the province of the control of the quality of a medically rendered service in the private sector, such a reaction seems wholly reasonable.

To the credit of the authors of this new form of public intrusion into what had heretofore been a private interest, it can be said that their motivation was rational even if their premise was not. The cost of medical care was, indisputably, increasing at a rate that was unacceptable. Because an increasingly large expenditure of public funds was involved, this was thought to justify a solution that was publicly contrived. The alternative, to retard the rate of increase in medical care costs by cutting back federal expenditures for health care, was politically unacceptable.

If such reasoning was politically rational, however, the premise on which it was founded was not. There is little evidence that cost and quality rise or fall in parallel. Better quality frequently costs more. Recognizing this, American medicine responded to the arrival of the PSRO by noting that to adopt standards is to adopt minimums. Consequently, any cost savings that may result from the adoption of standards can occur only once; thereafter, any justification for the perpetuation of the PSRO program must necessarily reside in its capacity to upgrade quality, primarily through the continuing education of the health professional. There is every reason to believe that with the passage of time the essential correctness of this position will be affirmed. Meanwhile, however, the PSRO program was implemented.

John W. Bussman, a practicing pediatrician, wisely concluded that the time is propitious to assemble the widest possible compendium of information currently available about the PSROs, their history, their mode of operation, their problems, and their potential. He has chosen his contributors from among a growing field of experts, who as a group have no current equal. This book is the result.

Every chapter has merits of its own, but the perspective that history inevitably provides will likely highlight Harrington's superb description of the impetus given to the early establishment of the San Joaquin County Foundation for Medical Care, and its system of peer review, as a result of the threat that was posed to the status quo by the activities of the Union-Pacific Maritime Association, as well as Wallace Bennett's recognition of the danger to the excellence of American medicine that might attach to improperly structured review organizations. The response of the American Medical Association to the PSROs is aptly described by Claude Welch, a very substantial contributor in building a bridge of understanding between his profession and society. The difficulty in cajoling physicians into a posture of helpful participation is also aptly recounted by Kenneth Platt. The problems encountered by the first National Advisory Council as it came to grips with the implementation of the program are succinctly described by Alan Nelson, whose personal role in the entire movement was enormous. Jonathan Fielding sensitively portrays the complexities of the interfaces that have been created by the simultaneous implementation of health planning and professional standards review. Paul Nutting exhibits prescience in addressing the future of the measurement of outcome assessment, and Paul Sanazaro's thoughtful and insightful overview of both the strengths and the limitations inherent in any movement to control quality in medicine is outstanding.

A final note, the legislation that created the PSRO was introduced and enacted in 1972 while I was serving as assistant secretary of health in the U.S. Department of Health, Education, and Welfare. I was openly opposed to the legislation because I was convinced that its

price—the further intrusion of the federal government into the professional and technologic side of medicine— was substantially greater than its promise. Although nothing has yet happened to change my view, 5 years of experience as a member of the National Professional Standards Review Council have convinced me that, as is so characteristic of so much federal legislation, great benefits may yet result—benefits that were never anticipated. As Sanazaro has noted, "PSRO is the most valuable tool physicians presently possess to retain their historical right to self-regulation."

Merlin K. Duval, M.D.

Contents

I

THE PAST

1

The History of the Bennett Amendment

Wallace F. Bennett

The PSRO program is a natural product of the interplay of two powerful forces that came into being in response to two fundamental human needs: the physical need for medical care and the psychologic need for a sense of security.

In response to the need for health care, a system embracing scientific knowledge and professional skill has grown slowly over the centuries, supported by the establishment of hospitals and similar institutions and the development of medicines and scientific equipment. Today all of these have grown into a vast range of resources whose totality is beyond the capacity of any single physician to comprehend or use. In response to this, a tremendous pressure for specialization has arisen and continues to expand. This proliferation promises increased benefits to those needing medical care but also creates great risk for both the patient and the physician in that the physician may not select and use the best means of treatment. Making a wrong choice, of course, affects the security of the physician as well as that of the patient.

DEVELOPMENT OF ACCOUNTABILITY IN THE HEALTH CARE SYSTEM

The traditional relationship of patients and physicians has been like a closed circle. Physicians were accountable to their patients for the care they provided, and patients were accountable to physicians for payment. But in today's complex world this one-on-one relationship no longer exists. Both physician and patient have brought in outside allies who will accept part of their obligation and with whom they can share their risks.

Like other aspects of life, the practice of medicine has become institutionalized. In the past physicians probably shared their risk by calling in a single consultant, but now they have risk-sharing relationships with a number of health care services and institutions. These services assume part of the obligation owed to patients but also create new obligations that physicians owe to them. The list, headed by the hospitals in which they practice, also includes the group of physicians with whom they associate and the various professional organizations of which they are members.

Patients also share their risk with a number of institutions. The first of these was the private health insurance carrier. Today this includes the lawyer, who may sue the physician for malpractice. The most recent and significant, however, is the federal government. Ostensibly the federal presence is the counterpart of the private health insurer, but actually it brought into the picture the factor that when government is involved, it can exercise the full power of its sovereignty.

3

When both sides brought in these new allies to help share their risk, they created the requirement that their obligation for accountability also had to be shared. Patients were no longer accountable to physicians for payment for services but accountable to the insurance company. Physicians were no longer accountable only to the patients but also to the institutions in which they practiced for the maintenance of its standard of quality. When the federal government became involved, both the patient and the physician became accountable to it and through it to the taxpayer.

As our health care system developed in complexity, the need for accountability grew with it. Originally it was probably expressed when the attending practitioner, whether witch doctor, faith healer, or embryonic physician, called in another practitioner for the reassurance of a second opinion. Then as the system of consultation became institutionalized, definite programs of review developed.

No specific dates are available to help us trace the very early beginnings of formally organized review mechanisms. One authority has suggested that this process began about 60 years ago. An older retired physician friend told me that he helped start such a program in Salt Lake City's largest hospital about 30 years ago. When the first private medical foundation was established in 1954, it set up a review system that could be considered a prototype PSRO. Certainly by the middle 1960s, some types of review were being carried out in many large hospitals. Unfortunately, most of these were postaudits and were of no value to the patients involved because they were performed after they had left the hospital.

CREATION OF PSRO

Now that the flow of forces that led naturally to the congressional action creating the PSRO have been described, it is time to identify events that are significant to the creation of the PSRO program.

During the Great Depression of the 1930s, the federal government moved into the field of social services and committed its funds to support welfare programs for the indigent. On August 14, 1935, benefits for the aged were added when President Roosevelt signed the bill creating the Social Security System. Although financial support for medical care was not provided in either system at the start, it is easy to look back now and realize that both programs would some day be expanded to include this added protection.

In 1965 Medicare coverage became available to all Social Security beneficiaries. In 1967 the Medicaid program extending medical services to welfare recipients became law. When Medicare and Medicaid became operative, they took their place alongside existing privately financed health insurance programs, of which Blue Cross and Blue Shield are the largest. The extent of the coverage provided by this combination of public and private health care insurance services has grown until it now protects approximately 90% of the American people.

The bills that created the Medicare and Medicaid programs also established in federal law the principle of the review of the quality of medical services provided in hospitals that were to be paid for in whole or in part with U.S. funds. Unfortunately, the original laws did not spell out the pattern of organization for the review systems they required, and it was not until 1969 that Congress moved to correct this deficiency. On May 20, 1969, the *Chicago Sun-Times* published a series of articles that revealed many improprieties in the use of Medicare funds by physicians on the staff of the Cook County Hospital. Both the medical profession (represented by the American Medical Association) and Congress thus recognized the need to develop a specific review program.

On July 1, 1969, a hearing began in the Senate Finance Committee on the abuse of the Medicare program in the Cook County Hospital. My interest in finding a successful and reliable review system was generated by that hearing.

In the spring of 1970, the American Medical Association (AMA) distributed to some members of Congress a detailed proposal for a federally financed system of review of the medical care provided under Medicare and Medicaid, which it called PRO (Peer Review Organization).

The PRO idea was a good one, but it had one fatal flaw. It would have given a private organization the right to administer a federal law, and it put limits on federal sovereignty in a program financed by federal taxes. Moreover, this power was to be lodged with an organization that operated primarily for the benefit of its members rather than the public, an organization with the power to deny membership to any physician it chose and to which only about half of the physicians and surgeons in the country belonged. When I studied the PRO proposal, I recognized that the system was in itself basically sound and practical and could be adjusted to fit into the reality of the federal role. Thus the AMA's PRO proposal became the source of the Bennett Amendment, which when signed into law by President Nixon on October 30, 1972, created the PSRO program.

The following essential differences between the PRO proposal and the PSRO program are worth noting.

First, the AMA's proposal limited the review to the actual services provided directly by the physician. This would account for a relatively small part of the total cost of institutional care.

Second, the pattern of organization differed. The PRO proposal required the secretary of the Department of Health, Education, and Welfare (DHEW) to contract with each state medical society for the establishment of local peer review organizations in that state, leaving the medical society free to control them in a number of ways. For example, each constituent state medical society would have had the privilege of naming the members of a statewide PRO commission of five doctors of medicine or osteopathy. The commission would have: (1) designated the local areas in which review systems would be set up in the state; (2) selected the physicians who would participate in the review; and (3) reviewed and decided all disciplinary actions recommended by the local groups, with the provision that the secretary of DHEW would have had the power to reduce the penalty imposed by the state commission but no power to increase it.

The review process would be brought into action only in response to a complaint bearing on the necessity of services, the quality of services, and the reasonableness of charges made by consumers, institutions, providers, carriers, or government agencies, except that the state commission might recommend random sampling under some circumstances.

Third, the PRO proposal contained no criteria to be used in review.

Finally, under the AMA recommendation, the records, evidence, and findings of the commission acting as a review panel would not be available for civil or criminal action.

The Bennett Amendment made the following changes to provide for proper federal administration. First, the PSRO program would require review of all services rendered to the patient, not just those services provided by physicians. Second, instead of forcing the secretary of DHEW to contract with only state medical societies, it permitted the secretary to designate appropriate local review areas. Third, in each area so designated, the local physicians would be encouraged to organize themselves into independent PSRO units and to take the initiative in applying to the secretary for the right to conduct the reviews. This would eliminate any risk that either the state society or the secretary would control the selection of the reviewers. Fourth, because the PRO proposal failed to establish norms and standards against which to judge the quality of medical care, the Bennett Amendment drafted the law to allow each local PSRO to take the initiative in developing its own criteria. Fifth, under the PSRO program, the local review organization would retain the authority for disciplinary action and could send its recommendations directly to the secretary of DHEW. In addition, the PRO proposal did not contain any detailed specifications for the disciplinary actions that could be used against a physician, whereas the PSRO program did. Finally, the PSRO law did not contain an absolute denial for access to records, because this would have made it difficult, if not impossible, for either the patient or the government to proceed successfully in the courts against a physician for good cause.

Thus the PSRO program was not just a creation of Congress or the brainchild of bureaucrats but a product of many trends and forces that had been moving toward such a result for a number of years. Peer review of medical practice had already been established and accepted within the profession, as had also the use of insurance to spread the financial risk. When the federal government became a provider of insurance for certain groups of its citizens, a law requiring review was a logical consequence. Because the basic pattern for in-house review had already been developed in many private hospitals and accepted by the AMA, it was also logical that it should suggest a national private program and equally logical that this should be modified into a federal review program consistent with federal sovereignty.

On July 1, 1970, I announced to the Senate that I was preparing an amendment to the Social Security

Act that would create the PSRO system. In that speech I acknowledged my debt to the AMA-PRO proposal.

On August 20, 1970, the Bennett Amendment was introduced and immediately referred to the Finance Committee, which was then considering other amendments to the Social Security Act. The amendment, with some modifications, was approved by the Committee and became a part of HR 17550 on October 10, 1970.

On December 18, 1970, while the bill was before the Senate, a motion was offered to strike the Bennett Amendment from the bill but failed to carry by a vote of 18 to 48. Although the Senate approved HR 17550, there was no time for a conference with the House before the end of the Ninety-first Congress, and the whole bill, including the Bennett Amendment, died.

The PSRO proposal was reintroduced on January 25, 1972, this time as an amendment to a bill called HR 1. The Bennett Amendment was added to HR 1 by the Finance Committee in March, and on October 3, HR 1 containing the Bennett Amendment, was approved by the Senate.

Because the Bennett Amendment had been a part of the House version of HR 1, it had to be approved by the Senate-House Conference and was, in fact, accepted with minor modifications on October 17. HR 1, including the Bennett Amendment, was signed by the President and became Public Law (PL) 92-603 on October 30, 1972.

When the AMA proposed its PRO program, the Utah State Medical Association created the Utah Peer Review Organization (UPRO) and made contracts to review services covered by private insurance. When the PSRO program became law, the same group applied for recognition, and on June 18, 1974, it became the first in the nation to receive a conditional contract. Today this organization has two functions. As UPRO it continues to serve its private clients, and as PSRO it reviews all Medi-care and Medicaid patients. It has created its own set of standards, which apply to both services, and the same staff of nurse coordinators and reviewers covers both review systems with the same programs and procedures.

This, then, is the history of the Bennett Amendment up through its adoption into law. How it has been interpreted, translated into regualtions, and reflected in administrative decisions is discussed in other chapters.

2

From Development to Performance:
A Federal View of PSROs

Michael Goran
Dorothy N. Moga
Dennis Siebert

The PSRO program represents an unprecedented nationwide effort to control the medical necessity, appropriateness, and quality of health care services through peer review and a new form of public-private partnership. From its inception, the PSRO program has been controversial. Attitudes of the medical profession, other health professionals, government, and the public have changed dramatically as the program has developed during a period when pressures for cost containment and national health insurance continue to build. This environment, changing in character as the program matured, dictated certain management approaches. It is this changing environment and how it affected the federal management of the PSRO program that is described in this chapter.

DEVELOPMENT OF PSRO

The concept of reviewing health care practices for quality assurance and utilization control had evolved over a period of 60 years. The pioneering work of medical care foundations (begun in 1954), the efforts at utilization review as a result of the

Medicare and Medicaid legislation, and the EMCRO (Experimental Medical Care Review Organizations) program led directly to the 1972 amendments to the Social Security Act creating the PSRO program. Despite this history, the approaches selected by the Congress were unfamiliar to most segments of the society, including those who would be required to implement them. In addition, evidence that the methodology to be used would accomplish what was expected was insufficient. Notwithstanding these inherent limitations, a nationwide effort to blanket the United States with new organizations was begun.

In those early years of the program, progress was slow and difficult. There was no ready pool of knowledgeable, trained people to manage the program either at the federal level or the local level, and it took several years to develop such capacity. The policy development and administrative responsibilities of the program were split among several agencies within DHEW. The Bureau of Quality Assurance (BQA) in the Health Services Administration of the Public Health Service finally became the focus of PSRO management; however, policy development and implementation that was critical to the progress of the program required the involvement and concurrence of the older established HEW agencies administering Medicare and Medicaid. This became a slow, drawn-out process often involving considerable conflict. An atmosphere of uncertainty and concern about adequate funding of the program existed and consumed extensive energy until a legislative amendment in 1975 allowed automatic support of hospital review costs through the Social Security Trust Funds. This difficult developmental phase of the program was also affected by the complexity and enormity of the task. There were few precedents to use in developing policy and administrative mechanisms, and the issues to be resolved were not only numerous but also complex. Accordingly, federal administrators were particularly cautious to assure thoroughness and appropriateness of promulgated policy. This developmental phase of the program was also lengthened by the unexpected time it took local PSROs to develop. The environment in local communities was not always supportive of developing PSROs, and thorough and sensitive planning was required to develop support of physicians and establish all the necessary relationships with hospitals, payment agencies, and community organizations.

INITIAL RESISTANCE TO PSRO

Throughout this developmental period there were elements of resistance that, perhaps more than any other factor, affected the course of this program and how it was managed. Four distinct groups can be identified as components of this resistance.

Physicians are the foremost of these groups. A basic premise of the PSRO program is that effective peer review requires broad physician commitment and participation. Physician support is essential for PSROs to have even a chance of success.

The program was initiated in an atmosphere of active physician opposition and hostility. Organized efforts to repeal the legislation and lawsuits filed to test the constitutionality of the program were tactics used to delay progress and register disapproval. In local communities, a handful of supportive physicians often had the task of convincing the majority of their colleagues that PSRO offered an opportunity not to be ignored.

Hospitals were another critical group that contributed to the resistance. Concerned about an external organization determining matters that had been previously within their province, many hospitals greeted PSROs with suspicion. Delays in signing working agreements and outright refusals to cooperate slowed PSRO progress and contributed to an atmosphere of conflict.

Also significant in this conflict atmosphere were states, particularly state Medicaid agencies. Concerned about rising state expenditures for Medicaid, state administrators were wary of these autonomous new physician-run organizations that were supported by federal dollars and controlled by federal statute and administration. Some states had already put in place their own mechanisms for utilization control and were reluctant to relinquish those. This opposition, present in most of the larger states, manifested itself in outright refusal or delay in negotiating necessary agreements, and in a few instances, the setting up of duplicate mechanisms.

The fourth and equally important source of resistance in the early period of the program was DHEW itself. With administrative control splintered in the department and acknowledged opposition in the more established agencies of the Social Security Administration (administering Medicare) and the Social and Rehabilitation Service (administering Medicaid), bureaucratic warfare and delays created an internal atmosphere of tension and crisis. This resistance within the government in turn contributed to the reluctance of outside groups, such as state Medicaid agencies and Blue Cross, to work cooperatively.

PURPOSE OF PSRO PROGRAM: QUALITY OR COST CONTAINMENT?

These first years of the program were years of growth and change despite the resistance present and the magnitude of the task of developing such a nationwide activity. Policies were developed; PSROs did organize themselves and begin to carry out their statutory responsibilities; and the environment surrounding the program changed, too. Increasing impatience for results along with new and greater expectations of their role created new pressures for PSROs.

Illustrative of this changing environment is what might be called the contrasting government-private perspective on the purposes of the PSRO program, or the long-standing debate of quality versus cost. The statute is very precise about the role of the PSRO: to assure that health services are of acceptable professional quality and that they are delivered effectively, efficiently, and economically. Through these years those closest to the program have stressed its dual role in assuring quality and controlling utilization. Yet, it is an historical fact that PSRO was originally passed by a Congress very much interested in containing health care costs, and it looked to the medical profession to help the government do that. Confusion about the ultimate purposes of the program has been present from the start. Concerned congressional committees emphasized PSRO's direct effect on costs, whereas the administration took a narrower view, emphasizing the PSRO's potential direct effect on the utilization and quality of health care services, which in turn would result in indirect short- and long-term effects on cost. In the early years the

medical profession tended to polarize the issue. If the PSRO program were to enlist the cooperation and support of the profession, the purpose of the program would have to be the enhancement of quality of care to the exclusion of concern about costs.

Cost-quality debate has persisted, but it has become more sophisticated and complex as the years have passed. During the period (1972–1976) when the program was struggling to develop, other approaches were devised to influence costs of health services. The more significant approaches were hospital cost containment measures, reimbursement reform, certificate of need programs, and rate setting. What part the PSRO was to play among these approaches was not at all clear. The result is a variety of federal expectations for PSRO success. Today the program is expected to reduce costs, yet there is little recognition of its legislative limits or definition of its role in relation to these other mechanisms.

In the early days of the PSRO, the private sector viewed quality as the purpose of the PSRO. The notion that PSRO was a cost containment program was rejected outright, and some believed that quality assurance and cost containment activities were contradictory and could not exist together. Recognition of the clear statutory mandate has gradually come as well as recognition that reducing unnecessary and inappropriate utilization has an indirect effect on costs.

This diversion of views on PSRO role, and ultimately on PSRO success or failure, is an important factor in the changing environment of the program.

Today the PSRO program is entering a mature phase in terms of its development. Virtually the entire nation is covered with PSROs. The developmental phase of putting together a viable organization is past for all but a few; instead the PSROs are immersed in the taxing job of making their review systems effective and extending them to other settings and kinds of health services. The resistance of the past has changed. The majority of physicians now support the program and believe it is a viable mechanism for self-regulation. Many now also see it as a valuable mechanism to relate to government, the principal payor of health care. Hospitals have become more cooperative and, in most areas of the country, work effectively with their PSRO. Resistance of a few state governments continues to be a problem in the present environment; however, a legislative amendment in 1977 (PL 95-142) provides a framework for working together while it gives a stronger voice to states in PSRO operation and evaluation. An important factor in the current environment is a unified program administration within DHEW. The PSRO program, which is a part of the Health Standards and Quality Bureau, is now an equal partner with Medicare and Medicaid in the Health Care Financing Administration, which was organized in 1977 to bring together in one organizational unit all activities that affect the financing of health services. Finally, contributing to this state of program maturity is the fact that basic and essential policy development for the program has been, for the most part, accomplished.

This program maturity occurs, however, in a changed public atmosphere. The concern that existed previously about rising health care costs has now turned to alarm. Costs continue to rise unabated, and virtually all segments of society call for control. There is increased public interest and receptivity on the part of Congress and the executive branch in national health insurance, and coincident with this interest is concern about how to control costs and assure quality under any such system. Although the PSRO seems to be a critical component of national health strategies, the public in general seems to know little of PSRO activity, and voices can be heard questioning whether the medical profession can effectively regulate itself.

Superimposed on these concerns is a growing displeasure with the cost of government programs.

With program maturity and a public concern about costs has come a mounting expectation for results from a Congress and an administration that have been eager for program payoff since passage of the legislation. Early efforts at evaluating PSRO impact provided mixed results, which gave additional impetus to those critical of the program. Evaluation, which has been seen from the beginning as absolutely critical to validate methods or point to needed changes in them, is now being viewed as a means by which decisions can be made about the program's very existence.

Demands that the program demonstrate its worth have become more insistent, yet there is no consensus on how "worth" should be defined. To many in the Congress and the executive branch it seems to translate into reduction in health care costs despite the PSRO's insistence that the quality aspects of the program are also worthwhile. Over the years, it has become clear to those involved in this program that PSRO activity only indirectly effects cost changes. The expectation that by influencing utilization the program would directly influence costs has been shown by experience to be an oversimplification. Fewer days in the hospital for a patient are not always translated into dollars saved in the total system. Fewer laboratory tests do not reduce costs if technicians continue on salary. The problem of measuring impact is complicated further by the lack of knowledge of existing patterns of care. Until relationships between PSRO activity and the efforts of others charged with cost control responsibility, such as Health Systems Agencies, are clearly defined and understood, and until there are effective ways of relating all of those activities to costs of the system, the effect of PSRO activity on cost of health care will not be known.

The costs of conducting PSRO review are also under attack. Pressure is likely to continue for reduction in the cost per review while calling for increased activities at the same funding level.

The current environment thus places the PSRO program in a dilemma: how to prove itself when there is no consensus as to what it should accomplish and when there is insufficient evidence about the effectiveness of its methods. The environment today can be summarized as an atmosphere of judgment for each PSRO and for the program in its entirety.

EVOLVING MANAGEMENT APPROACH

In those early developmental years, DHEW's approach to managing the PSRO program was characterized by close administrative concern with details of PSRO organization and review methodology. This was the result of a number of factors, including the newness and complexity of the program, the shortage and inexperience of federal PSRO staff and PSRO staffs at the local level, and the generally unreceptive environment described earlier. It had value for only a short period of time, and as the environment changed, more permissiveness and flexibility were possible.

Policy direction for developing PSROs came in the form of chapters of the *PSRO Program Manual* and later as ''PSRO Transmittals.'' Regulations, the usual and preferred method of promulgating program requirements, had to come much more slowly because of the difficulty of developing policy in the existing DHEW structure and because of the expressed need for actual operating experience before finalizing rules. Manual chapters and transmittals discussed PSRO organization, planning process, relationships, and review methods in extensive detail, and PSROs were generally required to comply. The contract, which was the only readily available financing mechanism, facilitated compliance as vouchers of expenditures

were examined, deliverables reviewed, and progress reports scrutinized. In many instances, a new activity in the PSRO's development could not be initiated until prior approval was received.

The administration of this approach was centralized. Regional HEW staff served as liaison with no authority for decision making. Policy development and operational management was located in Rockville, Maryland, the office headquarters for the BQA. Each PSRO had a project officer and a contracts officer, both from the central office, and their primary role was one of assisting PSROs in complying with program requirements.

Again, because of such factors as staff inexperience, shortage of resources, and resistance of those agencies with which PSROs had to work, variation or experimentation in review methodology was not encouraged. Details of how to conduct admission certification and continued stay review were provided, and every PSRO was expected to apply them with only minor variations. Every federal patient admitted to a participating facility was reviewed.

Changes in this strict management approach began to take place as the program matured in both policy development and administrative capability, as more PSROs developed operating experience that indicated the value or worthlessness of specific requirements, and most important, as the political-social environment changed. It happened gradually at first and then more rapidly as the calls for PSRO performance became more insistent.

The current management approach is characterized by two interrelated goals: (1) to assist PSROs to set and meet their own performance objectives and (2) to monitor PSROs carefully for the purpose of providing them with feedback on their own performance and assuring continuing support to those that are effective. In contrast to the earlier approach of strict attention to the details of organization and process and the uniformity of review methods, this approach is concerned with results. It allows individualized operation of a PSRO, within certain limits dictated by statute and regulations, and it has the advantage of allowing a PSRO to demonstrate to its own local constituents accomplishment of objectives that make sense in that local environment and that represent effective use of scarce resources.

The most important component of this management philosophy is the setting of performance objectives by each PSRO. Objectives are selected according to local conditions but in a context of national concerns. Objectives related to both utilization and quality are required, and PSROs are evaluated in relation to their achievement. Accompanying the process of objective setting is the encouragement of local variation in review methodology, that is, modifying or tailoring the review system so that it works as effectively as possible on areas with maximum potential impact and accomplishes review objectives with the minimum possible investment of review dollars. Local PSRO calculation of the cost effectiveness of accomplishing review objectives is a part of this effort.

Supportive of this individualized management has been a shift from contracts to grants as the method of financing PSRO activity. This became possible through the 1977 amendments (PL 95-142) that require the federal government's financial relationship with PSROs to be one of assistance rather than procurement. Prior approvals occur only infrequently now and primarily for those major new activities for which there are statutory or regulatory requirements. Many specific requirements have been relaxed or, in some instances, completely eliminated. Program requirements are now contained primarily in statute and regulations, and other formal communications from the department are generally considered to be program guidance. The administration of the program has become decentralized. The regional office Health Standards and Quality Bureau staff are responsible for both technical and financial program management, with central office emphasis on monitoring of regional performance, coordination, and determination of policy. The role of the project officer, now located in the regions, has changed to one of providing assistance in facilitating PSRO progress and monitoring performance. Compliance concerns are limited to those basic programmatic and financial areas where noncompliance will put the PSRO at high risk. New emphasis is being placed on careful financial management by local PSROs in order to keep down overall costs of the program.

Relationships with external groups are being given special attention. Because PSROs can only indirectly effect a reduction in health care costs, the development of a close working relationship with the Health Systems Agency in its area is required. There are many aspects of health planning that are effective only if PSROs provide them with information about malfunctions in the system. Another relationship that is being given extra attention in the current environment is the one between the state Medicaid agencies and PSROs. Because these agencies have been a continuing force of resistance in some states, renewed efforts are being made to develop cooperative working relationships. PL 95-142 places new requirements on PSROs to consult with states and gives states new roles in PSRO evaluation, but it also clarifies any ambiguity that states previously had used to ignore PSRO authority in review of Medicaid services.

The other critical component in the current management philosophy is monitoring PSRO progress and evaluating PSRO performance. The primary purposes of such activity are to feed information back to PSROs and to assess the effectiveness of the methods being used in the program. As discussed earlier, it is likely that results will also be used to determine the future existence of the program. The approaches used are multifaceted and involve many organizations inside and outside the federal government.

CURRENT MANAGEMENT

Communication of policy and advice to PSROs takes place through a variety of vehicles. As noted earlier, essential requirements for PSRO compliance are stated in either statutes or regulations. The developmental process for regulations assures extensive input and review by PSROs and the interested public before the time they are issued in final form and require compliance. Policy guidance documents also provide for the participation of PSROs in their development, because virtually all of them are submitted to the field in a draft form first, comments are received, and then final issuance is made. Communication of this kind takes place through the following vehicles, each having a different purpose: *PSRO Program Manual,* transmittals, general memoranda, and technical assistance documents.

The process of each PSRO setting objectives and targeting its review process to local needs is the cornerstone of the current management approach. Each PSRO must set annual performance objectives that are both facility specific and areawide specific and that are output oriented and quantifiable. An example is to reduce the length of stay for a certain diagnosis by a certain percentage. The success of the approach requires that the federal management supply each PSRO with current data describing health service patterns on a national, regional, and areawide basis. Each PSRO supplements this with its own hospital specific data and with every local source of available information bearing on local needs and problems in order to increase the accuracy and responsiveness of the objective-setting process.

With these data and other locally available information, PSROs can carefully examine their own experience and compare it with the rest of their region and the nation. Using their own data, PSROs will want to examine the comparative performance of each individual hospital in their area, extending the analysis of regional and areawide data to the hospital level to identify trends and extremes. The purpose of doing this is to try to pinpoint priority problem areas. The PSRO that finds it has an exceptionally high admission rate and a short length of stay, for example, will want to set objectives and establish review priorities related to admission review. Where the reverse is true, that is, low admission rates and long length of stay, the emphasis needs to be placed on the concurrent review system. In this instance, the PSRO would probably want to focus on those cases that constitute a high percentage of hospital use and also to examine the availability of nursing home beds in its area and strengthen its interaction with the Health Systems Agency. In those instances where there apparently is little problem in either area, the challenge for the PSRO is to set objectives and target their review system in newer areas (such as ancillary services or emergency room care) and to give more attention to issues of quality. These indicators, of course, are gross and do not provide explanations for the patterns. As part of their objective setting process, PSROs must use their own data capacity in profiling, for example, and they need to design specific medical care evaluation studies (MCEs) that will help provide the explanations. Objectives and change in review approach can then be more precise.

Linked with the objective setting process is the modification of review approaches. Once problem areas have been identified and causes determined or suspected, the review system can be modified to concentrate on those priority problems. For example, review can be intensified by subjecting certain cases to preadmission or preprocedure review. Similarly, where information indicates that a problem does not exist, in other words, that patterns of care are acceptable, the review system can be modified to exempt those areas from review. Modification of this kind is illustrated by automatic admission certification, or certification of an entire hospitalization, for specific diagnoses or conditions or exemption of an entire hospital from concurrent review. The process of identifying and implementing modified review approaches is an individual one, varying according to the PSRO's experience and the characteristics of its area. Consistent with overall management philosophy, no prior approvals by DHEW of such modifications are required.

The other major component of the current management approach is the process of monitoring individual PSROs and evaluating their performance. The process is intensive and involves many separate activities and strategies.

1. Project officers in the regions maintain close contact with PSROs through regular visits, informal and formal communication, and analysis of narrative and statistical reports supplied by PSROs and the external groups noted in this list. The central office staff oversees and coordinates these activities.

2. The PSRO Management Information System (PMIS) provides the mechanism for collecting, analyzing, and using a wide range of management, financial, and patient care data generated by the PSRO.

3. Medicare fiscal intermediaries perform postpayment review of a sample of PSRO determinations and compare PSRO performance with decisions the intermediaries would have made under the former utilization review requirements. Discrepancies are called to the PSRO's attention.

4. Medicaid state agencies are encouraged to monitor PSRO performance according to plans based on their particular capabilities and areas of interest; several states now have intensive monitoring systems in place. In addition, the state agency and the governor, through the provisions of PL 95-142, now have a role in the determination of PSRO effectiveness at all stages of PSRO development.

5. Comprehensive project assessments of PSROs are conducted by teams composed of members from both federal and nonfederal agencies, relying heavily on peers from other PSROs. The management of the review functions of the organization, the establishment of external relationships, and quantitative measures of program impact are carefully reviewed, and recommendations for improvement are provided to both the PSRO and DHEW.

6. Financial management of PSROs is assessed through periodic audits by the DHEW Audit Agency; independent auditors conduct annual audits according to guidelines prepared by the department.

Overall program evaluation is also pursued, and although some methodologic problems continue, there is increasing ability to assess certain aspects of the program's performance. Analysis of hospital utilization of federal beneficiaries in relation to PSRO activity is continuing to receive attention but with an expansion of capacity and technique over earlier efforts. For example, diagnosis-specific data are being analyzed using tracer diagnoses and surgical procedures to assess PSRO impact on previously identified problem areas, and the capacity is being developed to assess unnecessary hospital utilization. An increased emphasis is being made to assess PSRO impact on quality of care. As one part of this, PMIS data are analyzed for the number and nature of MCEs, and the effectiveness of MCEs is evaluated through the process of restudy. Costs of the program are also scrutinized as program component costs are analyzed, and projections according to various program variations are made. Information describing PSRO activities, the extent of program implementation, and changes in program direction and PSRO response continues to be collected and assessed as an aid to management.

SUMMARY

The PSRO program has moved from development to performance, and its administration has changed in character to support a more mature program. Yet it would be a mistake to suppose that the program is on firm ground and has a successful future ahead. Instead, the future is uncertain.

The environment for the program today is more unrelenting than it was in the beginning. The program is being forced to justify itself; yet the criteria on which it will be judged are not clear, and the review methods it relies on are not proved. The role of the PSRO in cost containment is indirect, and its relationship to the other agencies more directly involved in cost control efforts has not been adequately defined; nevertheless, decisions about the program's future are likely to be based on evaluation of results that address costs.

To counteract this uncertainty PSROs are being asked by the administration to demonstrate that they can effectively carry out the functions given to them by the legislation and that they can produce results that are relevant to their own local problems. Essentially, they are being challenged to be successful in their community despite the uncertainty in the national environment.

3

Foundations for Medical Care: A Stepping Stone to PSRO

Donald C. Harrington

BACKGROUND

The Great Depression was over, World War II had been terminated, and the returning physicians were anxious to get back to their private practices. Their experience in the military was not a happy one due to the restrictions in medical practice developed by the military, so they were eager to return to the freedom of their own offices. For the most part they were extremely uneducated in matters of medical economics, and as a matter of fact were not aware of three of the rather dramatic changes that had occurred during their absence.

The first was the increased activity between union and management in the development of collective bargaining methods.

The second was the new concept of fringe benefits conceived during the war because of the freeze on wages and prices. By the use of fringe benefits, rather extensive health and accident programs were made available to the employees of the larger corporations.

The third concept developed (primarily in California) was the concept of closed panel medical practice. Years ago Kaiser Permanente had developed an industrial accident program for its employees at the various dams it was constructing. Because of the distance from these dams to the nearest medical facility, the industrial accident program was rapidly expanded to include the care of the everyday illnesses of the employees and their dependents. This model was then replicated in Oakland, California because of the proximity to the large shipyards developed by Kaiser Permanente during World War II.

The decrease of employment in the Kaiser industries following World War II caused the Kaiser Permanente Foundation to open its membership to the community at large. This form of practice was attractive to certain physicians, and the security of the program was attractive to many consumers. The program, therefore, grew, prospered, and began to make itself felt by the physicians returning from military service.

SAN JOAQUIN FOUNDATION FOR MEDICAL CARE

In 1954, the Kaiser Permanente Foundation moved to Pittsburg, California, producing chaos in the medical delivery system. A ward of one of the community hospitals had to be closed, and a migration of physicians from Pittsburg to other communities occurred. Several migrated to Stockton, California. At about the same time, local labor leaders contacted the Kaiser Permanente Foundation about moving to Stockton and developing a Kaiser Permanente plan in this area.

The San Joaquin County Medical Society had developed a fee schedule approximately a year earlier. This fee schedule was a local statistical compilation of fees on the format developed by Alameda–Contra Costa County Medical Society. The fee schedule had been approved but had been placed in the vault of the medical society with the instructions that it was not to be used until authorized by the board of directors of the society. Concurrently the International Longshoremen's and Warehousemen's Union-Pacific Maritime Association (ILWU-PMA) Trust Fund had voiced its desire to have a closed panel program in Stockton, California. It worked both through Kaiser Permanente and through two local groups of physicians. With this stimulation, the medical society leadership decided that something needed to be done. The first idea was to approve all of the existing insurance plans as total coverage on a private practice fee-for-service basis. A committee was established, and this option was studied. However, it was found that the programs differed widely and that nine different methods of payment were in use by the various programs in the area. Because of this diversity, it was obvious that merely approving the existing programs would not produce the desired results and would be unmanageable. Therefore, the development of a separate organization was needed to produce the type of results that the Kaiser Permanente Foundation had produced but that would continue to maintain the free practice of medicine with fee-for-service and freedom of choice of physician and patient. A separate and new organization was then developed called the San Joaquin County Foundation for Medical Care. This organization had its own board of trustees, which in the beginning was elected by the board of directors of the San Joaquin County Medical Society.

The first two tasks of the organization were to reexamine the buried fee schedule and to develop a contract that would specify the ingredients of medical care to be insured. These two steps were carried out, and the health insurance industry was contacted, but only a minimal amount of interest was found. However, one insurance company agreed to participate.

The first contract was developed with the Lathers, Plasterers, and Hodcarriers Trust Fund. This contract contained primarily in-hospital medical services but did have out-of-hospital consultation and laboratory and x-ray services in a limited amount when referred by a foundation physician.

Thus, the first two responsibilities of the foundation were developed, namely, a fee schedule was set up (foundation physician members could charge their usual fee up to but not exceeding this level), and a set of minimum standards was incorporated. The insurance industry contracts were required to adhere to this set of minimum standards.

The foundation's second contract was developed with the ILWU-PMA Trust Fund. This contract was negotiated with Goldie Krantz, the secretary of the trust fund at that time. She insisted that the physicians should carry some portion of the risk. After considerable negotiation, the physicians agreed to carry risk on their own services, but hospital and ancillary services would be insured through the statewide carrier for the program. This then was the first partial Independent Practice Association and was followed after a period of some years by the federal employees' program, the state employees', and finally, the state Medicaid program.

The addition of peer review was a third responsibility. When first conceived, the foundation leadership felt that it was sufficient to develop a fee schedule and a set of service benefits. It was soon found with the first program that the leadership was aware of what the program entailed but that neither the physician members nor the patients had any idea as to what the programs involved. Further meetings were held with the trust fund executives in the Labor Temple in Stockton, and it was in this location that the Foundation leadership saw the first example of review for fee and overutilization.

Many of the claims were being reviewed directly in the Labor Temple. They were reviewed by claims examiners who had offices in that building and were hired by the labor unions. On the blackboards behind these examiners were such words as "don't go to so-and-so; he cheats the brothers," and listings of physicians who were being blacklisted were thus placed where they could be seen by all of the membership.

The foundation leadership soon found that claims were being administered in labor union halls, insurance brokers' offices, or insurance companies' offices, regionally or in the home office. It was suggested that with this diversification of claims administration, perhaps everyone would be better served by moving the claims administration directly to the foundation office, whereby proper payment could be assured. At that time no comments were made about the "fox in the henhouse." In fact, examination of the desires and responsibilities of each one of the administering groups reveals that the labor union people as well as the brokers and agents tended to overpay so that their membership would not be dissatisfied. The insurance companies, either regional or in the home office, tended to be strict and tried to disallow as many items as they could "by contract." The physicians made it clear to the insurers that their only interests were that the proper fee schedule be paid and that proper medical care be given to the patients under their supervision.

Local program growth was first stimulated by local agents, particularly by William Stemler and Chester Root, the group manager of a large insurance company. Both men have been closely identified with the foundation movement over the years. Growth covering approximately 25% of the population occurred rather slowly at first and then proceeded much more rapidly because of consumer knowledge and interest until approximately 60% of the insured population was covered.

RESPONSIBILITIES OF THE FOUNDATION PROGRAM

Fee Schedule

The fee schedules used by the various foundations vary from area to area. Usually they are developed by a local statistical study identifying the fee that would cover the services of at least 75% of the physicians. The benefit structure is then developed on the basis of this fee schedule, and the physicians who elect to become members of the foundation agree to accept the fee schedule and may charge their usual and customary fee up to the fee schedule.

Nonmember physicians will be paid according to the foundation fee schedule but are free to bill above this. Certain programs do not allow the payment of nonmember physicians except in certain emergencies. This fee schedule is revised yearly and has gone up markedly over the past 2 years, because of the recent tremendous increases in malpractice insurance premiums.

Schedule of Benefits

In general the schedule of benefits is similar among the various foundations. There is a minimum basic schedule to which all foundations adhere, but many foundations have increments over and above this basic schedule. The basic schedule usually covers all in-hospital care and all outpatient diagnostic services, consultations, x-ray charges, and laboratory fees. Many of the schedules also include home and office coverage and the use of pharmaceuticals. Coinsurance and deductibles are used.

Peer Review

As noted earlier, peer review was one of the early responsibilities assumed by the foundations for medical care. Foundations soon discovered that offering an extremely comprehensive program, one covering most of the services used by patients when ordered by physicians, and paying a fee schedule equivalent to that used by most of the physicians in the community was like giving many of the providers a blank check on the insurance company's account. Because of this, peer review was instigated and today is carried out similarly in most foundation offices. All claims are transmitted to the foundation office for payment, where claims examiners review them against a previously developed claims manual. The claims are reviewed using patient and provider profiles inasmuch as any one single claim might pass the restrictions in the manual, but if the total medical care of that patient is evaluated, it may be obvious that overutilization is present, and the claims would be remanded to peer review. These profiles are developed manually utilizing either a composite patient folder or a composite patient face sheet. Claims may be denied by the claims examiner if appropriate information is in the claims manual or, if not, referred to the peer review section for study by physicians or other providers practicing under the same discipline as the provider submitting the claim. If these peer reviewers cannot decide as to payment or nonpayment, additional information can be requested from the provider rendering the care, and if necessary the total claim can be referred to the review committee for group decision.

With the increasing practice of payment for ambulatory services, home and office call coverage, and pharmaceutical coverage, it has become necessary in larger groups and communities to use the computer as a method of remanding claims to review. Only a few foundation areas have carried on programs of this nature. They are the San Joaquin County Foundation for Medical Care, Santa Clara Foundation, and San Diego Foundation in California, Utah Foundation, and the New Mexico Foundation. (For further information about these programs, contact them directly.)

SPREAD OF THE FOUNDATION CONCEPT

New foundations were formed fairly rapidly as physicians became aware of medical economic forces. The first foundations incorporated the three original areas of responsibility. The Western Conference of Foundations for Medical Care was formed, which included in its annual meetings physicians, other providers, insurance representatives, and consumers. At these meetings medical problems, administrative problems, and peer review problems were thoroughly discussed and group solutions reached.

Some of the more notable solutions were the inclusion of therapy other than surgery in cases of malignancies, the incorporation of the intensive care unit and the coronary care unit, and methods of incorporating long-term care in lieu of acute hospitalization. As foundations spread across the country, the American Association of Foundations for Medical Care (AAFMC) was formed in 1971. This was patterned after the Western Conference of Foundations and has served as a stimulus to the development of foundations for Medical Care and for the necessary interplay between physicians and the various legislators, committees, and agencies in Washington, D.C. At the present, foundations seem to be going in two separate directions; one group is working toward PSRO development, and the other is working toward Individual Practice Association (IPA) formation. The two elements cannot be formed together, as this would constitute a conflict of interest—real or imaginary—and thus a legal constraint.

INCREASING AWARENESS OF THE NEED FOR PEER REVIEW

The discussion of the increasing awareness of the need for peer review is restricted to those foundation functions that led to the development of PSRO peer review. The early foundations were limited in their peer review activities to the contract responsibilities covered by the insurance companies. However, as the contract responsibilities became more comprehensive, including ambulatory care, pharmaceutical services, and long-term care, their peer review functions also became more comprehensive and more difficult.

Many of the California foundations developed contracts with Blue Shield of California for Medicare review. This program continued for several years and provided many benefits to the Medicare program and recipients of medical care. The impact of peer review on lengths of stay are shown in Table 3-1, produced by DHEW.

Three foundations grouped together to work with the Bureau of Retirement and agreed to go "on risk" for the Federal Employees Health Benefits Program. This program was greatly helped by Marie Henderson, Chief, Comprehensive Health Plans Office, Civil Service Commission, Washington, D.C. The peer review function in these programs allowed for the inclusion of extensive out-of-hospital care, resulting in a noticeable drop in the use of hospital services.

In 1968 greater interest in hospital utilization was demonstrated by several foundations, who through claims review analysis felt that lengths of stay could be changed and that unneeded hospital admissions could be monitored. Sacramento's Certified Hospital Admissions Program (CHAP) is the most prominent in this activity; other such programs are San Joaquin's Coordinated Medical Utilization (CMU) and the Illinois Hospital Admission and Surveillance Program (HASP).

The leaders of Kennecott Copper from Salt Lake City, Utah came to San Joaquin County and met with the leadership of the San Joaquin Foundation for Medical Care. Kennecott Copper brought administrators from the industry as well as labor union leaders. Their program stretched from Salt Lake City into Nevada and down into New Mexico. Their actuarial experience was getting progressively worse as their labor-management negotiations improved the comprehensiveness of the program. Considerable time was spent with them both in San Joaquin and in the field, and it became obvious that the foundation program was not the answer because of the geographic spread of both recipients and providers. What was needed was a restructuring of the existing program with their carrier to include adequate peer review.

Another example of this kind of activity occurred when the physicians in Kenosha, Wisconsin requested help from the AMA and were advised to contact the San Joaquin Foundation for Medical Care. American Motors had asked the Kaiser Permanente Foundation to consult in a feasibility study to determine whether a closed panel program would produce savings and improvement of care for the workers at the various American Motors plants. Members from the San Joaquin Foundation for Medical Care met with the physicians in Kenosha and with their Blue Shield program. It was obvious from a demographic study of the American Motors workers that a single closed panel program would not be effective and that multiple satellite clinics would be necessary. For the same reason a single foundation would not be satisfactory, and it was decided by all concerned that

TABLE 3-1.   Comparison of Average Length of Stay for Selected Diagnostic Groups During Fiscal Year 1974

DIAGNOSIS	LENGTH OF STAY		PSRO Federal No./City
All diagnoses	Low	7.2	PSRO 05001/Santa Rosa, Calif.
			05008/San Joaquin, Calif.
	High	13.8	33013/Kings Co., N.Y.
Malignant breast neoplasm	Low	7.2	PSRO 05001/Santa Rosa, Calif.
(174, ICDA-8)	High	16.2	33013/Kings Co., N.Y.
Diabetes mellitus (250)	Low	6.8	PSRO 27000/Montana
	High	15.4	33009/Purchase, N.Y.
Cataract (374)	Low	3.8	PSRO 41000/Rhode Island
	High	8.0	33011/New York, N.Y.
Hypertension (400-404)	Low	5.4	PSRO 32000/New Mexico
	High	13.6	23005/Flint, Mich.
Acute myocardial infarction (410)	Low	9.8	PSRO 05001/Santa Rosa, Calif.
	High	17.8	33010/Rockland, N.Y.
Chronic ischemic heart disease (412)	Low	6.8	PSRO 05001/Santa Rosa, Calif.
	High	15.1	33011/New York, N.Y.
Congestive heart failure (427.0, 427.1)	Low	6.8	PSRO 05001/Santa Rosa, Calif.
	High	14.9	33011/New York, N.Y.
Cerebrovascular disease (430-438)	Low	7.1	PSRO 05001/Santa Rosa, Calif.
	High	16.0	33013/Kings Co., N.Y.
Pneumonia (480-486)	Low	7.8	PSRO 27000/Montana
	High	15.6	33005/Adirondack, N.Y.
Ulcer (531-534)	Low	7.8	PSRO 32000/New Mexico
	High	16.4	33011/New York, N.Y.
Inguinal hernia (550)	Low	5.2	PSRO 05001/Santa Rosa, Calif.
	High	11.9	33013/Kings Co., N.Y.
Cholelithiasis, cholecystitis (574, 575)	Low	9.0	PSRO 38002/Portland, Ore.
	High	17.1	33013/Kings Co., N.Y.
Urinary tract infection (590, 595)	Low	4.2	PSRO 05001/Santa Rosa, Calif.
	High	13.2	33013/Kings Co., N.Y.
Hyperplasia of prostate (600)	Low	6.5	PSRO 05001/Santa Rosa, Calif.
	High	15.5	33013/Kings Co., N.Y.
Fracture of femur (820)	Low	11.2	PSRO 23001/Upper Peninsula, Mich.
	High	23.4	33011/New York, N.Y.

the main problem was that of peer review and that the physicians practicing in the American Motors programs should become more involved with Blue Shield in reviewing the claims submitted on the American Motors recipients.

FORMATION OF SUPPORT CENTERS

In recent years various regional and state foundations have in cooperation with the BQA become active in the formation of State Support Centers.

Their responsibility has been to assist the emerging PSROs in their attempts to become qualified as planning and as conditional PSROs. They are able to coordinate the statewide effort and to bring in consultants in the various phases of PSRO development.

OTHER PROGRAMS

With the passage of the law implementing PSRO, the AAFMC felt the need to experiment in this field. A program was developed for such a study with the approval of the Office of Professional Standards Review (OPSR) and the BQA. The Kellogg Foundation funded a grant proposal developed by the AAFMC in cooperation with the American Society of Internal Medicine, the American College of Physicians, the American Hospital Association and, for awhile, the AMA. Two members of the public were involved in the Management Committee; these were Dean Barr of the Northwestern School of Business Administration and Anne Somers, professor of Community Medicine and Family Medicine, College of Medicine and Dentistry of New Jersey-Rutgers Medical School. The purpose of the study, which was titled Private Initiative in PSRO (PIPSRO), was to review the successes and failures of the PSROs in various areas, namely, quality review, costs of review, and the relationship of consumers to the PSRO program. (For a detailed report of this program, examine the final report of PIPSRO.)

The rapid spread of PSROs throughout the country made it evident that an organization of the PSROs outside of the government was needed to allow for transfer of experiences and information, and thus the AAFMC proceeded to form a separate corporation, the American Association of PSROs (AAPSRO). AAPSRO, which for its first 3 years was headed by John Bussman, has been extremely active in assisting new PSROs in their problems

with the various departments of DHEW. They have also carried on training programs for PSRO staff, thus filling a vacuum with a much needed service.

RELATIONSHIP OF FOUNDATIONS TO THE DEVELOPMENT OF PSRO

With the implementation of the Medicare program and the Medicaid program, the government became involved in an extremely comprehensive set of medical care benefits. Though administered by separate agencies, both programs were rather disastrous financially, and over the years increasing cost overruns were encountered. Studies by various agencies revealed extensive areas of overutilization, great variation in lengths of hospital stay from region to region, and no apparent methods of control. The offices of the attorney generals in New York and California carried on investigations and later took legal action against certain providers who were shown to be overutilizing the program. These studies demonstrated the waste of many millions of dollars. It thus became obvious that some method of program control was essential. Senator Wallace Bennett and the Senate Finance Committee staffed by Jay Constantine, James Mongan, M.D., and others undertook a detailed study and developed the language for what ultimately became PL 92-603. During this study various foundation communities were examined in depth and their methods of peer review analyzed. The methods used by the state of Utah, Sacramento County, and San Joaquin County were integrated into the law, thus producing programs to control length of stay, develop peer review of provider activity by producing patient and provider profiles, and requiring the local PSROs to develop locally authorized criteria. Thus, certain of the major ingredients of PSRO responsibility were taken directly from the active functions of existing foundations for medical care. The adoption of these functions was not sought by the foundations involved but was developed by passive transfer to the individuals in charge of writing the PSRO program.

RELATED ORGANIZATIONS

Only a schematic description of foundation activities as they related to PSRO development has been sketched. The work of just a few foundations has been described, even though many foundations are carrying on similar activities. Many other organizations that have been devised by physicians throughout the country, but that have not assumed the exact administrative structure of foundations, have also been active in developing peer review programs. One such was stimulated by Paul Sanazaro with the implementation of the Experimental Medical Care Review Organizations (EMCRO) programs, notably in Multnomah County and in the state of Utah. The American Society of Internal Medicine and the American Academy of Pediatrics have also carried on voluntary programs for the study of quality of office practice. All of these organizations contributed to the recognition of the need for peer review, which is now reflected in our present PSRO law.

SUMMARY

A brief narrative of the development of foundations for medical care and their spread has been presented. The major function of foundations as it relates to the developing PSROs has been their development of peer review methodologies. This has been described in more detail because of the increasing interest in peer review by consumers, management, industry, and more recently, both the federal and state governments. Though peer review programs have been functioning for about 15 years, many of their administrative modalities are still primitive, and much needs to be done in the area of computerization, particularly with the increasing comprehensiveness of our medical care programs as they relate to outpatient care, pharmaceutical services, and long-term care institutions. Further, peer review in the past has been used primarily as a means of coping with problems of overutilization. Great interest has been developed in the review for quality in both the hospital and the ambulatory settings. A concern for underutilization of medical services is also growing, and methods of computerized identification of this problem need to be developed. One of the biggest problems in improving the techniques of peer review is a lack of funds for experimental programs and feasibility studies. It is my hope that this chapter will serve to heighten interest in the peer review program and allow private and public funding to develop to solve some of these rather difficult problems.

4

The National Professional Standards Review Council: Intent, Function, and Future

Alan R. Nelson

LEGISLATIVE INTENT

The anticipated role of the National Professional Standards Review Council (NPSRC), as perceived by Senator Wallace F. Bennett, was described by him in an interview in May 1977:

I was very anxious that the actual operation of the Professional Standards Review program be kept as far as possible out of the hands of the bureaucrats. As an extension of this thinking, I saw the National PSR Council as an instrument at the top level which would carry out that concept in a management and advisory capacity. The Council was to be an interpretive body, and an appellate body to solve local problems and not just to function under the direct authority of the secretary. I was striving to give as much responsibility as possible to the physicians at all levels of the program.*

The translation of this perception into statutory language is found in Section 247F of PL 92-603, which specifies the duties of the NPSRC (Section 1163):

1. Advise the secretary in the administration of Title XI, Part B of the Social Security Act relating to professional standards review.
2. Provide the development and distribution of in-

*From Bennett, W.F. 1977, personal communication.

formation and data among statewide Professional Standards Review Councils and Professional Standards Review Organizations that will assist such review councils and organizations in carrying out their duties and functions.

3. Review the operations of statewide Professional Standards Review Councils and Professional Standards Review Organizations with a view to determining the effectiveness and comparative performances of such review councils and organizations in carrying out the purposes of Part B.

4. Make or arrange for the making of studies and investigations with a view to developing and recommending to the secretary and to the Congress measures designed more effectively to accomplish the purposes and objectives of Part B.

In addition, Section 1156 requires the NPSRC, along with the secretary, to provide technical assistance to PSROs in "utilizing and applying norms of care, diagnosis, and treatment." Information about regional norms are to be distributed by the council to PSROs and local variations approved by the council.

FORMATION OF THE FIRST COUNCIL

The intent of the first council formation was to have multiple interests represented in the common good, but the practical outcome involved intense political push and shove as interest groups presented their candidates and applied pressures to have them named. Over 300 candidates were presented for the 11 positions on the first council. Some slots, such as that reserved for the AMA, were filled without contest. Other places were filled strictly through pressures on behalf of a candidate from strategically placed congressmen. All of those selected had solid credentials in peer review or continuing education.

The potential of the council as a shirt-sleeve working management committee was immediately lessened by the requirements of the Freedom of Information Act, which mandated open meetings, all of which were announced in advance in the *Federal Register*. The presence of an audience that exceeded 100, each of whom represented a special interest, muffled dissent among council members and occasionally led to grandstanding. In addition, from the first meeting the council chairman, the director of PSRO, and HEW staff appeared to conspire against a management-oriented council when they ruled against the council's right to set its agenda and call for meetings. The bureaucracy appeared to want a strong council as long as there was no question of who was in charge.

The second NPSRC, formed in June of 1976, again involved political maneuvering, with interest groups presenting candidates and vigorously promoting their selection. Since the statute did not call for staggered terms of council membership, it became clear that not all 11 members could be reappointed and still provide needed continuity with the third council to be named in 1979. Seven of the 11 members were ultimately renamed to the council; the remaining four were seated for the first time in July 1976. One-hundred and eighty-six nominations for 119 individuals were received from 96 outside organizations and sources. These were reviewed by a nomination committee, and the recommended list was approved by the secretary in June 1976. Merlin K. Duval, former Assistant Secretary for Health and for 3 years a member of the first council, was appointed as chairman.

The council, recognizing the need for continuity and having been advised by HEW legal counsel that a statutory change was necessary to provide staggered terms, recommended the introduction of a technical amendment. After receiving a differing legal opinion in June 1977, Secretary Califano abruptly terminated the appointments of the seven holdover members after 1 year (for four members), and 2 years (for the remaining three, including the chairman).

MOST SIGNIFICANT ACTIONS

The first annual report of the NPSRC, filed July 25, 1973, covered only a single meeting. That meeting was largely spent in familiarizing the council with the law, and only one action was recommended. A motion by the council was unanimously accepted:

If peer review is an instrument devised by the government to assure quality care while containing health care costs, then the government has a co-equal obligation to be sure that it conducts peer review in all federally operated establishments: i.e. military hospitals, VA hospitals, public health service institutions, etc. Federal institutions should be models of the system of Peer Review.†

That first recommendation is yet to be enacted.

Area Designation

For the first 3 months after the council was formed, area designation was a point of major discussion at

†From National Professional Standards Review Council, July 1973. *Annual Report*, Rockville, Md.: U.S. Department of Health, Education, and Welfare.

its meetings. The controversy centered around a guideline that specified minimum (300) and maximum (2500) limits on the number of physicians in a PSRO area. A hard line position by the bureaucrats signaled the beginning of the inflexibility that was to cause conflict between the council and HEW staff throughout the entire period of PSRO program development. Some compromise emerged when a council motion was approved that inserted the word "generally" into the guideline so that it read: "A PSRO area should generally include a minimum of approximately 300 licensed practicing physicians. While the maximum can be expected to vary with local circumstances, it generally should not exceed 2500 licensed practicing physicians."

In addition, the council adopted a position statement that read: "It is clear that area designation considerations within a state recognize that appropriate geographical sublimits within the state with a capability to develop a PSRO meeting law and regulatory requirements can seek, and can be expected to obtain, area designation."

The practical effect of this council position was to allow the formation of a statewide PSRO in at least two states that had previously been divided into more than one area.

Because of the determination of the Texas Medical Association and the Texas Institute for Medical Assessment to have Texas designated as a single state PSRO, a further concession was made by Deputy Assistant Secretary for Health Henry Simmons, M.D., which led to the development of the "statewide support center" concept. Ironically, although several support centers were subsequently developed, Texas steadfastly refused to accept that compromise and ultimately received a favorable ruling in the courts.

Some years later, the issue of area designation again surfaced in council deliberations when Health Systems Agency (HSA) areas were being

defined, and the council expressed the opinion that PSRO areas and HSA areas should be "coterminous when feasible." This advice was also largely ignored.

Norms, Standards, and Criteria

Logically, the council's first action regarding norms, standards, and criteria was to define the terms. On November 26, 1973, following a meeting in Salt Lake City in which the Norms Subcommittee of the council conducted hearings and developed recommended definitions, the NPSRC adopted the following:

Norms—medical care appraisal norms are numerical or statistical measures of usual observed performance.

Criteria—medical care criteria are predetermined elements against which aspects of the quality of a medical service may be compared. They are developed by professionals relying on professional expertise and on professional literature.

Standards—standards are professionally developed expressions of the range of acceptable variation from a norm or criterion.

Screening—screening is a process in which norms, criteria, or standards are used to analyze large numbers of cases in order to select for study in greater depth those cases not meeting the norms, criteria or standards.

Preadmission Certification

The appropriate place for preadmission certification in the review process was unclear in the early days of the PSRO program. The statute appeared to encourage preadmission certification, although it did not mandate this bureaucratic obstacle to patient entry into the hospital except in earlier drafts of the legislation. In 1974, the council clarified its position on preadmission certification and recommended that the PSROs be informed of acceptable, alternative review mechanisms for determining the medical necessity of admission to institutions and that the stated objectives of the national PSRO program recognize such alternatives to preadmission authorization. Following this statement, concurrent admission review emerged as the dominant certification process.

The NPSRC agreed that criteria should be developed locally, but it supported the provision of technical assistance for such development. Accordingly, it encouraged the national professional associations to develop model criteria that could be modified and used by the local PSROs. It was not generally recognized at that time that diagnosis-oriented process criteria would prove to be of relatively little value. Indeed, when the model criteria contract was awarded to the AMA, controversy arose because of the widely held view that such criteria sets would become "cookbooks" for the provision of medical care. Experience has shown that relatively few PSROs have actually used the process criteria sets in unmodified form in conduct of medical care evaluation studies.

Data Policy

The early expectations of the council were that data for reporting by the PSROs would come from the use of claims data collected by payment agencies. However, conflicts between Bureau of Health Insurance (BHI), Social and Rehabilitation Services (SRS), and the BQA gradually led to the formulation of a data policy by BQA, which provided for collection of the minimum data set (PSRO Hospital Discharge Data Set, or PHDDS) by the PSRO itself and for uniform reporting of aggregate data to BQA. The council had recognized the importance of data from the very beginning of the program.*

---

*Believing that "whosoever controls data will control PSRO and whosoever controls PSRO will control medical care."

Confidentiality

Early meetings of the NPSRC were attended by representatives of Ralph Nader's Health Research Group, who took advantage of the public comment to voice strong objections to a PSRO policy that did not call for full disclosure of physician profiles and the results of MCEs. However, with publication of DHEW's confidentiality policies, it became clear that identification of both patient and physician would be prohibited outside the PSRO, and with the recommendation of the NPSRC, this policy was extended to exclude hospital identifiers from the reporting requirements under PSRO. In 1977, the hospital identifier exclusion was reversed; however, since no physician may be identified "either explicitly or implicitly," the requirement for hospital identifiers becomes difficult for BQA to defend.

NPSRC and Role of Allied Health Professions

Nonphysician health care providers have periodically approached the NPSRC seeking an expanded role for nonphysicians in the PSRO program. The NPSRC has heard presentations from dentists, oral surgeons, nurses, and designated spokesmen for over 20 other health professions. In 1975, a staff paper was developed that considered four basic options: (1) establishment of a national committee of nonphysician health care practitioners advisory to the council as recommended in a formal proposal from the American Occupational Therapy Association, (2) establishment of an advisory council of nonphysician health care practitioners to meet separately from the council, (3) establishment of a liaison network of professional representatives from the major national nonphysician practitioner organizations, and (4) establishment of other less formal mechanisms such as the use of consultants or an invitational annual conference. After much

discussion, the council recommended the third option, establishing an informal liaison network, with
one spokesperson selected by all of the major
nonphysician practitioner organizations and representing the network at all council meetings and acting as a focal point for the program administrators.

In 1977 following a request for PSRO membership of dentists and for representation of dentists
on the National PSR Council and acknowledging
that legislation had been introduced that would afford similar opportunities to nurses, the NPSRC
passed a recommendation to the Secretary of
DHEW and to Congress that would permit nonphysician health care practitioners who held independent hospital staff membership and were independently licensed to become members of PSROs
at the option of the local PSRO.

Level of Care

The core issue of whether medical necessity judgments should be determined by covered benefits
was raised in NPSRC discussions regarding level
of care. It was the contention of BHI that PSROs
should guide their level of care determinations by
Medicare program coverage. The NPSRC, on the
other hand, held that the determinations of necessity must be independently considered apart from
the benefit package. Consequently, the council
agreed that PSROs should determine what level
of care is needed, and if hospital level of care is not
needed, the alternative level should be specified.
Should that level of care not be available, the
PSRO should advise the payment agency which
level of care is appropriate. This procedure would
be consistent with the proposed policy encouraging
the PSROs to work with state agencies and intermediaries regarding level of care determinations.
The council agreed that from a quality standpoint
it is not appropriate to have review efforts guided
by reimbursement policies.

Quality Assessment

Although the NPSRC has been concerned with
methods of utilization review, protection of confidentiality, the relationship of the PSRO program
with payment agencies, and with other governmental programs such as HSA's and end-stage renal
disease programs, the dominant theme throughout
the history of the council has been the concern with
the quality of medical care and with methods of
assessing and assuring that quality. This has been
expressed in a variety of ways, from the review
and critique of criteria sets submitted by national
organizations to the receipt of presentations on the
reliability and accessibility of clinical research literature. The NPSRC has also encouraged a variety
of technical assistance programs designed to assist
PSROs in conducting meaningful quality assurance
operations. A cautious cooperation with the Joint
Commission on Accreditation of Hospitals (JCAH)
was also a recognition of the need for all organizations and groups seeking to promote high-quality
medical care to work cooperatively. A review of
the evaluation protocol for PSROs also emphasized
the need to review and encourage medical care
evaluation. The council has recognized that part of
the program assessment will involve site visits to
PSROs for firsthand examination of the quality
assurance efforts. In this regard, one of the most
important activities of the council in the future will
be the refinement of its role in the actual review
and approval of PSRO norms, criteria, and standards. This will involve the difficult task of determining what is a significant deviation from
established models.

FUTURE OF THE NPSRC

The nature of the bureaucracy is such that programs become progressively more complex and
layered and the power of any individual segment

within the program becomes lessened. Advisory groups in particular seem to have a brief period of attention, then gradually recede within themselves, making decisions of no importance to anyone but the group itself. Reports are then filed and forgotten.

One might assume that the NPSRC would follow that pathway, except for the unique nature of the PSRO itself. The same partnership of public and private sectors that gives the PSRO program its promise makes the council unlike other advisory groups, and statutory responsibilities give the NPSRC a watchdog role over the bureaucracy that the Heath Insurance Benefits Advisory Committee (HIBAC), for example, never had.

Indeed, the second council appears to sense its authority more than did the first and derives substantial additional benefit from the experience and political skill of Dr. Duval, the chairman.

The next areas of immediate concern will be perfecting the procedures for assessment of individual PSRO capability before the designation of fully operational status and selecting alternate PSROs. The council will also concern itself with finding an effective linkage with Medicaid and Medicare in the recently organized Health Care Financing Administration, providing technical assistance to PSROs to help them develop methods of profile analysis and ancillary services review, and cautiously entering into a working relationship with HSAs.

Near the end of the decade after program design and implementation are complete, when all of the intricacies and burdensome processes that the bureaucracy demands are finally in place, the Bureau of Health Standards and Quality staff and regional project officers will wonder what to do next. The logical efforts will be toward tightening the screws, demanding more searching evaluation, permitting less local autonomy, expecting more proof of effectiveness, and allowing less experimentation except along approved lines. When this happens, the NPSRC will have as its major role the task of assuring equity and protection of the PSRO from unreasonable pressures from government.

II

PLANNING

5

Recruitment and Involvement of Physicians

Kenneth A. Platt

IMPEDIMENTS TO RECRUITMENT

The success or failure of the PSRO program nationwide lies in the individual PSRO's ability to recruit physician support. This support has to be not just tacit approval or reluctant acceptance but manpower willing to serve on committees, councils, and boards. Under the best of circumstances, such a task would be difficult, but it has been made incredibly so by the very nature of the program and the slowness of its implementation.

As one begins the task of physician recruitment, it would be of value, perhaps, to point out several general impediments. These range from the obvious constraints on physicians' time through the profession's intense suspicion of the governmental apparatus to the more practical economic concerns about time lost from more productive pursuits. Indeed, when one considers these problems in some detail, it is a tribute to the profession that so many have accepted this new and burdensome task.

Cost Containment

The historic and chronologic development of the PSRO program has been detailed earlier in this book. Spawned out of concern about overutilization of medical services, it was the government's first major attempt to address the containment of escalating costs. Certainly the aspect of quality of care was at least implied in the law, but preoccupation with cost containment was obvious. Since the signing of PL 92-603 in October, 1972, the concern about health care cost containment has intensified until it has become the central theme in almost all health care conferences, papers, or legislative endeavors. The preoccupation with cost to the apparent exclusion of concerns about quality has aggravated the problem of physician recruitment. Those members of the profession who have opposed the PSRO concept from its inception are using today's cost concerns and the governmental moves to address those concerns as a basis for continued opposition to the program's implementation. Equating cooperation with capitulation, they are turning to confrontation as the best means of meeting the perceived governmental threat. Indeed, even those who have worked with government for years in the implementation of this and other programs have to concede that the current problems faced by the profession in trying to retain certain freedoms and professional prerogatives is conducive to the development of a "siege mentality."

Public Accountability

Public accountability was always accepted by the profession when it had a simple clinical meaning. The outcome of a patient's clinical concerns and medical needs as expressed in terms of personal approbation or censure was an accepted part of medical practice. If one was not astute enough or skilled enough, one usually did not prosper either professionally or economically. When the relationship between a physician and patient was a simple one-on-one interface with an implied or agreed-on economic obligation assumed by the patient, such a simple outcome evaluation by the patient was probably adequate. Over the past several decades, however, much has transpired to complicate the task of public accountability and to propel us toward our current sate.

Third-party Payors

The most obvious advent was the appearance of third-party payors, such as the private health insurers and the government. By removing the direct contractual obligation between a physician and patient, they removed the potent economic lever the patient could exercise in holding the physician accountable. If the bill was rendered to a third-party payor who guaranteed payment regardless of outcome, then neither the physician nor the patient suffered economically if the procedure, process, or treatment was ill advised or unnecessary. No one complained as long as the economy was prospering and costs were merely passed on through higher premiums, increased taxes, social security deductions, or benefit adjustments only dimly perceived to be the direct result of individual decisions of the provider or recipient of health care services.

Increased Sophistication and Expense of Medical Technology

Paralleling the advent of the third-party payors has been the explosion in medical technology of increasing sophistication and expense. The litany of procedures now accepted as standard practice is staggering. Coronary bypass, renal dialysis, joint replacement, organ transplants, oncologic radiotherapy and chemotherapy, and computerized tomographic radiologic scanning are but a few. As technology has increased in sophistication and expense, the benefits of that technology have become increasingly limited to narrower segments of the population. Although not everybody will need these procedures, everyone must share the expense through increased taxes and insurance premiums. The rapid escalation of costs in recent years is bringing increased resistance to assuming the burden of paying for health care and a genuine concern about the ultimate capability of society to continue to bear the cost. That concern with cost lies behind most of the thrust of the PSRO program.

Medical Care as a Right

The current concept of medical care as a right granted by birth or citizenship must be discussed. This universal entitlement to medical care, promised by the political leadership and accepted by the public, has greatly aggravated the problems of access, cost, and accountability. When medical care was looked upon as a privilege, the inconveniences of limited access, geographic maldistribution, and economic barriers to care were tolerated, if not enjoyed. As the public attitude changed and medical care became a right, such inconveniences became unacceptable, and a resolution of these problems was demanded through the political process. Astute politicians have been quick to recognize the potential political mileage in the issue and have aggravated the situation by declaring a state of crisis in the system. Decrying the profession's attitudes as self-serving and archaic, they have labeled American medicine as a nonsystem; a "Maw and Paw Kettle operation" somewhat akin to the old corner grocery store. Using cost concerns as a base, politicians are mounting a wholesale attack on the profession to restructure the system, limit the growth of its physician plant, manipulate its manpower, and change its reimbursement mechanism. The outcome is yet in doubt, but change is occurring.

The net result of all of the current stresses within the medical care delivery system has been the development of a deep and abiding distrust of government within many physicians and physician organizations. It makes the task of physician recruitment for such programs as PSRO immeasurably more difficult and places the stamp of the "fed" on those who try to implement the program. If one is to be successful in interesting the profession in actively participating in the PSRO program, one has to keep in mind all of the ingredients previously mentioned that collectively arouse such distrust and resistance.

NATIONALIZED HEALTH CARE SYSTEM AND ROLES OF PHYSICIAN COMMUNITY

As a nation we are groping our way toward a nationalized health system. It is a hesitant, meandering movement full of bursts of activity, followed by lulls and even retrenchments. Because of the diversity of the nation's makeup, the process of reaching a consensus on the system is time consuming and evolutionary rather than abrupt and revolutionary. Let us take a brief look at the building blocks of the system and what role physicians will play in organizing and directing its implementation.

Manpower

Consideration of manpower needs is important in a discussion of the nationalization of the health care system. The problems being addressed at this time are largely in the areas of geographic and specialty maldistribution and in the concerns about the size of the medical manpower pool and its implications on costs. Traditionally medicine has accepted the role of knowledge transfer from the present to the succeeding generation. Through such devices as preceptorships, formal didactic education, and post graduate specialty training, the knowledge and skills of each generation of physicians has been passed on.

In a free society where individual decisions are cherished as expression of personal freedom, the choice of one's career training and location of practice has been left to each person to decide. That right is now being challenged as the concerns about the balance between society's perceived needs and individual choices are being voiced. The detractors of medicine's "nonsystem" state that the normal market mechanisms of supply and demand simply will not operate to arrive at an appropriate mix of primary care physicians versus the narrower specialties. Despite the fact that more of today's students and graduates are opting for primary care specialties, these critics continue to seek legislative answers to these problems. Using economic levers on medical schools to channel the medical manpower pool into areas of relative scarcity, politicians are succeeding in restructuring the system to a significant degree.

Thus the traditional role of the profession to train the germinating student body has been constrained to a significant degree by governmental action. It is unlikely that these efforts will diminish, and indeed, they will probably intensify with the profession's role increasingly relegated to knowledge transfer rather than manpower determinations.

Plant and Technology Expansion

Until quite recently no one thought it necessary or even sensible to question plant enlargement or technology acquisition. On the assumption that more was automatically better, the expansion of the physical facilities of the medical care delivery system proceeded at a frenetic pace somewhat akin to the pursuit of the Holy Grail. Each community and each facility judged its medical care delivery system by its size and technology rather than by its relationship to actual community needs. Competition for the latest technology between institutions often within a few blocks of each other and serving the same population base resulted in duplication and waste. This is an area in which physicians and hospitals must accept some responsibility for adding to the escalation of health costs.

The result of this largely uncontrolled expansion of plant and technology has been the loss of the profession's traditional role in deciding what is needed and where it should be installed. Through state and national laws, such mechanisms as certificates of need and consumer-dominated planning bodies have usurped the medical profession's prerogatives. Physicians are now relegated to advice and counsel while others make the final decisions.

Payment

For most of medicine's history, reimbursement for one's professional services was largely a direct contract between the physician and the patient. With the advent of the third-party payors, that direct contractual relationship has been increasingly displaced. As more money flows through governmental coffers and insurance companies, the constraints on cost have weakened, because both the provider and recipient of medical care are increasingly divorced from the payment mechanism. A secondary effect of this steadily expanding mechanism of funds transfer has been the loss of the profession's ability to set its own fees. The country is steadily moving toward negotiated fee

schedules, probably on a regionalized basis, that will likely cover the federal patient intially and then will spread into the private sector.

Paramedical Manpower

If manpower, planning, and payment are increasingly beyond the profession's ability to control or direct, what then is medicine's future? What will the medical profession's role in the medical care delivery system be in coming years?

One obvious role of the physician community is that of actually delivering medical care. Of all the territorial imperatives, this is the most sacrosanct. Yet, it may well be that what was once considered inviolate may now be in danger. The most immediate threat may possibly be the increasing expansion of the paramedical manpower pools. Such physician extenders as midwives, pediatric nurse associates, physiotherapists, dietitians, and registered nurses are now beginning to look with favor on independent practice with direct reimbursement. Certain that their skills justify such a state, they are vocalizing before an increasingly receptive state and federal audience. Seeing the use of trained paramedical personnel as a partial answer to geographic maldistribution and cost containment by displacing more expensive, highly trained physicians, program developers and antitrust investigators are beginning to press for independent status.

Physician Surplus

At the same time that vast numbers of new medical personnel in supportive roles are being trained, the physician scarcity of the early 1970s is becoming the physician surplus of the 1980s. The physician-population ratio of approximately 1:620 of 1977 is likely to decrease to about 1:450 in the mid 1980s. Whether this represents an oversupply or not will depend to a great degree on what happens to the demand for physician services. If no new federal initiatives are forthcoming to stimulate demand, the resulting surplus will create a fascinating paradox. Medical care costs will likely rise significantly in direct patient care. Unlike some manufacturers, more physicians will not necessarily drive down unit costs. Although I do not believe in the "target income" theory, I do not question that more physicians stimulate more services. Some well-known economists, such as Uwe Reinhardt, of Princeton have estimated that each physician generates $200,000 to $250,000 worth of medical costs per year. If physician manpower is increased by 100,000 within the next 6 to 7 years, medical care costs could conceivably increase by around $25 billion per year just because of the increased manpower.

At the same time that increasing numbers of physicians are being trained, with all that implies in escalating costs, more support personnel, as previously described, are being trained. Many of the latter will ultimately seek independent status and direct reimbursement, which quite probably will aggravate cost escalation.

Both physician surpluses and competing independent paramedical practitioners threaten the actual delivery of medical services. The secondary and tertiary levels of medical care will continue to depend on highly trained physicians, but the primary care or point-of-entry sector is threatened. If the country is going to have one practicing physician for each 450 persons, with an ideal closer to one per 600, something will simply have to give. Either these expensively trained physicians will be used in areas now thought to be somewhat inappropriate for their skills, or physicians will be grossly underutilized or patients overutilized to a degree unthinkable in today's concerns about cost escalation, fraud, and abuse.

Peer Review

It is in the evaluation of the appropriateness of the care they render that physicians can find the logical complement to their professional skills. Who are more competent to judge the quality of care and the appropriateness of the setting than one's peers? This is the underlying premise behind the PSRO program and the justification for the physician dominance in its control and implementation. The PSRO program is one that despite initial professional opposition and political reservations has survived and is steadily improving. This is a formalized expansion of the long-standing belief in peer review, which has been a professional hallmark. From the first few years in medical school through the more complex training during internship and residency, physicians have been willing to accept the critical evaluation of their peers. Hospital staff physicians have long been willing to work on audit committees, tissue committees, utilization review committees, and so forth. The PSRO program extends the scope of this activity and through its reporting and evaluation requirements provides the profession with a mechanism for public accountability.

IMPORTANCE OF LEADERSHIP IN PSRO RECRUITMENT

A more detailed look at physician recruitment and involvement in the PSRO program is necessary to portray the concerns that affect the attitudes of the physician community regarding recruitment. Recruitment is not a simple task! The ability to persuade one's fellow practitioners to devote time and energy to a project they only mildly approve, or even oppose, requires a knowledge of the forces molding their attitudes and a great deal of sympathetic understanding of their fears. The psychol-

ogy of recruitment is a fascinating subject and justifies separate consideration on its own. Little can
be gained by simply reading the law or conjuring
up the specter of "if we don't do it, they will,"
with the "they" being some ethereal, evil force
composed of equal parts of politicians and consumers. To persuade busy medical practitioners to
participate in the PSRO program, one has to be
able to convince them that it will be of ultimate
benefit to that vast majority of physicians who are
honest and hard working and to the public they
serve. Issues such as quality assessment versus
cost containment are gut issues and must be
analyzed in depth rather than rendered simple lip
service. It is only through honest analytic evaluation of the program with the extolling of its potentially positive impact on utilization and quality that
one can gain the physician support that is absolutely vital to its success.

GOALS IN RECRUITMENT

Once the knowledge needed to launch a recruitment program is acquired, how does one begin?
What jobs need filling? Where is the natural talent
and political savvy that must be tapped? Who
should assume the task of recruiting, and what
should the qualifications be?

It has been said that change is the only constant,
that societies respond to the efforts of the yeasty
10% who ferment the other 90% and through their
activist role motivate change. There is some element of truth in this, and it applies to the PSRO
program. Most successful PSRO organizations
have been largely the result of the activities of a
handful of men. It is this small nucleus of activist
leaders that one must identify and use as the base
on which to build a functional program. One of
them will usually surface as the acknowledged
leader and will frequently become the medical director of the fledgling PSRO. Although their

backgrounds may vary, such physicians frequently
have a history of multiple professional activities
outside of the scope of their day-to-day practice.
They may have been presidents of their local or
state medical society, the chiefs of a medical staff,
or the chairmen of a local hospital or medical society peer review committees. Whatever their background, they are the key members who spark their
fellow practitioners to form and staff the organization. Thus the first effort at recruitment must
be to identify and utilize these members. It is the
medical director's responsibility to spearhead the
membership drive that is essential for program viability and to aid in recruiting the professional
members on the boards, councils, and committees,
whose input is vital.

Once the key member has been identified and
entrusted with heading the organization, the following goals should be addressed to provide the
professional component to the PSRO:

1. General membership
2. Board of directors
3. Councils
4. Committees
5. Physician advisors

Each of these is unique and deserves separate
consideration, both as to the recruitment effort involved in staffing and the individual responsibilities and scope of work.

General Membership

In a discussion of the general membership drive, it
would appear logical to work through the appropriate medical society structure. This may be a single
county or a combination of several county or local
societies or through the state medical society, depending on the area involved in the PSRO designation. This is a time of great stress on the structure
of medicine. Significant outside forces are debat-

ing the role of medical organizations and their role in fee setting, potential activities for antitrust action such as the relative value scale (RVS) and personnel limitations, and professional ethical restrictions, such as advertisement. With such negative forces at work, it makes little sense for an organizing PSRO to bypass or ignore the existing medical organizations and their expertise in professional organization and activities. Often those men or women who have displayed leadership and interest in political activities within the medical society can be of great assistance with general membership recruitment once they have been convinced of the potential value to medicine in the PSRO program. The reverse is also true. If these people are ignored or antagonized, they can exert that leadership ability in opposing the PSRO within their areas of influence and make the general membership drive immeasurably more difficult. Such divisiveness within the ranks of medicine can only aid the detractors, fragment our energies, and splinter the medical community into groups of feuding malcontents that are totally ineffectual. Unfortunately, throughout the history of the PSRO program, some of the more powerful medical organizations have delayed its implementation significantly through their reluctant support.

The first move in working through the local medical organizations is to recruit first their leadership and then their members, letting the leaders spearhead the drive. This serves two useful purposes. It puts a stamp of approval on the PSRO organization, and it also provides the key physician and that person's original supporters with greatly needed additional manpower. No one individual or even several, no matter how dedicated, can carry the message to every medical society member, every medical staff, or every isolated hospital or community within the PSRO area, especially in some of the large and sparsely populated western states.

The goal should be to recruit at least 25% of the licensed physicians within the PSRO area, both allopathic and osteopathic. I would like to stress that this is an absolute minimum, and preferably the goal should be higher. The more members one has, the more effective is the organization's ability to deal with the multitude of political and professional problems it will face.

This is especially significant when one broadens the PSRO review activity into the private sector. Insurance companies, self-insured companies, and fiscal intermediaries are all interested in the degree of local support the PSRO enjoys, and one of their key indices is the membership roster. The credibility and effectiveness of the organization rises geometrically with the size of the membership. When one is marketing peer review to the private sector, this is a key issue.

Local Control of Peer Review and Quality Assurance

A major issue in general membership recruitment is the issue of local control of peer review and quality assurance. One of the most frequent criticisms leveled at those who urge participation in the PSRO program is that they are merely setting up a mechanism that ultimately will be taken over by the federal government. It is important, therefore, when addressing local medical societies and medical staffs to reassure them on the question of local control and local participation. This must include not only the utilization review with local physician advisors but also the development of criteria for the MCEs that take place within local institutions or among multiple institutions; nothing is more politically sensitive than this issue. That territorial imperative attitude extends not only to that polyglot group known as the "fed" but also to the central staff of the PSRO, especially at the state level. Given the chronic problems of communication that plague all such organizations, it is common for the general membership to feel uninformed and therefore at a loss adequately to evaluate actions taken by the board of directors or central staff. Since all physicians feel varying degrees of paranoia in these difficult times, it is natural for them to react with varying degrees of hostility when confronted with the implementation of rules and regulations. This hostility can be minimized if they are assured of local control of peer review and criteria development.

Reimbursement

Another key issue is reimbursement. Busy physicians are being asked to devote a great deal of time and energy to implement this program. They expect and are entitled to reasonable recompense for their time. In prior years, the time spent on tissue or audit committees was donated as an accepted responsibility of the active medical staff. When utilization review became a requirement under the Medicare law of 1965, this relationship and responsibility underwent a subtle change. No inordinate amount of additional physician time was actually required under the generally pro forma compliance with the utilization review requirement of Medicare, but that has drastically changed under the PSRO requirements. The implementation of this law demands a significant amount of professional time and effort. Some say that it is going to create a new career opportunity for a limited number of physicians and offer part-time work to a great many more. Whether that materializes is unimportant. What is important is that the physician effort in this program must be adequately compensated, either through a full- or part-time salary for the medical director and associates or as an hourly fee for physician advisors, peer reviewers, committee and council members, and eventually the board of directors.

Confidentiality

Another issue of great concern is the problem of confidentiality. Spawned by the inborn urge for personal privacy, it has been intensified by the malpractice crisis of recent years. This fear of personal disclosure is also reflected in the attitudes of hospital administrators and patient advocates. The conflict between individual privacy and the public's right to know could potentially result in a PSRO facsimile of the Good Housekeeping Seal of Approval being stamped on the forehead of each individual practitioner or on the door of each institution. To prevent such a dismal outcome of PSRO activity will require reassurance that the PSRO will resist such an eventuality. This is an important point to make in the membership drive.

Board of Directors

I have already mentioned the medical director as the key professional within the organization. Of equal importance is the physician membership that sits on the board of directors, councils, and the key committees of the PSRO. These key professionals are both elected and appointed and serve not only as the repository of authority but also as resource personnel who generate new initiatives and new policies for the organization to pursue.

Physician Dominance

The board of directors is an elected body that is by law physician dominated. Before discussing its role and makeup, I want to reemphasize that key issue of physician dominance of the governing board of the PSRO. In all the major governmental programs, such as health planning agencies, statewide health coordinating councils, and departments of health boards, physicians serve in a minority role. The minority role is important, but it does not allow the profession to set key policy for these agencies.

The reverse is true in the PSRO. Recognizing that only true peers can adequately evaluate a physician's performance, the authors of the PSRO provision in P.L. 92-603 deliberately set a policy of physician dominance of the governing body of these organizations. That policy was not universally accepted by Congress at the initiation of the program, and indeed, it still is not. Many seers predicted that physicians would either refuse to accept the responsibility for judging their fellow practitioners or do only a perfunctory, self-protective job of it. It is to the credit of a large segment of the profession that they have accepted this responsibility and have worked hard to implement it. Such acceptance is, of course, fraught with the potential danger of failure and all that would imply. Failure would provide additional ammunition to those detractors of our medical system who state that only governmental controls independent of the profession can curb excessive utilization and costs. Despite the possibility of failure, it is better to try than to concede the battle from the outset!

Election

Let us consider the makeup and function of the governing board of an individual PSRO. Because this is the authoritarian body of the organization, it is an elected one. The election comes from the general membership and should reflect the geographic and philosophic makeup of the electorate. Although it cannot be automatically synonymous with the governing boards of the local medical societies, there is frequently a significant degree of overlapping. This is quite understandable considering the fact that the leaders of organized medical societies are frequently the professionals who also have accepted the challenge of organizing the

PSRO in their area. That activist role places them before the general membership, who will often recognize their expertise and interest in this endeavor and elect them to the governing board. Since the role of PSRO is complex and constantly changing, the position of a director cannot be considered an easy one. Far from being a static, honorary position, it requires a great deal of study and effort to keep abreast of all of the nuances of the program. When members are recruited to serve on the governing board of the PSRO, recruiters must stress the effort and sacrifice it will demand. When the job description is presented to prospective candidates, the positive aspects of serving in such a position of trust must be emphasized as well as an honest evaluation of time and effort requirements.

Councils and Committees

Once an adequate general membership is developed, a medical director is hired, and the board of directors is elected, the next step is recruiting and appointing physicians to the councils and committees needed actually to oversee the various activities of the PSRO program on a day-to-day basis. The actual makeup and nomenclature of the various councils and committees will vary from PSRO to PSRO depending on its geography and scope of work, but some generalities can be made.

Councils

The council structure is seen more often in areas where the geographic boundaries are large. A typical example of this structure is the Colorado PSRO, which has a regionalized makeup in order to allow for more effective local control. Faced with a single, statewide PSRO and a large geographic area, the Colorado organization created five regions under its board of directors, each of which reflects both medical catchment areas and adequate physician population to do effective peer review. Each region has its own council, elected by the general membership. The council's makeup reflects both in number and professional representation the makeup of the board of directors. It is responsible for implementing the policies approved by the board of directors within its own region. That implementation includes the professional management of the PSRO program, to include acute care review, MCE, private review, ambulatory peer review, and long-term care review where implemented. These regional councils are active, functioning extensions of the board of directors and require time and effort from their members. If one's particular PSRO requires that type of organizational component, one should look to the local medical societies within the area for suggested nominees. One should emphasize that service on this type of council allows the elected member an opportunity not only to oversee program implementation but also frequently to be elected to the board of directors as a regional representative. The position of director allows a physician not only to serve in the role of program implementation as a regional council member but also to be a maker of policy through the physician's role as a director. That dual challenge and responsibility are often stimulating, and the prospect of meeting that challenge can serve as an inducement in the recruitment of prospective council members.

Committees

In addition to the council structure in Colorado, a number of fairly specialized committees were needed. Again, using the Colorado experience as a model, let us discuss the potential committee structure of a fully operational PSRO.

Committees are usually appointed bodies and serve at the discretion of the board of directors. They often have a specialized duty or interest and frequently require some degree of special expertise of their members. Because these committees are not policy-making bodies, the time spent in committee work is usually reimbursable, and this is an aid in recruiting members. Generally they will have a chairman who may be appointed by the board or elected by the committee members. The chairman's duties are to chair the meetings and coordinate the committee activities. The role of chairman may demand special knowledge or leadership ability, or both, and frequently requires a certain degree of motivational skill as well. Since committee meetings are frequently called at odd intervals by the chairman and do not carry with them the added stimulus of policy setting or implementation, it is frequently difficult to obtain an adequate representation. That is when the motivational skill of the chairman comes into play.

One of the most important committees that a PSRO must form is the one that serves as the criteria and standards committee. The duty of this committee is to set the criteria and standards for utilization review and MCEs, thus its role in the program is very significant. Its actual duties will vary from one PSRO to another depending on the decision by the board of directors as to how to derive these criteria and standards. If the decision is made merely to modify accepted sets obtained from other PSROs, BQA, or the AMA, the task of the committee is relatively simple. The other alternative is for the committee to create its own criteria, starting from scratch, and that increases the complexity of the committee's task immeasurably. If the latter course is chosen, this committee must be composed of recognized experts in many disciplines who are willing to serve in establishing the criteria and standards by which the PSRO will judge the reasonableness of program utilization and the quality of care rendered.

The criteria sets may ultimately encompass not only review within the acute care institutions but also ambulatory care, long-term care, and outpatient care as well. They will have to address such factors as the utilization of ancillary services, the justification for admission, the appropriateness of the care rendered or procedure performed, and the level of care that the patient needs after acute care, for example, skilled nursing, intermediate facility care, home care with assistance, or discharge to full duty. MCEs require criteria development within the PSRO in multi-institutional studies as well as in multidisciplinary and interdisciplinary areas. Many single institutional MCEs may be assisted with criteria development by this committee.

Since the role of the criteria and standards committee is so broad in scope and so vital to the effective performance of the PSRO, membership recruitment is of utmost importance. Top-notch people who are accepted by their peers as being both knowledgeable and pragmatic must be chosen and treated well. If they are challenged intellectually, complimented on their output when deserved, and reimbursed adequately, they will serve well.

There are other significant roles that the committee structure can assume in aiding the PSRO to fulfill its tasks. Since there are significant variations in the individual PSROs, one can expect variations in the number, size, and function of committees. In the Colorado PSRO, additional committees were formed to fulfill specific tasks vital to program implementation. The acute care institutional review is overseen by the Colorado Admissions Program (CAP) Steering Committee, composed of physicians, hospital administrators, and a consumer. The Medical Care Evaluation–Continuing Medical Education (MCE-CME) Steering Committee has the responsibility for overseeing the MCEs and continuing medical education. The Information Advisory Committee deals with the evaluation of the data system and interpreting its results. The Physician Advisor Committee works with training the physician advisors and aids

in evaluating their performance. This is merely one individual PSRO's committee structure and is presented merely to emphasize committees' roles in aiding a PSRO to function. Each plays a unique role and requires a certain interest and expertise from its individual committee members. Recruitment is not as difficult in forming this type of committee structure, probably because the role they play is easy to define and the work load is more limited.

Physician Advisors

Physician advisors also perform an absolutely vital role in any successful review program. If I were asked to name the most critical position one must fill in recruiting physicians for work in the PSRO program, I would say the role of physician advisor. To most physicians, physician advisors represent the PSRO program at this state of its implementation. If a question is raised about the justification for the patient's admission, the length of the hospital stay, or the quality of care rendered, it is the physician advisor who must make the initial professional judgment. For the program to be successful, they must be willing conscientiously to evaluate the patient's status and render whatever judgment seems appropriate under the circumstances. This will often necessitate direct consultation with the attending physician before arriving at a conclusion. This type of one-on-one discussion requires tact and diplomacy, with full awareness of the sensitivity of the situation. Physician advisors who disagree with the attending physicians must be willing so to state and to act in accordance with their personal beliefs. Depending on the attending physician's personality, this can create an awkward situation that many might find uncomfortable. Given the delicacy of the job, it is no wonder that the performance of physician advisors varies considerably from institution to institution.

A few suggestions are in order regarding physician advisor recruitment. It is best to choose physician advisors from physicians in private practice and preferably in primary care. There is always the possibility of a conflict of interest if the physician advisor is a salaried or full-time, hospital-based physician, such as a director of medical education, a pathologist, or a radiologist. In the majority of cases, such a charge would be totally unfounded, but even the suggestion of such a conflict of interest should be avoided. It is also best to avoid recruiting physician advisors from among physicians who are dependent on direct referrals for their primary source of income. This would include such specialties as general surgery, gastroenterology, neurosurgery, and orthopedic surgery. Again, this is to avoid even a semblance of conflict of interest that could conceivably arise should a physician advisor have to make an adverse finding on a case involving one of the physician advisor's referring physicians. Although it is not an absolute necessity, it is advisable to recruit physician advisors from the ranks of physicians who have had some experience with utilization review. This seems to be a natural tendency among hospital staffs, but it deserves mentioning.

Finally, it has been profitable to try to recruit physician advisors who are experienced practitioners, sound in their clinical judgment, and respected by their peers. Their role is difficult at best and occasionally controversial, and thus a stable, experienced background is invaluable.

SUMMARY

The success of a PSRO is inextricably tied to its ability to attract and motivate solid physician membership and direct physician participation. I have attempted to point out some of the concerns that will color the attitude of prospective members. It is incumbent upon all recruiters that they are well grounded in the facts underlying these concerns and can respond to questions in a concise, authoritative, and factual manner. Nothing is more reassuring to a concerned physician who is seeking an answer to a real or imagined problem than to have the problem analyzed in an articulate and reassuring manner.

Physicians in private practice today are insecure, confused, and irritable individuals. They feel threatened by their patients, constrained by their government, and politically impotent as the role of government in the medical care delivery system expands. In the government's bureaucratic regulatory activity, they see the opportunity for freedom of choice of specialty, location of practice, mode of therapy, and reasonable fee for service being limited. The result of this could be a polarization of attitudes between the government and the physician community that may lead to direct confrontation. Believing that force can be met only by force, the physician community may conceivably be treated to the unhappy experience of shout replacing dialogue, fear replacing reason, confrontation replacing cooperation, and the final sorry spectacle of the profession striking against the government. As long as it is humanly possible to avoid such a situation, it must be avoided. Those who are involved in the implementation of the PSRO program have an invaluable opportunity to bridge this widening gap. Accepting the responsibility for peer review and establishing a mechanism for public accountability can do much to defuse some of the biased rhetoric that is voiced too freely today.

Let me close with a quote from Plato, "The penalty for wise men who refuse to partake in government is to live forever under a government ruled by unwise men!"

6

Hospital Review Plans

Faye Gilbarg

As soon after conditional designation as possible, the local PSRO must involve area hospitals in planning for implementation of the review programs. A large part of this effort is the development of a review plan for each hospital once the hospital has expressed interest in seeking delegation for certain review functions and the PSRO staff has performed an initial assessment of the hospital's capability to perform any one or all of the review functions.

The development of the review plan is perhaps the most critical and the most time-consuming part of the delegation process and requires close cooperation and participation by both PSRO and hospital staffs.

PURPOSE OF THE REVIEW PLAN

The process of developing hospital review plans can serve several purposes, all of which should work toward the goal of implementing a review program in the PSRO area that not only is consistent with federal requirements but also meets the needs of each hospital's medical staff, administration, nonphysician personnel, and most important, the patient.

Through wide participation of the medical and hospital staff in this developmental process, the plan becomes an educational tool to inform participants directly about the goals and objectives of the review program and about the local PSRO in general.

The developmental process serves to increase communication between the hospital and the PSRO and is an opportunity for the PSRO staff to provide technical assistance and support, thereby establishing a close relationship, which is very important to the overall success of the program.

The content of the plan is a description of the hospital's intent to perform certain review functions and forms the basis for assessment of the hospital's capability to supervise or perform those functions requested for delegation. The review plan is also a useful document in the formulation of the memorandum of agreement and in the implementation stage guides staff in translating those functions that the PSRO has agreed to delegate into operational terms. Finally, the review plan is the reference document for PSRO staff in monitoring and evaluating the review process and procedures once the program is operational.

It is important to note the statement in the PSRO transmittal on PSRO/hospital relationships and delegation of review functions:*

The PSRO hospital review system, within which delegation may occur, builds upon the existing capabilities of hospital review systems now operational including those established pursuant to requirements of the Joint Com-

*From U.S. Department of Health, Education, and Welfare. Dec. 1974. *The PSRO–short stay hospital relationship and delegation of review functions.* PSRO Transmittal No. 11. Rockville, Md.: Bureau of Quality Assurance, Health Services Administration, p. 2.

mission on Accreditation of Hospitals (JCAH), Title XVIII, Title XIX, and recommendations of the American Hospital Association (AHA). Each hospital will thus require individual evaluation and consideration according to its experience and capabilities for review.

Obviously then, any plan developed and implemented should reflect each hospital's existing system of review as well as the federal and local PSRO requirements.

ELEMENTS OF THE REVIEW PLAN

The plan must include a detailed description of procedures for carrying out the requested delegated review functions, all of which must be based on the requirements for review by DHEW. Accordingly, this requires that the plan include:

(a) Description of the hospital's proposed organization of the review effort indicating the extent of hospital physician membership in the PSRO and participation in review will be communicated to Title XVIII, XIX, and V Agencies; (b) Description of the review components for which delegation is being requested, e.g., full delegation of all three components, or partial delegation of medical care evaluation studies with PSRO management of concurrent review; (c) Description of the methods for using PSRO norms, criteria, and standards in concurrent review and plan for adapting criteria and standards for MCE studies; (d) Description of methods for generating reports for PSRO monitoring and evaluation and how information required to manage or monitor review will be integrated with hospital record abstracting and claims activities; (e) Description of methods by which review findings will be linked with continuing medical education programs.*

In addition to these elements, the nonphysician review component in concurrent review and in medical care evaluation should be described. An

*From Goran, M.J.; Roberts, J. S.; Kellogg, M., et al. 1975. PSRO hospital review system. *Med. Care* 13 (suppl.):20.

explanation of the support services (such as the discharge plan and procedures and the admitting, business office, and medical records functions important to the process) and an explanation of the hospital's confidentiality policies with respect to the data collected on behalf of the PSRO are required.

INITIATION OF THE PLANNING EFFORT

Initial meetings with the hospitals in the PSRO area should be arranged according to a master time table developed by the PSRO staff to assure that all steps are followed and that the appropriate sequence of events takes place for each hospital. Figure 6-1 is an example of the type of chart that can be used as a control.

It is important to have wide participation by the medical staff. For example, the chairman of the utilization review and medical audit committees and any other appropriate medical staff committees, such as the executive committee, should be present. In addition, administrative staff, medical record personnel, the controller or business office department head, admitting personnel, nursing service, and representative from the review staff, if available, should attend.

The initial meeting is actually an orientation session; it is at this meeting that federal requirements for review and local PSRO requirements are presented and discussed in depth. The steps necessary to seek delegation, important elements of writing a review plan, and the process of evaluation and final approval should also be outlined and discussed.

The types of technical assistance that can be provided by the PSRO should be explained, allowing hospital representatives the opportunity to analyze the kind of assistance being offered and that which is required to complete the plan.

	Hospital A Date	Hospital B Date	Hospital C Date	Hospital D Date
1. Letter contact—PSRO				
2. Letter of intent—hospital				
3. Initial assessment—PSRO				
4. Initial meeting—hospital and PSRO				
5. Development of plan stages I–X—hospital and PSRO				
6. Plan submitted—hospital				
7. PSRO evaluation of plan				
8. Revisions required—hospital				
9. Summary to hospital and PSRO				
10. Decision to approve, disapprove plan—PSRO				
11. Decision on delegation—PSRO				
12. Implementation date—PSRO				

FIGURE 6-1. Sample schedule.

A model plan specifying the structure and content of the review plan and the type of detail required should be available to the hospital for use in preparation of the plan (see pp. 51–55).

Finally, the person or persons who will be responsible for coordinating activities on behalf of the PSRO and the hospital should be designated, in other words, one should identify the contact persons to spearhead activities and the completion of task assignment.

Most important, the tasks to be accomplished to produce the plan should be identified by both the PSRO and the hospital, ranking the tasks in sequential order. Resources (time, money, people, and materials) needed to accomplish the task also must be identified and a timetable for completion of each task specified. An example of such a matrix is given in Figure 6-2.

JOINT DEVELOPMENT OF THE PLAN

With the support and assistance of PSRO personnel, the hospital interested in delegation of certain review functions is required to develop a plan that at a minimum includes the seven major areas outlined in the transmittal on hospital/PSRO relationships (see Figure 6-3).*

1. Description of organization of the review effort including:
   a. Number and types of *personnel* to be used for each type of review.

*Adapted from U.S. Department of Health, Education, and Welfare. Dec. 1974. *The PSRO–short stay hospital relationship and delegation of review functions.* PSRO Transmittal No. 11. Rockville, Md.: Bureau of Quality Assurance, Health Services Administration, pp. 8, 9.

Task description	Prime responsibility	Resources required	Start date	Due date	Date completed
I. Hospital review plan					
A. Develop a detailed PSRO review plan					
1. Outline steps					
2. Establish time table					
3. Indicate priorities					
4. Determine division of responsibilities					
B. Reach agreement with affected parties					
C. Monitor plan progress					

FIGURE 6-2. Hospital/PSRO planning matrix.

    b. *Level of review* (such as review coordinator, review physicians, review committee(s) for each type of review.
    c. Current relationships with Titles XVIII and XIX claims payments agencies (such as waivered status, type of claims payment system).
    d. Current relationships with data collection agencies (such as forms to be used, aggregation of data, supply of data to the PSRO for federal reporting purposes).
    e. Review functions to be performed by PSRO personnel.
  2. Description of the types of review to be performed by the hospital, including the following for each type:
    a. Phasing in schedule.
    b. Methods for focusing concurrent review.
    c. Nature and source of data to be collected.

3. Use of PSRO norms, criteria, and standards, including:
    a. Use in admission certification and continued-stay review with justification for any proposed deviations from PSRO-approved norms, criteria, and standards.
    b. The organizational focus and the method of development of criteria and standards for MCE.
    c. Mechanisms for hospital to modify its norms, criteria, and standards.
4. The content and frequency of reports to be generated for:
    a. PSRO evaluation and monitoring.
    b. Hospital internal monitoring and management.
    c. PSRO use in modification of norms, criteria, and standards.

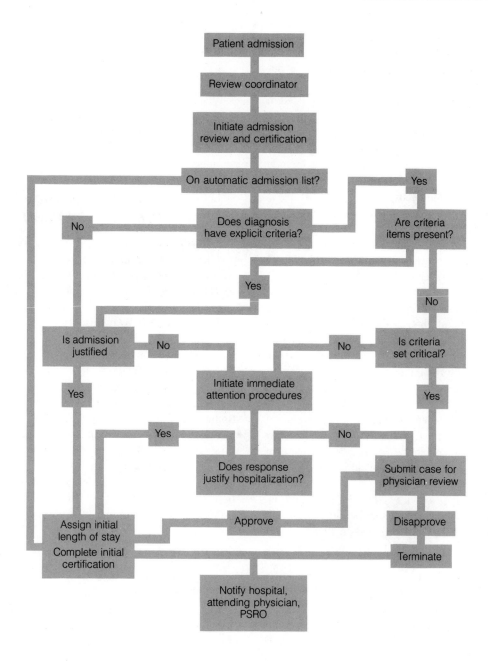

FIGURE 6-3.   Process diagram for admission certification.

5. Methods by which review findings will be used to develop continuing education programs (for example, it must include a description of how the hospital intends to assure the review findings will be utilized in staff education).
6. Types of technical assistance and education needed to implement the proposed review system (for example, it should include names of individuals or organizations that will meet the needs).
7. The number of physicians on the hospital's medical staff eligible for PSRO membership, the number of PSRO members, and the number who will be participating in PSRO review activities.

In addition to the specific requirements in the PSRO transmittal, the PSRO may wish to incorporate the following descriptive information to assure that all areas necessary to the smooth functioning of the review program are covered:

1. Nonphysician involvement in peer review activities. This should include a description of the involvement (of nonphysicians) in concurrent review and in the MCEs, development of screening criteria and norms to be used and the review methodology.
2. Support services. The function of discharge planning services and coordination, admitting, business office, and medical records procedures necessary to the review system should be described.
3. Confidentiality of data procedures. The hospital should describe policies and procedures with respect to the security of data collected, codes that are specific to patient, provider, or practitioner, or special codes specific to the area PSRO; policies and procedures governing personnel responsible for collecting data.
4. Implementation schedule. A time table

for implementation of the requested delegation functions should be described.

When the plan has been completed, it should be submitted in a timely manner to the PSRO by the hospital's medical staff, carrying an official stamp of approval by the governing board and administration.

EVALUATION OF THE REVIEW PLAN BY PSRO

The PSRO staff must establish criteria for evaluation of the review plan, which are also based on the criteria for delegation previously established by the PSRO. A very workable method for technical review of the hospital's review plan is the checklist developed by DHEW for use by the PSROs (see Figure 6-4).

After the technical review by staff, the PSRO may request modifications, to be worked out with the hospital staff person responsible for coordinating plan development activities. A summary of the findings should be distributed to the board of directors, to the committee within the PSRO responsible for evaluating review plans and for recommending delegation status, or to both. To be certain the hospital is informed about all aspects of this evaluation, the PSRO should establish a time by which official response to the hospital will be made.

APPROVAL OF PLAN BY PSRO

Once the decision is made by the PSRO regarding approval or disapproval of the review plan, a written evaluation should be delivered to the hospital. This notification should be sent to the hospital medical staff, administration, and board of trustees. If approval is granted, notification of the Medicare, Medicaid, and Title V agencies should also be initiated. If the plan is not approved, the notification procedures must specify the hospital's right of appeal, and the written summary should indicate what steps can be taken by the medical staff to correct procedures that would eventually allow for approval of all functions.

IMPLEMENTATION OF PLAN

Once delegation of the review functions requested is granted, the PSRO should provide assistance to the hospital in defining the steps in implementation and the roles and responsibilities of the different review participants in the implementation process. A system to monitor implementation in each hospital setting should be established so that the time table approved in the review plan can be realized.

Outline for Model Hospital Review Plan

The following illustrates a suggested format and content of a plan for performing concurrent review (admission certification and continued-stay review) and MCEs. This format may have to be abbreviated to avoid undue demands on smaller hospital staffs.

Review Plan for _____ Hospital

I. Organization (should include chart)
  A. Review committee(s)
    1. Composition, size (including specialty and nonphysician representation)
    2. Method of selecting membership, officers
    3. Terms of office
    4. Frequency of meetings
  B. Review staff
    1. Method of selection and functions of:
      a. Physician advisors
      b. Review coordinators
      c. Data and records personnel
      d. Supporting staff (clerks)
    2. Specification of means of training and supervising the review staff and whether or not the hospital wishes to use PSRO personnel if available for training, supervising, or performing parts of the review process
  C. Facilities
    1. Forms, software—use of PSRO versus hospital materials and printing facilities
    2. Computer resources (if planned)—use of in-house versus PSRO or subcontracted resources
II. Norms, criteria, and standards
  A. Source of norms and criteria for admission certification and continued stay review (PSRO or other source if not yet available from PSRO—include sample criteria set)
  B. Mechanism of development of criteria and standards for MCEs
III. Concurrent admission certification (Figure 6-3)
  A. Describe the process to be used for admission certification, including:
    1. Method of certifying admission for *all* patients
    2. Method and basis of selection of elective and emergency admissions for in-depth review using criteria, and list of diagnoses or problems to be covered initially
    3. Method of notification of review coordinator of patient's admission
    4. Timing and procedures for performance of review, including:
      a. Collection of data
      b. Assigning of initial length of stay (norm percentile used)

Element	Yes	Acceptable alternative	Deficiency or status unclear	No	Comments or explanations
Hospital _____ Date review plan received _____					Reviewer _____ Date of review _____

Concurrent admission certification
 	
*A. Will *all* elective, semiurgent, urgent, and emergency admissions undergo admission certification for patients eligible under:
 	
  1. Medicare
  2. Medicaid
  3. Title V
  4. Other (explain)
B. Will selected diagnoses/problems be subject to in-depth review using criteria?
*C. Will explicit written criteria be used to determine the medical necessity and appropriateness of admission?
D. Criteria used initially will be:
 	
  1. From the PSRO
  2. From other outside source (identify)
  3. From in-hospital source
  4. Other (identify)
E. Will reviewer be notified promptly of a patient's admission to the hospital?
*F. Will admission certification or in-depth review using criteria take place on or before the first working day following admission and before elective surgery occurs?					

*Indicates elements required by regulations.					

FIGURE 6-4. Partial work sheet for assessment of hospital applications for delegation. The complete review plan work sheet includes not only concurrent admission certification, which is shown here, but also concurrent continued-stay review, MCEs, and other material.

c. Notification of certification of admission (for example, stamp on chart)
d. Review coordinator notification of physician advisor for

peer review when criteria not met
e. Peer review by physician advisor when necessary
f. Notification of attending phy-

Hospital _____

Date review plan received _____

Reviewer _____

Date of review _____

Element	Yes	Acceptable alternative	Deficiency or status unclear	No	Comments or explanations
G. When reviewer finds an admission that may not be medically necessary:					
*1. Is the attending physician notified within one working day of admission?					
2. Is notification of a peer reviewer accomplished within one working day of admission?					
H. Peer review is done by:					
1. Whole committee					
2. Committee chairman					
3. Physician advisor					
*I. Will peer review be timely? (within two working days following admission)?					
*J. Will the peer reviewer consult with the attending physician before making a final decision on a denial of certification?					
*K. Will written notification of denial of certification be timely (within two working days of admission)?					
*L. Will written confirmation be sent to:					
1. Patient					
2. Attending physician					
3. Hospital					
4. State agency, if Medicaid or Title V					
5. Medicare intermediary, if Medicare					
*M. Will decisions denying certification be made only by peer physicians?					
*N. Is there a written procedure for reconsideration of decisions?					

sician, patient, hospital, and fiscal agent of noncertification (verbal and written procedures)

g. Reconsideration and appeals of adverse decisions

IV. Concurrent continued-stay review

A. Describe the process to be used for continued-stay review, including:

1. Method of notification of patient's presence in hospital at end of initial length of stay

2. Timing of first and subsequent continued-stay review (identify means of assigning continued-stay review checkpoint for patients with multiple or uncertain diagnoses)
3. Description of the procedures and timing planned for:
   a. Collection of data
   b. Notification of certification of continued stay (such as stamp on chart)
   c. Assigning of extended length of stay (norm percentile used)
   d. Notification of physician advisor of need for peer review
   e. Peer review by physician advisor when necessary
   f. Notification of attending physician, patient, hospital, and fiscal agent of noncertification (verbal and written procedures)
   g. Reconsideration and appeal of decision

V. Medical care evaluation studies
   A. Project the number of MCEs to be carried out during the first year of review delegation; include specific topics planned for study if known
   B. Describe the process for:
      1. Selection of study topics
      2. Development of study design, including criteria and standards (as well as criteria sets already prepared)
      3. Collection and display of data
      4. Analysis of results, including reporting of results to medical staff, administration, and governing board

5. Development of corrective actions
6. Implementation
7. Evaluation of corrective actions
8. Cooperation with the PSRO and other hospitals in performing area-wide MCEs

VI. Data
The hospital plan for an ongoing information system should:
   A. Briefly specify the scope of the system—objectives or functions to be served.
   B. List and justify those data elements that will be added to the uniform hospital discharge data set.
   C. List other kinds of information to be collected to manage and measure performance, cost, and impact of the reviewing process in conformance with the PSRO reporting system. (This should be done with the understanding that the PSRO Management Information System was developed as a model for PSRO use and is the basis for federal reporting requirements. The hospital may need assistance in this area to assure conformance).
   D. Identify the sources of data.
   E. Describe the process for collecting the data, such as who, when, where, and how.
   F. Outline projected steps for testing and modifying forms, procedures, and reports, and for assuring data quality.

VII. Continuing education
   A. Resources available for use in continuing health education programs
   B. Description of the hospital organization and process for:
      1. Assurance of the development of appropriate educational programs

and introduction of corrective measures for problems identified by review
  2. Interface with available existing programs of continuing health education
  3. Evaluation of the effectiveness of the health education program
VIII. Plan for involving nonphysician health care practitioners in review functions
  A. Outline the mechanism and process for including nonphysician health care practitioners in hospital review activities, including:
    1. Establishment and ongoing modification of criteria, norms, and standards for their disciplines
    2. Development and implementation of review for assessing their peer's performance
    3. Development and implementation of appropriate continuing education programs for their disciplines and participation in hospital or areawide programs
IX. Timetable for implementation of review
  A. Describe the time table for phasing in each component of review, including:
    1. Time when concurrent admission certification and continued-stay review will begin, if not already started
    2. Schedule for MCEs
    3. Date for submission of first report to the PSRO and intervals between subsequent reports

X. Technical assistance
  A. Identify in as much detail as possible areas in which the need for technical assistance is anticipated if available from the PSRO or other source. Include assistance in training, supervision of review personnel, design, and evaluation of review activities, and include other resources, such as forms or data processing capabilities needed.

SUMMARY

The importance of a well-defined, thoroughly detailed review plan cannot be overemphasized. The PSRO board of directors' decision whether or not delegation of review functions can take place will in large part be based on the hospital medical staff's documentation of the resources and procedures necessary to carry out these functions.

Implementation and actual operation of the program become easier if the plan has been well defined. Most important, the PSRO staff will rely on the plan for monitoring the review process; thus, it becomes the checklist against which the PSRO will evaluate the hospital's compliance during the first months of operation. With this thought in mind, it behooves a hospital to allocate time and personnel to the creation of a plan that reflects the hospital's intent, that is, a document that can realistically be used for evaluation purposes, such as the work sheet in Figure 6-4.

7

Review Coordinators

Sue Christofferson

Writing a chapter on the review coordinator for a book on PSRO initially seemed like a relatively simple, straightforward task—a task that could be completed in a couple of days by systematically cataloguing commonly held information. Not so!

The greatest fallacy is that there is any commonly held information. Reflection on the articles read and the conversations held remind me that I have yet to discover two people in the PSRO system who agree on the definition of the title "review coordinator," to say nothing of the role and functions.

The phrase "review coordinator" evolved, no doubt, from Medicare's "utilization review coordinator." Review coordinator as used in the PSRO system generally takes on a broader definition that encompasses involvement in quality assessment as opposed to the more narrow utilization review definition of Medicare. However, some in the PSRO system refer only to utilization review when they speak of the review coordinator. Perhaps this stems from the original cost containment emphasis of the federal government, or it may stem from a general lack of clarity surrounding the role of the nonphysician facilitators in the peer review process. In any case, common terms are used in uncommon ways.

In an effort to discuss the varied roles of the nonphysician facilitators of peer review, I have chosen to dissect the review process into several common functional areas:

1. Concurrent review
2. Data abstraction
3. Medical care evaluation studies (MCEs)
4. Program management

The functional descriptions that follow are not intended to be all inclusive but are intended to describe the basic tasks to be performed by nonphysician personnel.

CONCURRENT REVIEW

Concurrent review involves the assessment of the medical necessity of admission and continued stay for all Title V, XVIII, and XIX patients. The nonphysician screens the documentation in the medical record of each patient against physician-generated criteria. If the documentation meets the criteria, the nonphysician assigns the next review point, usually based on diagnostic-specific norms. If the criteria are not met, the case is referred to a physician advisor who determines whether or not the hospitalization is necessary. This process is repeated at regular intervals throughout the patient's stay in the hospital. In PSROs assessing concurrent quality, the process looks not only at the appropriateness of hospitalization but at various quality of care elements as well.

The majority of the nonphysician's time is involved in the process just described, but many additional tasks of equal importance must be done. These include patient and family education, participation in physician advisor orientation and training, development of attending and reviewing physician profiles, presentation of review information to physician committees, identification of problems in the review system, interface with physicians on a one to one basis and in committees, and interface with other departments affected by the review process (such as nursing service, admitting department, billing department, and social service).

The actual review of patient records can require a varying degree of skill depending on the type and complexity of the criteria used. At the very least it requires skill in the understanding and use of medical terminology and advanced skills in communication.

The other tasks require skill in training, problem identification, problem solving, data use, and committee facilitation.

DATA ABSTRACTION

In the most basic sense, the future of the PSRO program will depend on the analysis of the data collected. PSROs have invested a good deal of time and money in developing effective systems for concurrent review, valid criteria, meaningful norms, workable standards, and significant medical care evaluation study topics. But have they invested equivalent amounts of time and money in developing quality control systems for data collection? Some have. Many have not. Since future planning for focused review, quality assessment, and problem identification as well as PSRO program assessment will result from the profiles developed, the accuracy of the data collected is of utmost importance.

In many data collection systems, the people with the least knowledge of the information being collected and the most distance from the impact point of the data are the people selected to abstract it. In these cases it is not surprising that there is frequent criticism about data inaccuracy and subsequent reluctance to accept the data as a measure of anything.

One wonders how many data abstractors realize that the data they abstract will be used by physicians to assess other physicians, by hospitals to assess themselves, by PSROs to assess physicians and hospitals, by DHEW to assess PSRO effectiveness, and by Health Systems Agencies to assist in long-range health care planning, to name a few. The people who collect the data must understand the importance of completing their task accurately, and they must recognize the potential impact the data may have.

MEDICAL CARE EVALUATION STUDIES

Nonphysician functions in MCEs include the day-to-day operation of the Medical Care Evaluation Program. This involves assisting physicians in medical care evaluation study topic selection, study objectives and design, and criteria development. Nonphysician functions also include data collection and display, assisting physicians in variation analysis, corrective action, and restudy.

In addition to having skills in the exacting process of MCEs, people carrying out these functions must be able to train others, often physicians, in the necessary skills of MCEs. Most physician activity in this area is carried out in committees, thus another function of the nonphysician is that of committee facilitator.

The medical care evaluation process, the training process, and the committee facilitation process each require very separate sets of skills. To assume that people who are skilled in the technical MCE function are also skilled in training others to do MCEs may lead to ineffective training. To assume that people with skills in the technical medical care evaluation function can also effectively facilitate committee meetings may lead to chaotic, unproductive meetings.

It is wise to bear in mind that some college curricula devote the bulk of their course work to developing training skills and that others emphasize skills in group process. To expect people who are involved in MCEs automatically to bring these skills to their jobs is unrealistic.

PROGRAM MANAGEMENT

Program management is perhaps the least well defined of the nonphysician functions. Ideally this function is carried out by physicians; however, most often the function is carried out by nonphysicians—if it is carried out at all.

Program management involves the overall coordination and management of all aspects of a peer review program. It includes supervising all nonphysician personnel, linking the concurrent and retrospective components of the program, planning programs, assuring accurate data, coordinating physician involvement and training, reporting review program patterns to physician committees and administration, coordinating the training of other hospital personnel, budgeting, staffing, coordinating the hiring and training of personnel, evaluating personnel performance, and performing countless other tasks.

Clearly, program management requires a high degree of management skill. Once again, to assume that people who have the skills necessary to carry out the three other functions described will also have the skills necessary to manage the program may lead to a poorly managed, ineffective program.

Whether in a delegated or nondelegated system, concurrent review, data abstraction, MCEs, and program management are necessary functions and skills of the review coordinator that must be performed by nonphysician personnel. They can be, and are, performed in various combinations by people with differing backgrounds, who may be employed by a PSRO or a hospital.

QUALIFICATIONS

From the beginning of the PSRO program, there has been controversy over the qualifications necessary to be a review coordinator. There are those who think review coordinators must be registered nurses. Others think registered record administrators (RRAs) and accredited records technicians (ARTs), make good review coordinators. Some think it is a fine position for former military corpsmen. Still others think clerks can do the job.

Everyone has known of registered nurses who were poor nurses, RRAs who were poor administrators, teachers who could not teach, and attorneys who practiced poor law. To equate educational background with competence can be a costly mistake in any system.

Perhaps the most satisfactory answer to the question of which background turns out the best review coordinators is "none of the above." One should ask, "What kinds of competencies are necessary to be a review coordinator?" If job descriptions described the skills necessary to carry out the tasks and prospective employees were required to demonstrate competence in each of the necessary skills, the controversy over educational background would disappear.

This is not to say that certain disciplines do not make a better starting place than others when looking for people with particular skills. To locate someone with skills in the technical process of MCEs, it is logical to begin looking at medical records professionals. If job descriptions and advertisements describe necessary skills, however, the field of potential employees may be broadened considerably. To hire an employee with a background that is not customary for the position often provides the bonus of a fresh and different perspective.

TRAINING

It is a rare occasion indeed to be able to hire personnel having all the skills necessary to perform a given job. More often people are hired because they have most of the necessary skills, and employers expect to train them in the remaining areas. Using the earlier functional descriptions, I developed the following list of skills necessary for nonphysician facilitators of peer review.

1. Ability to understand and use medical terminology
2. Ability to understand and use medical criteria and norms
3. Ability to understand and apply the review processes
4. Training skills
5. Skills in profile development
6. Skills in data use
7. Problem-solving skills
8. Communication skills
9. Conflict management skills
10. Group process skills
11. Data abstracting skills
12. Committee management skills
13. Management skills

An impressive list, is it not? It is impressive enough to make one wonder how any organization could ever provide training in such a wide variety of skills. The answer, of course, lies in the use of external resources.

Most colleges and universities offer courses in many of these areas. In addition, organizations such as the American Management Association offer short-term intensive seminars in conflict management, communication, problem solving, and many other.

The PSROs should not forget that other PSROs are frequently excellent resources. Many have developed training programs in a variety of areas and have personnel able to serve as trainers.

REVIEW COORDINATORS WITHIN THE HOSPITAL

Despite the fact that PSROs are directed by physicians, review coordinators are the heart of the system. Without them, the PSRO would not be a viable concept.

The job of the coordinator is a frustrating one that has not received the attention it deserves. The quality of the relationship between the coordinator and the physicians on the staff of a hospital is critical to the success of the review program. The coordinator can set a tone of cooperation or hostility. Each will most often evoke a similar response from physicians, and it is only through cooperation that review programs will succeed.

Although it is essential that coordinators do the initial screening and make positive decisions based on physician-generated criteria, it is equally necessary for physicians to make all negative decisions regarding care given by their peers. The coordinator must walk that fine line between assisting the physician and overstepping the scope of the job. If this fails to happen, physicians are no better off than they would be with nonphysician organizations carrying out the review responsibility.

REVIEW COORDINATORS WITHIN THE PSRO

Good coordinators may know more about the patterns of medical practice in hospitals than anyone else. In addition, good coordinators are more knowledgeable about the review process and its strengths and weaknesses than anyone else. To exclude them from PSRO boards of directors or their committees is to say that their knowledge and expertise is not valued by the PSRO. It may not always be feasible for coordinators to be voting members of boards or committees, but it is possible for them to be (ex-officio) members. Their early input into decisions that affect them is likely to ensure their support of the decisions and greater ease of implementation.

REVIEW COORDINATORS IN THE NATIONAL SCENE

It was not until 1977 that much attention was given nationally to the special educational and support needs of the coordinator, and then it was not the government or the AAPSRO that responded to the needs but the National Association of Utilization Review Coordinators (NAURC), an organization developed by a private enterprise. By October of 1977, the NAURC still was not universally recognized as the organization to speak for coordinators. In fairness to the AAPSRO, it must be said that efforts were made to develop a section for review coordinators; however, lack of adequate funds and staff time interfered with the effort.

The lack of a national forum has certainly been felt by review coordinators during the frustrating implementation phase of the PSRO. Their emotional survival has been largely the result of local support groups that have emerged. The future in the PSRO program points to additional involvement of coordinators in long-term care, ambulatory care, alternative methods of evaluating the quality of care, preservice education for health professionals, and continuing medical education. With these new frontiers in view, the need for a national forum, where educational programs can take place, ideas can be exchanged, and problems can be shared, will continue to grow.

For coordinators to grow effectively into their emerging expanded role with the help of a national peer group, it will be necessary for PSRO physicians and executive directors to provide the necessary funding and time for them to be involved.

8

Discharge Planning

Dorothy Archer
Sharon V. Davidson

DISCHARGE PLANNING
AND THE PSRO

The efficient and effective movement of patients along the health continuum is based on the correct timing of discharge planning between various levels of health care facilities. Since concurrent review occurs during the hospital episode and relies on personnel trained in assessing the quality of patient care and the need for hospital level of care, the PSRO coordinator provides a natural and important link to discharge planning. As the PSRO coordinator assesses the level of care and identifies potential discharge problems or patients that could benefit from a different level of care, contact with the discharge planner is indicated.

The PSRO's responsibility is to provide information and monitor the discharge planning process, and the reviewers should not perform the total discharge planning function. The PSRO's responsibility need not extend to the actual conduct of discharge planning.

The PSRO's involvement in discharge planning is set forth in the *PSRO Program Manual,* Section 705.29, which states:

Where problems in post-discharge care or discharge placement are anticipated, discharge planning should be initiated as soon as possible after admission to the short-stay hospital. Discharge planning should include both preparation of the patient for the next level of care and arrangement for placement in the appropriate care setting.

Information needed for the discharge planning process include:

(a) prior health care status of patient (i.e., was patient receiving care in his home or in some type of long-term care facility?)

(b) current level of care needed

(c) projected level(s) of care needed

(d) projected time frame for moving patient to next level of care

(e) therapy(ies) and teaching that must be accomplished prior to hospital discharge

(f) available resources for post-hospital care

(g) mechanisms for facilitating transfer to other levels of care.

PSRO coordinators can identify patients with anticipated problems, provide information to the discharge planner about average lengths of stay, encourage discharge planning, and monitor the success of discharge planning as it might affect the length of stay. The demand of the consumer for further help on his discharge should help to boost the role of the discharge coordinator into proper perspective.

Because of the advantage of patient placement in the appropriate level of care facility, the PSRO should encourage comprehensive discharge planning units within health care facilities, which will also help to ensure continuity of care to the patient and his family.

DISCHARGE PLANNER

A comprehensive discharge planning unit encompasses the entire health team, with one key person to initiate and coordinate the discharge plans for the patients so that the best of care is provided in an unbroken sequence. This key person should be a registered nurse, because nursing is the service that is characterized by a 24-hour vigilance over patients. This in itself will make nurses the experts in determining the continuing needs of patients. The nurse will closely coordinate planning with medical social workers who have the ability to identify appropriate community agencies to meet the continuity of care needs assessed by the registered nurse.

There are many titles for those who are discharge planners. Some of these are: liaison nurse, coordinator of discharge planning, public health coordinator, and discharge planning nurse. Discharge planners have many functions, but most of all they think first of how patients can get "there from here," and usually there is a way, tough though it may be. Therefore, those planning for discharges of patients must be problem solvers, persons who do not possess the word "no" in their vocabulary. Additional requirements for discharge planners are background in nursing and experience in the clinical setting of a hospital as well as in the field of public health nursing.

Functions of the Discharge Planner

The functions of the discharge planner include:

1. Visiting patient and family to assess the total needs of the patient (such as psychologic, social, economic, physical, and health education needs).

2. Educating the family and patient in the areas of need so that continuity of care is assured.

3. Attempting to involve other members of the health team, especially the medical social workers.

4. Consulting with the physician regarding the type of continuing medical and nursing care the patient will require.

5. Working with the utilization review committee.

6. Working with community agencies to coordinate community resources with patient needs.

7. Identifying all of the health disciplines involved in the care of the patient and determining patient need for continuation of services (such as continuity of physical therapy or speech therapy after discharge).

8. Providing education for the hospital staff to encourage their participation in discharge plans and to increase their awareness in assessing areas requiring continuity of care.

9. Establishing a multidisciplinary planning committee for the planning of care for the patient anticipating discharge.

Hospital policy and size will dictate the functions of those who coordinate discharges. As the emphasis on continuity of care increases, those planning for discharge will be required to devote all energies to discharge planning. One must remember that the patient does not miraculously appear at the hospital door; the patient comes to the health team members from the community with physical, mental, social, or economic problems. This same patient goes back to the community with a need for further assistance with his problems;

there must be a link to ensure continuous care. This link is the discharge planner.

At one time "discharge" meant to many health care workers that their responsibility for the patient's care had been completed. Current philosophy assumes responsibility for continuity of health care for the patient and his family. Emphasizing continuing care increases the possibility that the patient may return to society having made the best possible adjustment within his capability.

Approximately two out of three patients will require additional treatment, equipment, instructions, or other care upon discharge from a health care facility. Discharge planners can cross agency lines and assist in providing for the care so necessary to restore the patients to their maximum potential as members of society.

DISCHARGE PLANNING PROGRAMS

The patient has certain rights as set forth by the American Hospital Association in 1972. One of these rights is the right to expect reasonable continuity of care. The patient will no longer be blindfolded to prevent him from acquiring knowledge about his treatment and condition.

Some health care institutions have already established discharge planning programs because of their philosophy and commitment to patient care. The PSRO can assist and encourage additional institutions to add this type of care for their patients because of the federal government's mandate on discharge planning, especially for the Medicare patient.

Physicians must also be familiarized with the need for and availability of discharge plans to better serve their patients in this area. A survey of physicians in the St. Louis area indicated that 84% of those surveyed knew about the Visiting Nurse Association and realized they provided nursing care to the patient in the home, but only 16% were aware that speech therapy was also available in the home.

RESPONSIBILITIES IN DISCHARGE PLANNING

To achieve maximum benefit in discharge plans, the health care team should assume the following responsibility:

1. Initiating discharge plans on the first day of the hospital stay or when a handicap is identified.

2. Matching the needs of the patient to community resources.

3. Educating the patient and family in the care of the present illness as well as prevention of other illness or injuries.

4. Applying a working knowledge of utilization data.

5. Identifying needs for new community resources.

6. Communicating openly with all disciplines for implementation of effective discharge plans.

7. Selecting the best discharge plans for each patient.

8. Providing appropriate referral information.

For the health team members to be successful with discharge planning, the hospital and community should assume responsibility for:

1. Establishing an effective and organized program of discharge planning.

2. Providing an assessment of the level of care, with placement in the appropriate care setting.

3. Establishing criteria for the assignment of patient care to the community resource most appropriate for providing for the individual's needs.

4. Assuring the wise use of the dollar for patient care.

A plan for the patient's discharge requires the assumption of responsibilities by the members of the health care team, the health institution, and the community agencies involved in continuity of care.

PATIENT ADMISSION AND TIMELY DISCHARGE PLANNING

The right plans at the time of a patient's admission to a health care facility will determine whether a referral is to be completed. All patients should be assessed for possible identification of needs that will require a referral for continuation of care after discharge. The intensity of needs will depend on such factors as the disease process, the type of surgical procedure performed, diagnostic measures utilized, or specific treatment regimens. For the professional working with hospitalized patients, a definitive action plan for discharge should be available on all patients.

The assignment of the average length of stay for acute-care or long-term care facilities has resulted in a fairly rapid movement of patients along the health continuum. A decrease in hospital or other institutional cost can be realized with effective discharge planning that helps to decrease the length of stay by transferring patients to proper levels of health care facilities. A decrease in length of stay in acute-care facilities may result in an increase in the length of stay at skilled nursing facilities; however, the overall cost in the lower level of care facility is considerably less than cost in an acute-care facility.

Certain groups of patients have definite potential for accurate discharge planning. To plan for discharges, admissions should be screened with identification of patients for assessment based on diagnosis. Conditions frequently requiring discharge coordination and planning include the following:

PEDIATRICS

Battered child syndrome
Burns
Children in body casts
Congenital malformations
Disabling birth injuries
Leukemia
Positive PKU
Weight of baby below 4½ pounds

MATERNITY

Age 16 years or younger
Delivery of stillborn
Drug or alcohol abuse
First baby past age 40 years
Hypertension
Multiple births
Obesity
Postpartum psychosis
Preexisting physical handicap

MEDICAL AND SURGICAL

Aged
Amputation
Arteriosclerotic heart disease
Arthritis
Battered adult syndrome
Bronchitis
Burns

Cancer (such as colostomy, mastectomy, laryngectomy)
Cerebral vascular accidents
Chronic obstructive lung disease
Colostomy
Congestive heart failure
Decubitus
Dehydration
Diabetes
Drug and alcohol addiction
Emphysema
Fractures
Head injury
Hypertension
Malnutrition
Myasthenia gravis
Neurologic disorders
Parkinson's Disease
Spinal cord injury with paralysis
Tuberculosis

In addition to the pediatric, maternity, and medical-surgical conditions listed, emotionally disturbed patients constitute another group that usually benefits from discharge assessment and planning. The needs of the emotionally disturbed patient upon discharge are much the same as those of the medical and surgical patient. The plans for these patients might include outpatient treatment, continued medication, and possibly rehabilitative services for training in marketable skills of employment.

CONTINUING PATIENT CARE

The patient and his family are more than anxious at the time of discharge, and even the simplest information about a procedure of care may be viewed as an insurmountable situation. The patient's anxiety level determines the effectiveness of verbal interactions. The health team members should understand the types of care that can be provided after discharge, provide written instructions, and assure that health teaching has been completed before the day of discharge. Continuing patient care frequently revolves around the continuity of nursing care.

The types of nursing skills that can be required after discharge include the following:

Activities of daily living
All phases of diabetic care
Bed positioning
Bowel and bladder training
Brace application
Care of the teeth
Care and safety of blind person
Care and use of oxygen in home
Colostomy care (includes teaching irrigations, skin care, changing bags, dilation)
Crutch walking
Decubitus care
Deep breathing exercises
Diet supervision, instruction, or both
Dressing change
Elevation of head of bed
Evaluation of shunt functioning
Evaluation of bladder control
Evaluation of home situation and environment
External catheter care
Family planning
Financial aid
Foley catheter care (includes catherizations and irrigations)
Follow-up for suspicious chest x-ray film
Gastrostomy care and feedings
General care—taking vital signs, observing symptoms
Heat application
Homebound teacher
Hydration and nutrition

Ileostomy care

Infant care (instruction in feeding and general care)

Injections given by nurse

Intake and output

Laryngectomy care

Maximist nebulizer

Nephrostomy care

Paraplegic care

Perineal irrigations

Placement of a congenitally abnormal baby

Prevention of contractures

Progressive ambulation

Quadriplegia care

Range of motion exercises

Regulating insulin

Rehabilitation

Rental equipment ordered for home nursing care of patient

Sitz baths

Skilled care—extended care facility

Skin care (includes supervision of family giving care)

Social service

Speech therapy

Spica cast care

Strict bed rest

Suctioning

Supportive care

Suprapubic catheter care

Teaching and supervision of family member (such as, changing a tube)

Teaching and supervision of medication

Teaching and supervision of postural drainage

Teaching sterilization of home equipment

Temporary breast prosthesis

Terminal cancer care

Tracheostomy care

Transfer techniques

Transfer to chair

Transportation

Tuberculosis contact, follow-up in home

Walker or cane, use of

Wound irrigations or cleaning

Patient Referrals

When a discharge planning system is in operation, the health team member who assumes responsibility for discharge coordination identifies patients for assessment of potential care needs after discharge, formulates a discharge plan, identifies appropriate community resources, and communicates the patient's needs to community agencies. This communication is achieved through the completion of a referral form and verbal communication with community agencies. A written referral should include the patient's name, diagnosis, location after discharge, description of services rendered, analysis of present condition, medical treatment plan with medications and treatments, appliances or equipment, dietary restrictions, level of activity, physical, occupational, or speech therapy orders, and any other pertinent information that will serve to assist the person receiving the patient referral in providing the required continuity of care. The utilization of a checklist referral form can expedite the preparation of the written communication. A physician's signature is always required.

SUMMARY

Discharge planning has multiple advantages, including the improvement of the overall care of patients, reduction of cost to the patient and to the health care facility, a decrease in the readmission rate, and compliance with one of the criteria established by the JCAH.

Encouragement of health care facilities by the PSRO to establish comprehensive discharge planning units will recognize that for effective continuity of care, discharge planning must take place on a day-to-day basis by setting priorities to sustain the quality of care that recognizes the needs of every patient. By executing high-quality discharge planning for continuity of patient care, the health care team, institutions, and community agencies express their awareness of their responsibility to the citizens.

BIBLIOGRAPHY

A fond farewell to patients shouldn't mean goodby to care. June 1977. *RN* 40:33–41.

Beaudry, Sister M.L. Dec. 1975. Effective discharge planning matches patient need and community resources. *Hosp. Prog.* 56:29–30.

Cucuzzo, R.A. Jan. 1976. Method discharge planning. *Supervisor Nurse* 7:43–45.

Davidson, S.V.S., editor. 1976. *PSRO: utilization and audit in patient care,* St. Louis: The C.V. Mosby Co., pp. 65–67.

Furbanks, M.E. 1976. A nursing referral system: admissions, transfers, and discharge to and from hospital. *Nurs. Times* 72:41–44.

Hicks, A.P. and Ashby, D.J. 1976. Teaching discharge planning. *Nurs. Outlook* 24:306–308.

Jennings, C.P. March 1977. Discharge planning and the government, *Supervisor Nurse* 8:48–52.

Leanitt, M. Jan.–Feb. 1975. The discharge crisis: the experience of families or psychiatric patients. *Nurs. Res.* 24:33–40.

Liaison nursing service at BMH. Jan. 1971. *Baptiscope* 23:6.

Nursing service hears about discharge planning. Nov. 1976. *Tex. Nurse* 50:10.

Riley, M. and Moses, J.A., Jr. April 1977. Coordinated care: making it a reality. *Nurs. Admin.* 7:21–25.

Schuman, J.E., and Willard, H.N. Feb. 1976. Role of the acute hospital team in planning discharge of the chronically ill. *Geriatrics* 31:63–67.

Stevens, P.F. 1974. Discharge from hospital, the problem of adjustment. *Nurs. Times* 70:700–702.

Weber, C.E., Jr., and Sather, M.R. Nov.–Dec. 1976. Discharge medication counseling. *Hosp. Top.* 54:39–42.

9

Physician Advisors

Daniel J. O'Regan

One of the most important personnel in the daily operations of the PSRO program is the physician advisor (PA). Smooth operations of review functions in the hospital, whether delegated or not, will depend greatly on how the physician advisor interacts with other participants in the system. The number of physician advisors will obviously vary with the size and complexity of the hospital, and this is discussed later in the chapter. This chapter is written with the delegated acute-care hospital in mind. The duties in the nondelegated hospital would be the same except for the chain of command.

EVOLUTION OF UTILIZATION REVIEW

The physician advisor and the review coordinator (see Chapter 7) personify part of the evolution of utilization review. The early utilization review committees (URCs) usually consisted of a few dedicated members of a hospital's medical staff. They met periodically and reviewed charts referred to them for a variety of reasons. As the pressures on paying agencies increased, the demand for more frequent and more intensive review of lengths of stay also increased. It was often necessary to review charts on a daily basis, increasing the demands on the time of physician reviewers. The use of review coordinators was developed as a way to conserve physicians' time; the latter would review

only those cases where professional peer knowledge was essential. Such cases were selected by the screening procedures of the review coordinator. This system has resulted in the PSRO review coordinator selecting cases for physician review according to norms, criteria, and standards selected by the utilization review committee (or the PSRO). The demands for efficient and timely review meant that the coordinator could not wait a week or more for meetings of the utilization review committee. The result was the designation of a physician who could consult with the coordinator on a daily basis to consider those situations that failed to meet the applicable standards. This individual became known as the physician advisor.

Levels of Review

The idea of multiple levels of review is thus established. The first, or primary, level is that done by the review coordinator, who can certify an admission or continued stay. If unable to do so, for whatever reason, the review coordinator refers the problem to the physician advisor, who represents the second level. The third level, if the physician advisor cannot decide, will be either an additional physician advisor or the URC, depending on the utilization review plan in effect. Reconsiderations and appeals may be considered the fourth level of review.

QUALIFICATIONS OF PHYSICIAN ADVISORS

Physician advisors require considerable talent for their tasks. They must understand the operations and objectives of the PSRO procedures and regulations, including the reasons for their existence. Practicing physicians with knowledge of the hospital, its personnel, its patient mix, and its socioeconomic environment make a valuable contribution to utilization review. They must bring this knowledge and experience into the practice of quality assurance. Diplomacy, patience, and tact are also requirements. Physician advisors should be neither policemen nor rubber stamps. Each situation must be honestly and fairly evaluated. Consideration should be given to the individual patient but also to the effects of decisions on numbers of patients and on the hospital's overall efficiency. The latter can be a problem in orientation; physicians usually consider patients one at a time, whereas fiscal agents regard them collectively. Some adjustments in attitudes on both sides are necessary.

To itemize some of the suggested requirements for the task, physician advisors should:

1. Be practicing physicians.
2. Have the respect of their colleagues.
3. Have good relationships within the hospital.
4. Have patience, tact, and understanding.
5. Keep the problems of patients in mind.
6. Be familiar with the *PSRO Program Manual,* regulations, and requirements of the PSRO plan in their area.
7. Be members of the URC.
8. Understand the role and procedures of the review coordinators.
9. Understand the role of discharge planning, social service, medical records, and other departments involved.

10. Have good relations with other physician advisors.
11. Be familiar with the operative norms, criteria, and standards.
12. Be familiar with all forms in use.
13. Be familiar with procedures for reconsiderations and denials.
14. Be decisive and willing to make decisions.

A suggested sample of a job description for this important position follows.

PHYSICIAN ADVISOR (PA)
JOB DESCRIPTION
Overall Responsibilities

Contribute to the provision and maintenance of quality medical care in the hospital under the direction of the utilization review committee (URC) and the PSRO operative in the area.

Nature and scope of work

Review on a regular and timely basis those cases referred by the review coordinator (RC) for the decision of the PA. The PA is accountable to the URC (delegated hospital), PSRO (nondelegated hospital), or both.

Job Requirements

Be a licensed physician.
Be a member of the PSRO.
Be a member of the URC.
Attend all meetings of the URC.

General Qualifications and Responsibilities

1. Become familiar with all rules and regulations that govern the PSRO program.
2. Learn the procedures and methodology adopted by the PSRO and the policies and procedures of the URC.
3. Learn the utilization review plan operative in the hospital.
4. Review on a day-to-day basis the quality, medical necessity, and appropriateness of the care rendered in the hospital.
5. Contribute to the improvement and updating of the norms,

criteria, and standards, plus other suggestions to improve the system.

6. Suggest topics for medical care evaluation studies and continuing medical education studies on the basis of experience in the review process.
7. Use the PA activities as a means to familiarize other medical staff members with the principles and purposes of utilization review.
8. Make high-quality medical care the main objective while assessing the efficiency of that care through concurrent review.
9. Emphasize the need for clear, legible documentation on charts.
10. Submit regular reports of his or her activities as required by URC/PSRO.

Specific Duties

1. Establish efficient and smooth working relationships with the RC.
2. Review all cases that the RC is unable to certify for admission or continued stay.
3. Discuss all questionable cases with the attending physician.
4. Consult with another PA or appropriate specialists on unresolved matters.
5. Refer unresolved matters to the URC/PSRO.
6. Initiate the issuance of letters of denial to all parties involved where appropriate.
7. Notify the attending physician of denial decisions (PA must not delegate this duty to the RC).
8. Review samples of all review by the RC on a periodic basis; monitor the usefulness of forms, stamps, filing system, and other parts of the RC's methodology.
9. Review all continued stay cases before the date specified by the URC/PSRO.
10. Maintain effective liaison with the discharge planning and social service departments, including the availability of alternate levels of care.
11. Fully document decisions made in the established format.
12. Notify the RC of all of his or her decisions, as well as those of other PAs, the URC, or the PSRO, in each case.
13. Where cases are admitted without specific diagnosis, be sure that specific diagnoses are identified as soon as possible.
14. Observe the influence of ancillary services, including laboratory, radiology, pharmacy, and operating room, on the efficiency of care in the hospital.
15. Consult with nonphysician health care providers where appropriate in accordance with URC/PSRO rules.

16. In hospitals that frequently admit Title V (Maternal and Child Health) patients, a PA who is familiar with Crippled Children's Services (CCS) and other Title V cases should be available.
17. Notify the URC and RC of his vacation schedule, and so forth, so that coverage is not interrupted.

SELECTION OF PHYSICIAN ADVISORS

To identify enough individuals with the attributes just discussed to fill all the billets in all PSRO areas is a formidable task. It will require time for a sufficient number of medical staff members to become familiar with the review functions. Those with knowledge and interest will no doubt quickly rise to the occasion. Some programs may prefer to use such individuals exclusively. It may be more desirable as time goes on to provide the medical staff with wide exposure to the PSRO system. This can be done by rotating physicians through the URC at first and then selecting those who are willing and capable to serve as physician advisors. They will become familiar with the principles of review and the levels of decision making. As more staff members participate, those who are more capable and effective will be identified. A small group serving on a permanent basis should be avoided, because it may be identified with administrative and bureaucratic structure. This can promote resistance and friction between medical staff members.

TRAINING OF PHYSICIAN ADVISOR

The foregoing discussion indicates the need for technical knowledge about the PSRO program in general and utilization in particular. A good deal of homework is indicated. Some of the methodology will be best understood by on-the-job, or apprenticeship, experience. An outline of topics to be covered follows. How this is done will depend on local circumstances. It is not easy to assemble busy physicians for lengthy orientation instruction.

Broad-based PSRO areawide seminars should be supplemented by sessions involving smaller groups at the hospital level. Participation by review coordinators and PSRO representatives as faculty is very helpful.

SUGGESTED SYLLABUS
Role of the physician advisor in the PSRO utilization system

I. Origins of PSRO
   A. Development of quality assurance programs since 1910 (Flexner, Codman, American College of Surgeons, JCAH, AHA, and so forth)
   B. Development of utilization programs (such as Blue Cross, Medicare, Medicaid)
   C. Public Law 92-603
      1. Legislative intent
      2. Basic provisions
      3. Utilization sections other than PSRO
II. Structure of a (the local) PSRO
   A. Organization
   B. PSRO area
   C. Stages of development—planning, conditional, operational
   D. Responsibilities
   E. Staging of review coverage: acute-care, long-term care, ambulatory, ancillary, private sector
III. PSRO relationships
   A. Organizational framework of DHEW, Health Care Financing Administration, regional offices, and so forth
   B. Relationships with other PSROs and, where applicable, state Professional Standards Review Council
   C. Relationships with hospitals, delegation and nondelegation
   D. Relationships with Medicare, Medicaid, and Maternal and Child Health agencies and fiscal intermediaries
   E. Relationships with Health Systems Agencies, state Health Coordinating Councils, and so forth
IV. Levels of responsibility
   A. PSRO level
   B. Hospital level, delegated and nondelegated
      1. Governing board
      2. Administration
      3. Medical staff
      4. Utilization review committee
      5. Audit committee
      6. Admitting office, nursing, social service, discharge planning, and medical records
   C. Nonphysician health care practitioners
V. Components of the PSRO review system
   A. Concurrent review—admission certification and continued stay review
   B. Medical care evaluation studies
   C. Profile development
   D. Overall purposes: medical necessity, quality, and appropriateness
   E. Continuing medical education
VI. Utilization review process
   A. Utilization review plan
   B. Utilization review committee
   C. Physician advisor
   D. Review coordinator
   E. Levels of review
   F. Norms, criteria, and standards
   G. Comparison of screening criteria and standards for utilization review with those used for retrospective medical care evaluation studies
   H. Use of percentiles, length of stay data, and coding
VII. Physician advisor and review coordinator roles in the utilization review plan
   A. Step-by-step description of the plan and the procedures of review; use specific examples of actual cases
   B. Review of all appropriate forms, stamps, and so forth
   C. Problem-solving exercises on all aspects of review process
   D. Physician advisor relationships with medical staff, utilization review committee, other physician advisors, specialty consultants, and so forth
   E. Review of the procedures for reconsideration and appeals
VIII. PSRO information requirements
   A. PHDDS—uniform hospital discharge data set, with PSRO elements added
   B. Need for accurate documentation at all levels
   C. Responsibility of physician advisor in recording his decisions
   D. Confidentiality of identifiable information
IX. Review of other informational materials
   A. Coverage codes of Titles V, XVIII, and XIX
   B. Applicable regulations regarding long-term care, level of care, and so forth
   C. Applicable rules of local state agencies and fiscal intermediaries
   D. Regulations of local state department of health

This syllabus is a suggested outline; topics can be added or deleted as necessary. The amount of time devoted to each of the major headings should be varied. The majority of time should be devoted to the practical aspects of the review methodology, because the accuracy of the determinations will be vital to the program. Much of the background material can be summarized in prepared papers and supplemented by references to the literature. The need for review of portions of the syllabus will become evident as the results of the review process are fed back to the PSRO and the hospital. No attempt should be made to cover all of the items suggested in a single session. A series of presentations is best. The problem usually is how to gather a physician audience for subject matter that is not of scientific interest. The leadership of the medical staff and the various departments can be essential in stimulating interest and attendance.

Once the physician audience understands the role of the physician advisor, they should be advised to avoid certain problems when in that position to function as effectively as possible. The development of a small clique of physician advisors is to be avoided. Also, the tendency of a review coordinator to deal selectively with a particular physician advisor, to the exclusion of others, is not good practice. Although it is comfortable to deal with those who frequently agree with us, this can give the appearance of favoritism and bias and disturbs the objectivity of the review process. Such appearance of bias must also be avoided in the case of professional corporations, partnerships, deference to department heads, and the like. Physician advisors obviously must not make decisions on their own patients. To be effective, the review procedures must be applied equally to all. The only bias should be in favor of the patient who is in need of hospital care.

NUMBER OF PHYSICIAN ADVISORS

The number of physician advisors required depends on the size and character of the hospital. A basic rule may be one physician advisor for each 100 beds. In larger hospitals one physician advisor might be assigned from each of the major departments (medicine, surgery, and so forth). A high admission rate or busy ambulance and emergency services may call for more physician advisor participation. Decisions by the PSRO to focus review on particular physicians, departments, or groups of patients may also indicate a change in the number of physician advisors. A sufficient number should be available to provide coverage when illness or vacation schedules might interrupt surveillance.

SUMMARY

The PSRO program brings together concurrent utilization review and retrospective analysis to produce an integrated quality surveillance and assurance process. Information gathered will be referred back to physicians and other providers and will indicate topics for continuing medical education. The resultant improvements in the quality and efficiency of medical services will be the real benefit of this peer review system. The usefulness of information will depend on the accuracy of the initial record (the patient's chart) and how this record is used for utilization and abstract purposes. The attending physician bears primary responsibility for the medical record, but the physician's closest peer, the physician advisor, is in the best position to assess the faithfulness of the original record to the actual events.

The physician advisor, then, is not merely an overseer of lengths of stay but is one of the key figures in this entire peer review process. Interest of physicians in physician advisor duties and training programs can be sustained if the peer review aspects are stressed.

BIBLIOGRAPHY

Colonial Virginia Foundation for Medical Care. 1976. *PSRO Handbook for Physician Advisor.* Norfolk, Va.: The Foundation.

Colorado Foundation for Medical Care. 1976. *Physician advisor manual.* Denver: The Foundation.

Davidson, S.V.S., editor. 1976. *PSRO: utilization and audit in patient care.* St. Louis: The C.V. Mosby Co., pp. 34–36.

Decker, B., and Bonner, P. 1973. *PSRO: organization for regional peer review.* Cambridge, Mass.: Ballinger Publishing Co.

Greene, R. 1976. *Assuring quality in medical care: the state of the art.* Cambridge, Mass.: Ballinger Publishing Co., pp. 213–239.

Houston, P. 1976. *PSRO manual for the review coordinator.* Trenton, N.J.: New Jersey Foundation for Health Care Evaluation, Sections III and IV.

Newmark, G. Dec. 1976. The PSRO physician adviser: who he is, what he does. *Hosp. Med. Staff,* 5:8–11.

Office of Professional Standards Review. 1974. *PSRO program manual.* Rockville, Md. U.S. Department of Health, Education, and Welfare, Chapter 7.

O'Regan, 1976. *PSRO manual for the physician advisor.* Trenton, N.J.: New Jersey Foundation for Health Care Evaluation.

U.S. Department of Health, Education, and Welfare. *Suggestions for monitoring PSRO functions delegated to hospitals.* Technical Assistance Document No. 8. Dec. 27, 1976. Rockville, Md.: Bureau of Quality Assurance, Health Services Administration, p. 5.

10

Potential Roles of Nonphysician Health Care Practitioners in the PSRO Program

Geraldine L. Ellis
Rebecca R. Sadin

The role of health care practitioners other than physicians in the PSRO program has posed a perplexing dilemma since the passage of PL 92-603. The statute includes the requirement that services provided by practitioners other than physicians are to be reviewed under the aegis of the program.* It also stipulates that the PSRO is authorized to make arrangements to utilize the services of health care practitioners other than physicians engaged in the practice of their profession within the PSRO area to undertake professional inquiry in the review for which the PSRO is responsible.† Programmatic questions arising from those rather general directions include: (1) which practitioners other than physicians should the PSRO include in its review system; (2) where in the review system is it appropriate for those practitioners (once identified) to participate in review; (3) when should evidence of such review be required for a PSRO to be considered in compliance with those sections of the statute; (4) are the physician members of the PSRO sufficiently supportive of the

concepts inherent in the referenced sections of the statute to foster any, a token, or a comprehensive effort in implementation of peer review of services provided by health care practitioners other than physicians; (5) what are the budgetary ramifications of such effort; and (6) what are the professional interests and the experiential base in PSRO-type review among the various disciplines?

Since 1974, the BQA (now the Health Standards and Quality Bureau) has been able to glean some tentative, but far from conclusive, answers to those programmatic questions. Each question is addressed from the base of knowledge available and extent of the program policy and guidance developed to date.

Which health care practitioners other than physicians should the PSRO include in its review system?

Based on the goal of the PSRO program— establishment of effective local peer review systems to assure that federal expenditures for beneficiaries of Medicare, Medicaid, Maternal and Child Health, and Crippled Children's programs are spent on medically necessary, high-quality care— the programmatic definition of health care prac-

*PL 92-603, Section 1155(a)(1).
†PL 92-603, Section 1155(b)(1)(2).

74

titioners other than physicians specifies three characteristics of such practitioners:

Health care practitioners other than physicians are those health professionals who (a) do not hold a doctor of medicine or doctor of osteopathy degree, (b) meet all applicable State and Federal requirements for practice of their profession, and (c) are actively involved in the delivery of patient care or services which may be paid for, directly or indirectly, under Titles V, XVIII, and/or XIX of the Social Security Act.*

Whereas it is instantly clear to any reader that a doctor of medicine or a doctor of osteopathy is a physician, individuals using this definition have had difficulty identifying precisely the professional disciplines meeting the three characteristics of health care practitioners other than physicians. Therefore, it has required further interpretation of the specific health care practitioner disciplines covered and the meaning of "paid for directly" versus "paid for indirectly."

A search of documents published by Medicare, Medicaid, Maternal and Child Health and Crippled Children's programs, and the Bureau of Health Manpower as well as consultation with representatives of health care professional organizations permitted identification of 15 generic disciplines whose practitioners provide health care services that may be paid for either by direct payment to the practitioner by at least one of the three funding programs or by the employing institution, which, in turn, is reimbursed by at least one of the three funding programs.

Within the 15 generic disciplines there are more than 1.5 million practitioners, with a wide range of educational requirements for professional qualification and with varying levels of responsibility for

*From PSRO advisory groups, rules, and regulations. July 12, 1976. Federal Register. 41:134.

patient care. Minimum professional requirements may be completion of a post-secondary education diploma-awarding program and successful performance on a licensing examination, whereas the maximum professional requirement may be possession of a doctoral degree and completion of an internship experience. The levels of responsibility for patient care range from those practitioners who are initiators of care, that is, they serve as independent primary points of entry into the health care system in hospitals, in out-of-hospital settings, or both, to those who require physician referral or order but have independent functions, to those who work under order, supervision, or direction of a physician most of the time.

Table 10-1 identifies each discipline by generic name, its number of active practitioners, and the level of responsibility for patient care held by the majority of practitioners in the discipline.

Just as the term "physician," as used in various documents dealing with the PSRO program, is inclusive of all physicians regardless of their specialty areas of practice, the generic term for each discipline (such as dentist, nurse, and social worker) cited in this chapter includes those in specialty areas of practice. Concern has been raised about elimination of other categories of allied health professions that have been recognized in such documents as the Health Manpower Source Book. Some of the 125 professions identified in such references are those in specialty areas of practice but are here included with the generic discipline. Others either are not actively involved in the delivery of patient care or services, such as a medical illustrator or an environmental aide, are not recognized by the payment programs, or would not have professional responsibility for review of patient care or services.

However, persons working in the PSRO program need to be alert to legislative action that may

TABLE 10-1.   Health Care Practitioners Other Than Physicians Meeting the Characteristics
of the PSRO Program Definition

DISCIPLINE	NUMBER OF PRACTITIONERS	INITIATORS OF CARE	PHYSICIAN REFERRAL PLUS INDEPENDENT FUNCTIONS	PHYSICIAN ORDER, SUPERVISION, OR DIRECTION MOST OF THE TIME
Clinical laboratory	1,055,000			X
Clinical psychology	19,000	X		
Dentistry	125,000	X		
Dietetics	16,400*		X	
Medical records	21,000			
Nursing	961,000		X	
Occupational therapy	12,000		X	
Optometry	21,000	X		
Pharmacy	120,000		X	
Physical therapy	30,000		X	
Podiatry	7,200	X		
Radiological technology	125,000			X
Respiratory therapy	55,000		X	
Social work	50,000*		X	
Speech-language pathology and audiology	11,000*		X	
TOTAL	1,697,100			

*Number practicing in the health care system only.

change the status of currently identified disciplines or create new categories of health care professionals who receive recognition by the Social Security Act. For example, podiatrists currently may not certify the medical necessity for hospital admission of a Medicare beneficiary, but a legislative amendment to the act has been introduced in Congress to amend Section 1861(i)(3) to enable the podiatrist to certify or recertify a patient's need for hospital care. An example of a new category to be recognized by the act is the physician's assistant group named in PL 95-210.

Where in the PSRO review system is the participation of health care practitioners other than physicians appropriate?

To discover where the participation of nonphysician health care practitioners is appropriate, it is necessary to consider the goal of the PSRO program, the components of the PSRO review system, and the scope of responsibilities for patient care assigned to health care practitioners other than physicians. Another factor that greatly influenced bureau policies is that the legislative history indicates that Congress intended the PSRO program to be based on the concept of peer review. Therefore, where the PSRO is assessing the necessity, appropriateness, or quality of patient care or services provided by health care practitioners other than physicians, it is appropriate that peers of those practitioners participate in the review.

Three basic policies encompass the considerations just presented and are intended to assist a PSRO in determining where health care practitioners other than physicians may properly become involved in its hospital review system.* These are:

1. Where health care practitioners other than physicians are accorded active staff privileges and have responsibilities for hospital admission, continued stay and discharge, review for admission certification and continued stay should involve such practitioners.

2. Participation of health care practitioners other than physicians in MCEs and profile analysis shall be similar to that of physicians when care provided by other practitioners is being reviewed. This policy applies to all categories of health care practitioners other than physicians who are authorized to perform review under the act and to the conduct of any MCE study or profile analysis that includes the review of patient care or services provided by peer practitioners.

3. Criteria, standards, and norms are an integral part of the peer review system, and must be developed by peer practitioners for their specific areas of practice.

*From U.S. Department of Health, Education, and Welfare. Jan. 25, 1977. *Policies applicable to PSROs involving HCPOTP in peer review in short stay hospitals.* Transmittal No. 44, Rockville, Md.: Bureau of Quality Assurance, Health Services Administration, Public Health Service.

Clearly the first policy should be implemented by the PSRO when it is performing review of titled patients admitted to hospitals by dentists who have been accorded medical staff membership and independent admitting privileges. At the present time, dentists are the only practitioners other than physicians who can qualify for full hospital medical staff membership as well as independently certify the necessity for hospital admission and continued stay. It is recognized that the number of dentists holding hospital medical staff membership within a given PSRO area may be relatively small, and the PSRO leadership may need assistance in identifying dentists who can be called on for the performance of peer review services. Where the PSRO has established either a statutory advisory group or an informal advisory committee, assistance in securing a cadre of dental reviewers may be obtained from that group. Another source of assistance could be the local dental society, because these organizations frequently have established peer review or quality assurance committees.

Participating in the concurrent review process may be appropriate also for those health care practitioners other than physicians who hold clinical privileges in hospitals and who play significant roles in initiating the hospital admission process even though such practitioners may not certify the necessity of the admission. Podiatrists and clinical psychologists are practitioners who may meet those characteristics. Podiatrists, for example, may participate in justifying the need for podiatric surgery in the hospital where the patient has a medical condition that precludes surgery on an outpatient basis.

Some professionals who do not initiate admission or discharge from a hospital are often in a position to provide information that is essential for the justification of certain hospital admissions or surgical procedures. For example, before a pharyngeal flap procedure to achieve appropriate speech and voice quality should be performed, there should be confirmation by a speech-language pathologist that there is a speech or voice problem requiring surgical correction. Another example relates to admission to skilled nursing facilities or rehabilitation facilities. Justification for admission is frequently dependent on the need for skilled nursing care or intensive rehabilitation care, which is determined collaboratively by physicians, professional nurses, and rehabilitation professionals. In both these instances, health care practitioners other than physicians serve a valuable advisory function to the physician regarding admission to the facility.

Continued-stay review should include those practitioners responsible for initiating patient discharge as well as those who impact on the patient's readiness for the next level of care. Dentists and podiatrists should determine when patients admitted for their care need to be discharged. Other health care practitioners, such as nurses, respiratory therapists, and those providing rehabilitation services, should be available to provide consultation to the review coordinator, physician advisor, or both at the time of continued-stay review and discharge planning when there are problems relating to their areas of practice. This may be a structured process whereby, before the expiration of the assigned length of stay, a team composed of all those disciplines whose care impacts on the patient being reviewed are brought together, or it can be unstructured, where the review coordinator consults with whomever he or she thinks appropriate to the case under review.

Where a PSRO is reviewing ancillary services and the referral for the service, type, frequency, and duration of treatment are determined by the physician in consultation with the health care practitioner providing the service, the development of criteria and the review of necessity and appropri-

ateness should be done collaboratively. For example, it is common for the physician to consult with the physical therapist, occupational therapist, speech-language pathologist, and sometimes the respiratory therapist when ordering the services and planning the treatment. Some of these health professionals have developed referral and discharge criteria for their services with the assistance of the PSROs. Another example of collaborative review of ancillary services is in the area of drug utilization review. Pharmacists can assist the medical staff by reviewing patients' medication profiles to monitor such items as appropriateness of specific drug usage, dosage, adverse effects, and interaction with other drugs.

In long-term care facilities, PSROs are required to develop an approach to concurrent quality assurance that will assess the necessity of services as well as the quality of services being provided to patients while they are in the facility. The process may include a review of patient care plans, prescribed medications, progress notes, and a bedside evaluation of the patient's condition. Since care in long-term care facilities is multidisciplinary, those health care practitioners providing the care will participate in the concurrent quality assessment process.

The major participation by health care practitioners other than physicians in the PSRO program will be in the retrospective review of the quality of care rendered utilizing MCEs. Since outcome of care is generally dependent on intervention by more than one practitioner discipline, it is logical to assume that medical care evaluation study topics selected by the PSROs will, in addition to physician care, address the care rendered by health care practitioners other than physicians. In those instances, the practitioners who have the professional responsibility for the care rendered by the disciplines involved in the study should participate in all phases of the study, including the development of criteria for assessment of their care, the identification of problems, the recommendations for follow-up actions, and the carrying out of these corrective actions.

Under the circumstances previously discussed, the PSRO or hospital delegated the medical care evaluation study function may apply either the interdisciplinary or the multidisciplinary approach to the conduct of the MCEs. The two approaches have been defined for program use as follows:

Interdisciplinary medical care evaluation study: the medical care evaluation committee, comprised of peer members of the disciplines whose care is to be reviewed (physicians along with other health care practitioners), develops or selects and agrees on a single set of criteria; those are applied against one set of patient records from which data are collected, and the analysis of the data, identification of variations and development of recommendations

are conducted collaboratively by the committee

Multidisciplinary medical care evaluation study: the study topic and patient records are the same, but each discipline develops or selects its own discipline-specific criteria, analyzes the data relevant to those criteria, identifies the variations, and develops its own discipline-specific recommendations for follow-up actions

It is necessary to point out that monodisciplinary, or single-discipline, MCEs dealing with the care or services provided by a health care practitioner discipline other than physicians, such as nursing audits or dietary audits, may not be applied toward the PSRO requirements for MCEs unless there is at least physician participation at the committee level. Moreover, the advantages of interdisciplinary and multidisciplinary MCEs seem to outweigh the advantages of monodisciplinary studies, as depicted in Table 10-2.

TABLE 10-2.   Advantages of Medical Care Evaluation Studies*

ADVANTAGES	INTER-DISCIPLINARY	MULTI-DISCIPLINARY	MONO-DISCIPLINARY
Communication among professionals	X	X	—
Team approach	X	—	—
Impact on total power structure	X	—	—
Cuts through formal structure	X	—	—
Economical	X	X	—
Clerical work done by medical records	X	X	—
Conflict resolution ⟶ change	X	—	—
Unification of evaluation activities	X	X	—
No duplication of efforts	X	X	—
Lower degree of coordination	—	—	X
Lower conflict	—	X	X
Open negotiation	—	—	X
Focus on single discipline concerns	—	X	X
Closer relation to criteria and audit results	—	X	X
Short lead time for topic selection flexibility	—	—	X

*From Donald A. Dennis, Ph.D., Director of Medical Education, Daniel Freeman Hospital Medical Center, Inglewood, Calif. 90306.

When should evidence of review by health care practitioners other than physicians be required for a PSRO to be considered in compliance with the statute?

Because it was realized that a developing PSRO had many complex problems to resolve in its early implementation of review, program guidelines regarding evidence of review by health care practitioners other than physicians have been flexible. However, the project assessment effort, currently underway, includes exploration of the mechanisms employed and the degree to which the PSRO has taken steps to include review of care or services provided by health care practitioners other than physicians. Some evidence of definitive action in this area is considered necessary for a PSRO to become eligible for operational designation.

The NPSRC has requested that the bureau implement a mechanism to encourage systematic reporting of activity in support of current policies dealing with peer review of care or services provided by health care practitioners other than physicians by PSROs. Changes in the contract management manual that will effect the council's request have been developed.

Advisory groups, composed of seven to 11 members who represent health care practitioners other than physicians, hospitals, and other health care facilities, are required by statute to be established by each Statewide Professional Standards Review Council and by PSROs in states without councils. The purpose of an advisory group is to advise and assist the council or the PSRO in carrying out its functions. The annual reports of the advisory groups, the first of which was completed in 1978, include information on measures taken by the advisory groups to assist the statewide councils or PSROs in carrying out their review functions that relate to health care practitioners other than physicians.

Evidence acquired at this time from a sampling of PSROs includes the following activities in review of services provided by practitioners other than physicians:

A. *PSRO activity in admission review by health care practitioners other than physicians*
1. Charles River PSRO. This PSRO has a dental committee for those dentists who have hospital admitting privileges. The chairman of the dental committee is a member of the board of directors and of the executive committee of the foundation. If a problem comes up regarding a dental admission, it is referred to the dental committee.
2. Hartford, Connecticut PSRO. The local dental society has developed criteria for dental review. If there is a question regarding a dental admission, the PSRO asks the dental society for three names of dentists and chooses one with whom to consult. The present PSRO policy is that an adverse determination is not made unless two physicians agree on it. With dental questions, one physician and one dentist are required.
3. Central Massachusetts PSRO. An oral surgeon is on the board of directors of the PSRO. When a dental problem comes up, the PSRO asks the oral surgeon for a list of consultant dentists.

B. *PSRO activity in continued stay review by health care practitioners other than physicians*
In the Southwestern Pennsylvania PSRO, most of the hospitals require patients subject to continued stay review to be reviewed by a patient care team. When the patient is reviewed at admission and a length of stay is assigned, a determination is made as to need for team review based on such variables as age, diagnosis, and associated problems, condition of patient at admission, living arrangements, location of residence, next of kin, and economic situation. Be-

fore the expiration of the assigned length of stay if it is more than 7 days, the patient is placed on the team agenda for review. The review team is generally composed of the review coordinator, social service coordinator, and representatives from those disciplines who have had responsibility for the direct patient care of this patient, as well as such out-of-hospital representatives as are needed, such as home health agency or nursing home personnel.

C. *PSRO multidisciplinary/interdisciplinary medical care evaluation activities*

1. South Carolina Foundation has conducted four regional medical care evaluation study workshops. A letter was sent to each hospital administrator asking him to send a physician and other health care professionals to the workshop. Cost to the hospital consisted of travel plus a $7.00 registration fee for each participant. There were 60–100 participants at each workshop, with hospitals sending 3–10 people each. The advisory group to the South Carolina Foundation has scheduled a statewide audit on cerebrovascular accidents. Each discipline on the advisory group will be responsible for the development of criteria, identification of problems, and recommendations for follow-up and corrective action, in other words, criteria will be developed by the committee members, reviewed by members of their discipline in the hospitals and state association, and then coordinated by the advisory group committee. The South Carolina Quality Assurance Committee has appointed a physician liaison to the advisory group, who will be responsible for the medical criteria for the study.

South Carolina pharmacists have written an article on pharmacy criteria and pharmacy activities under the auspices of the foundation for the *American Journal of Hospital Pharmacists*. In one hospital, for example, the pharmacists discovered problems in charting of medications, in patients not receiving drugs ordered by physicians, drugs that were contraindicated in combination with others, and so forth.

South Carolina intends to do an areawide study involving 15 nondelegated hospitals. The foundation also plans on developing an audit manual for all health professionals. The most active disciplines are dentists, dietitians, nurses, and pharmacists.

2. The advisory group of the Minnesota Foundation for Medical Care is participating in a regionwide interdisciplinary audit on cerebrovascular accidents. Three of the hospitals in that area are also doing multidisciplinary and interdisciplinary audits. The chairperson of the advisory group has been given official board status, and the board has appointed a physician liaison to the advisory group, and the liaison attends the group's meetings.

3. Colorado Foundation. Colorado has regional medical care evaluation study committees that review audits from hospitals in their region. The regional MCE committees are composed exclusively of physicians. As interdisciplinary audits increased, the regional medical care evaluation study committees called on health care practitioners other than physician consultants to review the audits. These consultants were suggested by the advisory group. In Colorado, the hospital medical care evaluation study committees generally include only physicians or both physicians and nurses, but depending on the study topic, they invite other disciplines to sit in. Generally, combined audits include physicians and nurses or physician, nurse, and pharmacist. However, hospital rehabilitation departments are doing interdisciplinary audits involving rehabilitation professionals.

4. Eastern Connecticut PSRO. The PSRO sponsored an interdisciplinary audit workshop for health professionals working in the seven

acute-care hospitals in its area. One-hundred fourteen people attended the workshop. These included hospital administrators, physicians, nurses, pharmacists, social workers, dietitians, physical therapists, respiratory therapists, and medical records administrators. The agenda included the history and theories behind MCEs and how to go about doing an interdisciplinary or multidisciplinary medical care evaluation. The medical care evaluation study topic chosen was diabetic amputee. Groups were first divided by discipline to develop discipline-specific criteria, they then returned to their own hospital teams to discuss these. Enthusiasm was very high. The evaluation forms filled out by participants showed that they were very "turned on" by the workshop and learned a lot. Eastern Connecticut PSRO has indicated that the hospitals are very eager to work on multidisciplinary audits.

5. Recent data from the PSRO Management Information System show that 80 PSROs have reported nursing participation in MCEs. Fifteen percent of the total number of completed MCEs reported in the first half of 1977 have nursing participation, representing an increase of 6% from the last half of 1976. Participation in MCEs by nonphysician practitioners other than nurses (pharmacists, respiratory therapists, social workers, and so forth) is 1% of the total number of completed MCEs reported and involves 13 PSROs.

Are the physician members of the PSRO sufficiently supportive of the concepts of peer review with respect to services provided by health care practitioners other than physicians to foster any, a token, or a comprehensive effort in implementation of such review?

This question can be answered only at the local level, but it is crucial to successful implementa-tion of a meaningful effort in reviewing services provided by practitioners other than physicians. Progress in this area may be slow and frustrating, because as cited earlier, the PSRO physician membership has many complex problems to resolve in implementing its responsibilities, and tackling those of highest priority may absorb all available energy. At the same time, the PSRO may be receiving overtures from a wide range of outside groups, not only professional groups but also planning, institutional, and consumer groups to implement activities specific to their interests.

Interdisciplinary relationships must also be considered. Where there is an existing team spirit across the various disciplines on which to capitalize, collaborative activity may be relatively easy. On the other hand, when turf battles exist, it may be tempting to take no action rather than to resolve the professionally sensitive conflicts that must precede reaching a decision on the issue.

There appears to be a positive correlation between the type of PSRO board membership and support staff and the degree of participation by health care practitioners other than physicians in its review program. Where the PSRO has included representatives of other than physician disciplines on its board, some review activity incorporating the represented discipline generally evolves. Likewise, where the PSRO has employed persons experienced in direct patient care among its key administrative or support staff, these individuals frequently help the PSRO membership to decide where review of services provided by other than physicians offers the potential for impacting on the cost or quality of patient care in the PSRO area.

Where the PSRO has established a statutory advisory group or some form of nonstatutory advisory committee, these groups can assist the PSRO to decide about the timeliness, type, and extent of emphasis that it should place on review of services provided by health care practitioners other than physicians. Such groups also can assist the PSRO in identifying qualified practitioners to participate in the review and in securing any available criteria for possible adoption for review.

Finally, the PSRO's experience in both its basic concurrent and retrospective review can sometimes result in identifying problems in care provided by health care practitioners other than physicians. This may prove to be the best way to convince the PSRO to begin implementing peer review by those disciplines.

What are the budgetary ramifications of implementing peer review of services provided by health care practitioners other than physicians?

The cost of expanding the PSRO program to incorporate review of the services provided by disciplines other than physicians is a natural concern. Obviously, if all services provided by all disciplines were under routine review, the cost would be prohibitive; however, this is not the case. Program policies require that participation by health care practitioners other than physicians in PSRO review is indicated when that review includes services provided by disciplines other than physicians. It is in those instances that peers of those practitioners whose care is being reviewed are to perform the review. This places the burden on the PSRO to ascertain where potential problems exist with respect to quality and cost of services provided by other than physician practitioners so that the result will justify expenditure of public funds. For example, if such effort has the potential for improving quality of nursing care or dietary services, increasing the efficiency of laboratory or diagnostic x-ray study reporting, curtailing unnecessary utilization of hospital facilities for dental or podiatric procedures, or increasing the effectiveness of drug utilization and use of respiratory and rehabilitation services, the cost of such review can certainly be justified.

Institutions striving to comply with standards of the JCAH are already accustomed to absorbing some of the costs for review of services provided by the various service departments. Since the reimbursement policies for PSRO review stipulate that the cost for MCEs is apportioned on the basis of the percentage of federally supported patients included in the studies, and since the major participation by health care practitioners other than physicians in the PSRO program is anticipated to occur in the conduct of MCEs, it is expected that cost of such effort will be reasonable in relation to the overall program costs. So far the major costs appear to be those incurred in criteria development, which may be time consuming. As efforts in criteria sharing among PSROs become more evident, this cost should decrease. There also is well-documented evidence that as groups become more familiar with the criteria development process, the time required for such development lessens.

Because the number of practitioners other than physicians who should be involved in the review of admission and continued stay in institutions will be relatively small, concern for costs in this area are insignificant. Present policies permit reimbursement for consultation in such review.

Considerable effort has been expended by the professional organizations of health care practitioners other than physicians in criteria development that may be adaptable to PSRO review as well as in training their membership in the techniques of criteria development and review methodology. These efforts should diminish the inflationary threat of incorporating into the PSRO's program the review of services provided by disciplines other than physicians.

What are the professional interests and what is the experiential base in PSRO-type review among the various disciplines?

Quality assurance has been of major concern to all the health care professions. Most of the national associations representing the other-than-physician disciplines identified in this chapter had at least one to several initiatives in assuring the quality of practitioner performance prior to the passage of the PSRO legislation. All have been working to resolve licensure or certification, recertification, and continuing education issues as mechanisms to assure quality. In addition, many have implemented programs to develop standards of practice, to prepare members for conduct of peer review, and to develop explicit criteria for use in assessing need and quality of their respective services.

The initial reactions of these professional organizations to the PSRO legislation covered a wide range: near apathy ("the program won't affect us because our discipline is not named"); expressed anxiety about the amount of effort that would need to be expended to prepare members for participation in the PSRO program; enthusiasm for the opportunity for their group to participate in the peer review process; resentment toward the Congress, the department, and the medical community because their profession was not given specific recognition in the statute; and concern that physicians would be reviewing their care. In the intervening years, most of those reactions were turned around or at least suppressed, with intensive programs spearheaded by the organizations to prepare their members for participation in peer review and quality assurance programs. The volume of literature about such activities from the various disciplines has increased markedly in the past 4 years. Today it is difficult to find an official journal issue or newsletter from a national organization of these health care professionals that does not have at least one news item dealing with some aspect of quality assurance activities and its relationship to the PSRO program.

In addition to the references made in previous sections of this chapter regarding examples of PSRO-initiated review of services provided by other than physicians, the new standards for accreditation of the JCAH dealing with patient/medical care evaluation has resulted in a significant base of experience in both criteria development and performance of audits among practitioners employed in hospitals. Although the JCAH standard specifically calls for nursing participation in patient/medical care evaluation studies, other hospital-based disciplines, such as dietitians, physical therapists, occupational therapists, and social workers, have begun to participate in such studies since the JCAH views patient/medical care evaluation studies as one way of assuring quality of care in a department.

The Health Standards and Quality Bureau has supported several programs relating to the PSRO effort with national health professional organizations, as have other components of the federal government. In addition, the national organizations have invested considerable resources of their own in similar programs. Listed below are the major examples of these activities:

1. The American Dental Association was awarded a bureau contract to develop models for review of dental care.

2. The American Nurses' Association under contract with the bureau produced a manual, *Guidelines for Review of Nursing Care at the Local Level,* which provides instructions to nurses on how to develop criteria that can be useful for other disciplines as well. The manual includes 15 sets of sample outcome criteria for assessing the quality of nursing care. This manual has been distributed to PSROs and hospitals. In addition, the American Nurses' Association has been actively conducting audit workshops throughout the country.

3. The American Podiatry Association under contract with the bureau produced a manual, *Model Screening Criteria for the Review of Surgical Procedures and Associated Care Ren-*

dered by Podiatrists, which has been sent to all PSROs. Podiatrists in the PSRO area may wish to modify these criteria to suit local needs.

4. The American Speech and Hearing Association on behalf of the Coalition of Independent Health Professions under a 6-month contract with the bureau developed and pilot tested a patient care audit workshop that was taught to selected representatives of each of the 11 member organizations.

5. The American Optometric Association established a quality assurance task force that has developed criteria sets for six diagnoses covering 80% of optometric patients.

6. The American Psychological Association has recently been awarded a 1-year contract by Civilian Health and Medical Program of the Uniformed Services (CHAMPUS) to develop criteria for review of ambulatory psychologic services. The American Psychological Association also has state professional standards review committees, which generally deal with review of claims questioned by insurance companies and would be more than happy to relate to PSROs.

7. The American Society of Hospital Pharmacists is working on a model quality assurance program for peer review of pharmaceutical services. Both the American Society of Hospital Pharmacists and the American Pharmaceutical Association are providing materials to their membership on drug utilization review.

8. The American Society of Medical Technologists under a training grant from the Bureau of Health Manpower presented six workshops on peer review for medical technologists in 1976. The American Society of Medical Technologists produced a set of model criteria for the evaluation of clinical laboratory services available in 1978.

9. The National Association of Social Workers has established the Health Quality Standards Committee to provide guidance to social workers.

10. The national organizations representing dietitians, physical therapists, speech-language therapists and audiologists, and occupational therapists have been conducting patient care audit workshops for their members throughout the country and have developed audit manuals with examples of discipline-specific criteria. They also have lists of people that could serve as resources to PSROs.

In general, it appears that when a PSRO is ready to incorporate review of services provided by health care practitioners other than physicians into its program, it will find not only a high degree of interest from the relevant disciplines but also practitioners who have some preparation in review. Where advisory groups or committees are not available to assist the PSRO in identification of practitioners knowledgeable in the peer review process, the state constituent of the parent national professional organization is usually prepared to assist the PSRO in that effort.

Summary

Since changing behavior of practitioners is the PSRO preferred method of improving care, it makes sense to assume that the chances for improving patient care will be greater if PSROs can effect changes in the practice patterns of all of those who provided the care being reviewed. Certainly when the PSRO identifies problems in care that involve services provided by health care practitioners other than physicians, the chances for success in eliminating the problems will increase if the involved practitioners participate in the review process, and if physicians and other health care practitioners collaborate in correcting the deficiencies.

11

Statewide Support Centers

Daniel J. O'Regan

An examination of the PSRO statutes will not reveal mention of statewide support centers. The idea of a statewide organization to assist and coordinate PSRO development evolved during the 1973 negotiations on PSRO area designation. In many populous states, foundations for medical care and other organizations applied for designation of those states as single PSRO areas. Practicality and the guidelines ruled against them, leading to the impression that statewide organizations would be prohibited from participating in the PSRO program. However, an HEW policy statement issued in the fall of 1973, said that the statute permitted the participation of "Statewide Resource Centers."[1] Although PL 92-603 did not mention such resource centers, the policy statement added, nothing in the legislative history or intent prevented it. OPSR Memo No. 3 of March 1974, announced that statewide support centers would be established, and projected activities included the assistance of planning, conditional, and operational PSROs as well as state PSR councils.[2] Eventually, support centers were established in 13 states: California, Connecticut, Indiana, Maryland, Massachusetts, Michigan, Missouri, New Jersey, New York, North Carolina, Ohio, Pennsylvania, and Virginia. States selected had five or more PSRO areas.

PURPOSE

The centers were designed to capitalize on the experience and knowledge of state professional organizations, particularly the state medical societies or foundations for medical care. Guidelines were issued as Chapter 3 of the *PSRO Program Manual* on March 15, 1974.[3] The general purpose was to stimulate and coordinate the development and operation of the program through a variety of services. The initial thrust was to educate physicians in PSRO principles and objectives. This was largely accomplished by physicians who gave freely of their time to acquaint their colleagues with the need for response by the medical community to the challenge of this new law. Such activities facilitated the emergence of many PSROs in the 13 states. As potential PSROs appeared, the support centers helped them to organize, recruit members, establish bylaws, qualify as nonprofit corporations, find staff members, write proposals, and learn how to deal with the federal structure. A variety of groups was brought together, with the support centers as the focal points: medical and hospital associations, Medicare, Medicaid, and Title V agencies, regional HEW staff, data processors, and others. In most instances, physician contact with the other parties involved had previously been minimal.

ROLE OF SUPPORT CENTER IN THE DEVELOPMENT OF PSROS

The development of the formal plan for operation by the PSROs was assisted by the support centers. In some instances, criteria and standards were developed by the center for local adaptation. Options for peer review techniques, evaluation of in-house review mechanisms, development of memoranda of understanding, and training methodologies for review coordinators and physician advisors were addressed. Seminars and workshops were conducted, and manuals for review personnel were developed. The local autonomy and authority of each individual PSRO was maintained.

As planning PSROs were designated, support center efforts were directed to helping them prepare for conditional status. Since the progress in the various areas in most states was uneven, the support center often found itself involved with conditional and planning PSROs as well as areas without funding. These presented a variety of challenges, as did the resistance of physicians here and there. Helpful activities had to be conducted at several levels.

The cooperation between the local PSROs and the support centers began to bear fruit as most planning contracts were awarded. Conditional PSROs became more numerous as budgetary restrictions were relaxed. As the PSROs gained experience, their staff capabilities improved, and their needs changed. The services they desired from support centers also changed. As the number of conditional PSROs increased, the future role of statewide support centers became questionable.

CHANGING STATUS AND OPTIONS FOR STATEWIDE ASSISTANCE CENTERS

The initial plans were for direct federal funding of centers to continue as long as there was a need for effective statewide groups. As the states became filled with qualified PSROs, direct funding would cease; further operations were to depend on subcontracts for specific tasks between the PSROs and the support centers. Similar options were to be available between the centers and the state PSR

councils, when operational. The combined support centers met with Henry Simmons in November of 1974 to explore their status and future options. A discussion draft was presented to the NPSRC early in 1975. Transmittal No. 18, issued April 23, 1975, was the result.[4] It stated that support centers that prove themselves to be useful and efficient should expect a long-term role in the PSRO program. By July of 1975, all 13 centers were continued in force because of the gaps in area implementation. Direct federal funding was scheduled to cease at the end of fiscal year 1976. It was later decided that Connecticut, Maryland, Massachusetts, and Missouri would cease direct funding after September 30, 1976. The remaining nine were to be continued for an additional 12 months.

The NPSRC considered a draft transmittal at its July 1977 session.[5] Because there were 43 relatively new planning PSROs in the states with support centers, direct funding was recommended for states where the PSROs and the centers so desired. The Virginia center elected not to continue. This policy was adopted for a period of 6 months or until March 30, 1978. Thereafter continuation in the program would depend on the subcontract route where desired by the PSROs and state councils and where the support centers remain effective.

SUMMARY

Support centers have played a useful role in the development of the PSRO program. Manned by dedicated core staffs, most have been effective in terms of the relatively small expenditures used. Many of their accomplishments are intangible, but the PSRO program development would not have reached its present level in the 13 states without the presence of the support centers. Several of these populous states are still the areas of contention between federal and state authorities over binding review decisions, particularly those involving Medicaid. Broad-based physician groups have been helpful in the negotiations on these matters.

Chapter 3 of the *PSRO Program Manual* states that renewal requests will be evaluated on the basis of (1) satisfaction of the organizations served by the support center, (2) the development of the PSRO program within the support center's geographic service area, (3) the operational success of individual PSROs served by the support center, (4) support center performance of original contract goals and obligations, and (5) projections for future support center progress in promoting development of Operational PSROs.

The 1977 draft transmittal concludes:*

Statewide PSRO Support Centers have played a valuable role and made significant contributions to the development and establishment of the PSRO program. The staff and resources of the Support Centers represent experi-

*From U.S. Department of Health, Education, and Welfare. Aug. 2, 1977. *PSRO support center policy.* Transmittal No. 56. Bureau of Health Standards and Quality, Health Care Financing Administration.

enced sources of services which PSROs and Statewide Councils should seriously consider utilizing as they progress in the implementation of their respective responsibilities.

REFERENCES

1. *Departmental policy statement on PSRO area designation.* Oct. 1973. Washington, D.C.: U.S. Department of Health, Education, and Welfare.

2. Office of Professional Standards Review. March 1974. *OPSR Memo No. 3.* Washington, D.C.: U.S. Department of Health, Education, and Welfare.

3. Office of Professional Standards Review. 1974. *PSRO Program Manual.* Rockville, Md.: U.S. Department of Health, Education, and Welfare.

4. U.S. Department of Health, Education, and Welfare. April 23, 1975. *PSRO support center policy.* Transmittal No. 18. Bureau of Quality Assurance, Health Services Administration, Public Health Service.

5. U.S. Department of Health, Education, and Welfare. Aug. 2, 1977. *PSRO support center policy.* Transmittal No. 56. Bureau of Health Standards and Quality, Health Care Financing Administration.

III

PERFORMANCE

12

Profile Analysis

Linda Jackson

What are profiles? For what purpose are they used? How are they developed? What do they contain? How are they evaluated? These are just a few of the questions asked when the topic is "profiles." All of these questions involve the same concern, which is, how can this new unique PSRO data base be used as a tool? The problem has been that the PSRO data, along with the PSROs, are whole new concepts in the medical field and require a new orientation in terms of application. Of course, the word "profile" has been around for a long time and in data analysis has developed a new meaning. The PSRO profile can be defined as a display of aggregate or individual data elements that portray particular subjects or topics. The subject of the profile can be anything that is related to the PSRO review system.*

Based on this definition, a profile can be anything as long as it displays some sort of data. Unfortunately, the mere act of displaying data does not necessarily result in a profile that is meaningful. Since the crux of profiling is the ability to use PSRO data as a tool in solving and identifying problems, profiles are developed with two basic constraints. The profile, or the display of data ele-

ments, must be based both on a purpose and a hypothesis. Simply stated, the purpose of a profile should be somehow related to the overall objectives of the PSRO, and the hypothesis is a statement based on the premise that specific data elements portray certain components or activities of the review system. As a result, it is not profiling itself but the ability to analyze and make observations from the profile that makes profiling so important.

PROFILE ANALYSIS SYSTEM

It is generally accepted that a profile is a potential mechanism through which the PSRO data can be applied as a problem-solving and identification tool. Yet, the question still remains as to how the PSRO data can be used most effectively. Effectively using the entire PSRO data base requires a "profile analysis system."

The purpose and objectives of a profile analysis system go hand in hand with the purpose for which PSROs have developed and evolved. Since the purposes of a PSRO are to (1) strive for the appropriate utilization of health care provider facilities and (2) assess the quality of the medical care that is provided, the ultimate purpose of this profile analysis system is to aid in the achievement of those PSRO objectives. To support these over-

---

*The PSRO legislation specifically identifies three types of profiles that must be reviewed: (1) patient profiles, (2) practitioner profiles, and (3) institutional profiles.

all PSRO objectives and use the PSRO data most effectively, a profile analysis system must consist of two components: (1) those profiles that are developed for problem-specific studies and (2) those profiles that provide a means for ongoing monitoring and evaluation of the review system and its activities. The profiles developed for problem-specific studies are called *supportive profile analysis* (SPAN), and the set of profiles routinely compiled for the ongoing monitoring and evaluation of the review system are grouped under the title *evaluative profile analysis* (EPAN).

EPAN AND SPAN AS A PROFILE ANALYSIS SYSTEM

EPAN and SPAN are two types of concepts through which profiles are developed. Together they create a profile analysis system in that they are complementary and interrelated as well as working concepts in and of themselves. Profiles developed in either of these conceptual areas are analyzed through asking a sequence of three basic questions. First, do the values or variances of the data elements appear to be appropriate for the circumstances? Second, if the values or variances of the data do not appear to be appropriate, are the problem areas identified and sufficiently defined so that action can be taken? Third, based on the values or variances of the data, additional questions are raised, and according to the degree of seriousness involved, are additional profiling and analysis necessary? This sequence of questions reveals that the profiles developed through EPAN and SPAN are used as problem-solving and identifying tools. It is when the third question is asked that the complementary relationship between EPAN and SPAN becomes apparent.

EPAN is the set of routinely compiled profiles developed for the purpose of ongoing monitoring

and evaluation of the review system. Because of this characteristic, it not only provides a means for making specific one-time analyses but also provides a means for identifying and analyzing trends. This ability to profile trends adds an additional dimension to profiling and allows for a more concise analysis because the knowledge of how a data element has behaved over time is provided. The analysis of EPAN profiles can result in a variety of conclusions; however, if the observation is made that additional profiling is necessary, that additional profiling falls under the heading of SPAN.

SPAN, the profiles used in support of in-depth analyses, is a set of profiles whose design is tailored to the purpose of the study. Because of this aspect, it is one of the most readily understood concepts of profiling and is often preferred by a PSRO in the initial phases of using profiles. Traditionally, topics for SPAN can be derived from a variety of sources (review coordinators, physician advisors, hospital administrators and staff, PSRO administrative staff, and so forth). EPAN provides an additional perspective in the list of SPAN topics in that they are specifically derived from the analysis of data. It is this complementary relationship between EPAN and SPAN that uses the PSRO data base itself as a problem-solving tool.

Once again, if the conclusions that are drawn from a SPAN study are of the third category (additional investigation or analysis may be necessary), and if there are questions that concern the quality of the medical care, the additional analysis may be a *medical care evaluation study* (MCEs). MCEs are not formally defined as part of the profile analysis system, but the relationships between MCEs, SPAN, and EPAN are such that MCEs must be included in the profile analysis system concept.

The description of a profile analysis system as a series of different levels of profiles (that is, from the very broad profile, EPAN, to the very specific profile, MCEs) only partially portrays the mechanisms involved in a profile analysis system. An interactive process also occurs between the different levels. For example, in the process of conducting a SPAN study or a medical care evaluation study, it may become apparent that additional aspects of the review system should be routinely monitored and evaluated. To be able to evaluate those aspects of the review system, additional data indicators (profiles) should be included in EPAN. (The levels of the profile analysis system and the interaction between them are displayed in Figure 12-1.) As a result, an organized profile analysis system based on these three conceptual levels will both monitor and evaluate the review system as well as respond to problem-specific studies. If in addition to these three basic levels of profiles the profiles themselves are based on a sound methodology that includes both a purpose and a hypothesis, the outcome will be the most efficient and effective use of the PSRO data base.

Evaluative Profile Analysis (EPAN)

As mentioned previously, SPAN and MCEs are the types of profile analysis most readily conceptualized and implemented because they are the result of specific questions or problems. On the other hand, EPAN by its very definition of being the broad, ongoing monitoring and evaluation of the total review system has the potential of becoming an overwhelming task. It need not be overwhelming if there is a well-organized methodology to give guidance for the development of EPAN profiles. This methodology, or plan, involves three basic steps: (1) formulating the objectives and goals of EPAN, (2) establishing a set of profiles in relationship to those objectives, and (3) generating a set of norms, standards, or criteria with which the

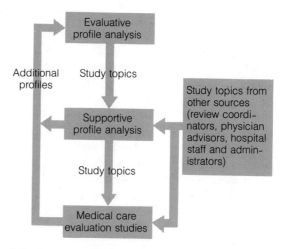

FIGURE 12-1.   Profile analysis system.

profiles are analyzed. The EPAN plan—how it evolves and what is involved—is described in the following sections.

Objectives and Goals

The objectives of EPAN, although more concise by necessity, must reflect the objectives of the PSRO. Based on the PSRO objectives, EPAN can be divided into two basic areas: (1) those profiles that monitor and evaluate the health care providers and (2) those profiles that monitor and evaluate the PSRO. With respect to the PSRO objectives, the reasons for monitoring and evaluating the health care providers are self-explanatory. On the other hand, why it is just as important to monitor and evaluate the PSRO may not be as clear. Two basic reasons for including the PSRO as an area for which EPAN is developed are: (1) how well the PSRO is operating directly affects how effective it is in achieving its goals and (2) the data, how and for what reasons they are collected, have an impact on the analysis of the data that are profiled to monitor and evaluate the health care providers.

Although the main objective of EPAN is to monitor and evaluate both the health care providers and the PSRO, it is necessary to divide this objective into some well-defined subobjectives. Based on the overall objectives of the PSRO, the subobjectives of monitoring and evaluating the health care providers can be broadly labeled as profiling: (1) the utilization of the health care facility, (2) the efficiency of the health care facility as well as the health care provider, and (3) the quality of the medical care. The subobjectives of monitoring and evaluating the PSRO are to profile (1) the efficiency and productivity of the PSRO, (2) the quality and accuracy of the data collected, and (3) the effectiveness of the PSRO in achieving its overall goals. It is for these six subobjectives that the EPAN profiles are developed.

Developing EPAN Profiles

Once the objectives and subobjectives of EPAN are understood, the next step in the plan calls for developing a set of profiles with respect to the stated objectives. Since a criterion for developing a profile is a statement of a hypothesis, the next stage in the development of EPAN is designing a systematic approach for the development of hypotheses. The hypotheses themselves are statements that refer to specific data elements and to what they may reflect in terms of the objectives of the profiles. To ensure that all areas of the health care providers and the PSRO are profiled, they are divided into separate components. The components that constitute the PSRO are: (1) the review coordinators, (2) the physician advisors, and (3) the catchall category of the administration of the PSRO. The health care providers are partitioned into the categories of (1) the administration of the

health care facility, (2) the medical staff, and (3) the patient. For each of these six components, hypotheses (and thus profiles) are developed for each respective subobjective. For example, a profile that might reflect the "effectiveness" of the "administration of the PSRO" might be the display of the average days of uncertified stay per patient who is terminated in each hospital.

It is important to mention that when a set of profiles is developed, the subobjectives to be analyzed and the different components to be represented may not be mutually exclusive. In other words, one profile may be applied to more than one component or to more than one subobjective. This is particularly true for the subobjective of effectiveness of the PSRO. As displayed in Figure 12-2, the effectiveness of the PSRO is evaluated and monitored not only through its own profiles but also through the profiles that are developed for the monitoring and evaluation of the health care providers. The above mentioned components and subobjectives are merely guidelines to ensure that the total review system as well as the goals of the PSRO have been considered in the development of EPAN profiles.

Developing Criteria, Standards, or Norms to Evaluate the EPAN Profiles

Once the EPAN profiles, based on specific hypotheses, have been developed, a set of criteria, standards, or norms should evolve to evaluate or analyze the profiles. Although the norms that are used to analyze a profile are related to the hypothesis that was used in developing the profile, three types of norms are used most often. The first type of norm is the evaluation of a profile in terms of the variance of the data with respect to the average for the total. In other words, the groups with the highest or lowest (or both) values are more closely analyzed to explain the high or low var-

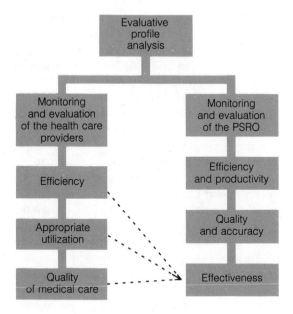

FIGURE 12-2. Evaluative profile analysis.

iance of those values. This type of norm might be applied to a profile that displays the number and percent of physician advisor referrals that occur during the review process in each acute-care facility. The hypothesis for this profile is based on the assumption that the concept of peer review means that there should be a certain amount of physician advisor involvement in the concurrent review process. The norm is supportive of the hypothesis in that it is based on the theory of the PSRO that the total review community will set the acceptable rate of physician advisor involvement.

The second type of norm is the analysis of the profile in relationship to a minimum or maximum acceptable value based on general consensus. A general consensus norm could be derived from the subjective judgment of the PSRO that with its knowledge of the review procedures, it feels there should be only a certain level of retroactive reviews taking place in each acute-care facility.

Another general consensus norm could be the subjective judgment of the medical community that only a certain percentage of postoperative complications should occur in surgical facilities. As a result, this type of norm could be a vehicle through which idealistic goals could be tested against reality.

The third type of norm is the most complex, yet the most important, because it complements the EPAN philosophy of a broad overall understanding of the data and what it may indicate. When this norm is used, the profile is analyzed with respect to the expected relationship when the profile is compared with another profile. A very simple application of the norm is the analysis of a profile that displays the percent of hospital certifications terminated in comparison with a profile that displays the percent of patients referred to a physician advisor during their acute-care stay. This norm is founded on the knowledge that a termination requires a consultation with a physician advisor; therefore, the percent of patients referred to a physician advisor should at least be equal to the percent of patients whose certifications were terminated.

Summary

EPAN, developed through the application of this methodology, becomes a set of data displays designed to depict the individual components of the review system in terms of the overall objectives of the PSRO. Through the analysis of the EPAN profiles, one gains additional knowledge about the PSRO data along with the ability to identify those situations that may be problem areas. Appendix B contains a sample of some possible EPAN profiles, the hypotheses used in developing them, and the criteria used for the analysis of those profiles.

Because EPAN is developed on the basis of the overall objective of the monitoring and evaluation of the review system, it is a flexible tool with a number of outcomes and adaptations that have an impact on a variety of PSRO activities. A discussion of some possible outcomes and extensions of EPAN and the role they play as part of a profile analysis system follows.

Outcomes and Adaptations of EPAN

The most extensive impact that the routine analysis of EPAN has is one that is not immediately recognized when compared with the broad definition of EPAN as a tool to identify and analyze potential problem areas through profiling data. This area of impact is related to the role that EPAN can play in providing input to the constant struggle to obtain reliable, consistent, and accurate data. Through the process of continually looking at the EPAN profiles, analyzing them, and feeding back the results, information as to how aggregated data are interpreted and used becomes readily available to those individuals who are involved in collecting the data. Therefore, EPAN becomes an educational tool through which guidelines can be developed to make the data more consistent and reliable.

Broadly speaking, part of the outcome of the routine analysis of EPAN is identifying study topics and providing support for SPAN and MCEs. Some of the topics and support that EPAN provides for SPAN and MCEs can be grouped under the PSRO function of focusing or waiving concurrent review. Although EPAN, along with SPAN and MCEs, can identify and produce supportive data for the decision concerning the waiving or focusing of the concurrent review process, more important, the flexibility of EPAN allows for additional profiles to be added, whose purpose is to monitor and evaluate over time the patient group whose review is focused or waived. For example, if normal deliveries were waived in the concurrent review process, a profile that might be included in EPAN would be the average length of stay and the variance of the average length of stay for all normal deliveries that were admitted to each hospital in the PSRO review area. Any abnormal fluctuation in the length of stay for those patients might be an indicator that the waived review process is not effective. In that case, additional analysis or investigation should take place to determine the reasons for the fluctuations in the data. This example shows that in the case of waiving concurrent review, EPAN can be used as a tool to monitor the patient group that was waived. If concurrent review is focused, EPAN can be used to monitor the patient group for any impact in the patterns of utilization and medical care of the patient group.

Traditionally, the basic unit for PSRO concurrent review and evaluation has been the health care facility. Because of this, a basic EPAN profile would be the comparison of data between individual health care facilities in the PSRO area. (Although some PSROs might be small enough to be able to compare all health care facilities at once in an EPAN profile, larger PSROs might be required to arbitrarily group the health care facilities by bed size, urban versus rural location, and so forth before profiling is feasible.) If the method of presenting the EPAN profiles is altered, their uses can be expanded. One possible result of the alteration of the EPAN profiles is the development of an "EPAN hospital profile." (See Appendix C for an example of a possible EPAN hospital profile.) Hospital profiles are developed by combining into one document all of the EPAN profiles for which a specific hospital does not meet the criteria for analysis. The original EPAN profiles are then altered to display only the individual hospital compared with the criteria for analysis. In the case of a variance analysis, the profile would display the data for the hospital, the community average, and the high and low values for each time period. As a result, an EPAN hospital profile is a comprehensive profile of an individual hospital that not only provides information as to how the data have described the facility but also provides information as to how well the review system is operating within that facility. The important concept of hospital profiles is that they break down the EPAN system into a document that is easily understood by an individual who may not be familiar with PSRO data and the EPAN concept.

Supportive Profile Analysis (SPAN)

In contrast to EPAN (the broad ongoing evaluation of the review system), SPAN is the title given to studies related to a specific topic. Although not discrete, there are two basic types of SPAN: (1) the study designed to gather specific information in support of PSRO activities and (2) the analysis process designed to verify and define "perceived" problem areas. Topics for both types of studies can be obtained from similar sources—review coordinators, PSRO staff, hospital staff, and of course, EPAN.

The first type of SPAN can be defined as merely an information-gathering process in which the PSRO data are the resource for descriptive information about hospitals, patient groups, physicians, and so forth. For example, before the implementation of a medical care evaluation study, it may be useful to the PSRO to identify in which facilities the patient group can be found and how large that patient group may be. This type of information may affect the design of the medical care evaluation in terms of sampling techniques and analysis resources. Basically, it is this type of SPAN that provides the PSRO with as much detailed information as necessary to facilitate the implementation of a variety of its activities.

The second type of SPAN can best be described as that investigative process concerning "perceived" problem areas, with the objective of verifying or defining the parameters of the problem area. Once a problem has been identified, it is important to define the problem specifically so that any resultant PSRO actions can be as effective as possible. Study design for this type of SPAN centers around the profiling of all relevant data based on those hypotheses that explain the characteristics of the problem area. For example, EPAN, in the process of profiling "quality of health care" indicators, might reveal a large number of postoperative complications in a particular facility. A SPAN study would then be designed to see if (1) the data reveal any patterns in postoperative complications with respect to diagnoses, operative procedures, surgeons, and so forth, and (2) the postoperative complications appear to be medically justified. As a result, a SPAN study of this nature would include profiles of data as well as consultation with physicians, review staff, and so forth to obtain additional information as well as their evaluation of the data. In the event that a problem area is identified and can be related to a specific operative procedure, a medical care evaluation of the operative procedure and any related activities should take place.

IMPACT OF A PROFILE ANALYSIS SYSTEM

A profile plan such as the design and interaction between EPAN, SPAN, and other PSRO activities is essential for the efficient and most effective use of PSRO data. A profile plan that is based on a comprehensive methodology and is regularly applied can serve a variety of needs. The use of a profile analysis system (particularly EPAN and SPAN) impacts in the four following areas:

1. Provides the capability to monitor trends and maintain a continuous overall perspective of the activities of the review system.

2. Provides information so that deficiencies, modifications, or both in the data can be identified.

3. Serves as a tool that can validate and define perceived problem areas as well as identify variances in the data that may not have been perceived.

4. Serves as a mechanism that increases the PSRO familiarity with the data and the knowledge of the relationships that exist between different data elements.

Special Considerations

Before a profile analysis system can be used as a monitoring and evaluative mechanism in the PSRO setting, several considerations that have an impact on the effectiveness of the profile analysis system must be studied. The first area of concern is the data.

A profile analysis system (made up principally of EPAN and SPAN) is primarily dependent on the PSRO data base. The first question concerning the data is, how accurate and reliable are they? Despite the fact that a PSRO may have a variety of edits for its data, some data elements exist that are virtually impossible to monitor for accuracy. As a result, an awareness of the data elements that have a reliability or consistency problem aids in the critical analysis of those profiles containing those data elements. A second consideration that must be made during the analysis of profiles is the question of whether or not the data are subjective or objective. Objective information is factual, whereas subjective information portrays a concern or judgment on the part of the individual who collects the data. In the case of analyzing a profile that contains subjective data, a conference with the individual who is responsible for abstracting the data is necessary before any final conclusions can be drawn.

In the process of developing a concurrent review system, many administrative decisions are made that result in procedural changes in the concurrent review process. These changes may result in specific data elements being added, omitted, or altered in the data collection process for portions of the data base. It is imperative that these changes are documented and that a profile be analyzed with respect to how any changes have affected the data within that profile.

A profile analysis system is largely made up of the data that are collected by the PSRO, and it logically follows that a comprehensive knowledge of the characteristics of those data increases the effectiveness of the analysis of profiles. In addition to the data quality, how the data are managed and provided by a data system also makes a large impact on the potential effectiveness of a profile analysis system.

The PSRO data base, because of the complexity of the basic data set that is required by the federal government, almost always requires some sort of computerization. How the computerized data system is designed and used depends somewhat on the size and needs of a PSRO. However, to increase the effectiveness of a profile analysis system, the data system must have three basic characteristics. The first characteristic is directly related to EPAN in that EPAN requires a basic set of routine reports. Without a basic set of information being supplied, the entire principle of EPAN as being an ongoing monitoring and evaluation of the review system is destroyed.

Second, in the course of conducting profile analyses through EPAN or SPAN, it may become apparent that specific data elements need to be added or deleted in the PSRO data base. The design of the data system must be flexible to allow for such modifications. Particularly when data elements need to be added, the data system should be able to include that data element in its reporting mechanism to support the outcome of the profile analysis.

The third characteristic of a data system must be the capability to access specific data elements quickly and efficiently. This type of data-accessing ability is crucial for the effective use of SPAN in that by its very definition it is the in-depth analysis of specific patient groups, diagnoses, and so forth. The optimum data-accessing facility would be one in which one can interact with the computer through a special program and define and analyze a variety of data elements within the topic of the SPAN study. This system must also be efficient, because the efficiency of the system defines the number and type of SPAN studies that can be conducted. In addition, an efficient data-accessing facility allows the PSRO to conduct exploratory analysis that can be just as fruitful as a study that has the problem well defined. In summary, the more thoroughly the data can be analyzed, the more well defined and action oriented the conclusion of the analysis will be.

SUMMARY

The data base and how those data are supplied affect the development of profiles and, more broadly, affect any application and analysis of PSRO data. If the basic requirements of the data base and the data system are met, it becomes most important how to use the data, because it is the use of data that justifies the collection of those data. A profile analysis system that includes both EPAN and SPAN uses the PSRO data as overall monitoring and evaluation tools as well as tools to analyze perceived problem areas. In addition, the design of the profile analysis system should be flexible, allowing it to grow and change with PSROs along with providing an opportunity to obtain a comprehensive knowledge of the new, unique PSRO data base.

13

Use of Outcome Measures in Quality Assurance

Paul A. Nutting

As conceptualized by Donabedian,[27] the quality of medical care can be assessed from the perspectives of structure, process, and outcome. The majority of quality assurance activities focus on structure and process, based on the assumption that adequate structure (resources, facilities, and competent providers) will lead to an adequate process of health care (compliance with acceptable standards) and in turn will result in acceptable outcomes (improved health status).

The first recognized attempt to base the evaluation of medical care on patient outcomes in the United States is generally attributed to E.A. Codman.[20,21] In the early part of this century, he advocated case by case review of patients following surgery to determine the final outcome. He further suggested that hospitals publish the results of such studies for a public accounting of the end results of their care. His suggestions created as much professional outcry at that time as they might today, and existing political pressures led to the use of structural criteria for hospital accreditation that have persisted into recent times.

Since 1952, the JCAH, which is a voluntary nongovernment agency, has been the major operational quality assurance program, accrediting hospitals based on both structural and process criteria. More recently, the JCAH developed a performance evaluation procedure (PEP), which had to be implemented by hospitals seeking accreditation. The PEP relied heavily on appraisal of health outcomes.[38]

Quality assurance activities are now mandated under two federal laws. In 1972 the PSRO legislation (PL 92-603) directed that medical care evaluations were to be prerequisites for reimbursement of costs payable under Medicare and Medicaid. Although PL 92-603 does not specifically require outcome appraisal, the BQA is encouraging the incorporation of outcome measures into medical care evaluation.[32] The Health Maintenance Organization (HMO) Act of 1973 (PL 93-222) requires quality assurance activities in all federally supported HMOs. In addition, the legislation specifies that quality will be appraised in part through the use of outcome measures that reflect both medical and consumer values.

Despite the policy demands that the quality assurance activities utilize outcome appraisal, many unanswered questions and tenuous assumptions surrounding the use of outcomes remain. A number of proposed methods exist, but none are yet commonly accepted as valid and feasible. Several noted research groups have recently reported on the state of the art of outcome assessment,[9,35,48] proposed a conceptual framework,[71,72] and formulated recommendations for further study.[9,34,35] In light of the current flux and continued testing of approaches to outcome appraisal, this cannot be an authoritative chapter on how to evaluate health outcomes. Rather, the chapter reviews some of the considerations relevant to outcome appraisal and attempts to put them into perspective for PSROs.

CONCEPTS OF OUTCOME

There are currently several differing concepts of health outcomes. Donabedian originally defined health outcomes as any good or bad state of a patient following care for an injury or illness, without any causal relationship implied.[25] Shapiro includes a causal relationship and refers to outcome as "some measurable aspect of health status which is influenced by a particular element or array of those elements of health care."[68] Bickner adds the concept of a change in health status and defines outcomes as a change in health status that can be attributed to the intervention of health care.[5] Other outcomes have also been proposed, including utilization, work loads, and waiting time as programmatic outcomes.[39,47,79] Decker terms these administrative outcomes and adds economic outcomes (cost benefit measures) to the list.[22] Densen has pointed out that outcomes are a function of viewpoint.[24] He suggests that morbidity, mortality, and function are outcomes from the medical perspective; accessibility of care is an outcome from the patient's viewpoint; and a measure of unmet health need is an appropriate outcome from the perspective of the community.

The dimensions of health outcome chosen for outcome appraisal also vary among investigators. They have been described as recovery, restoration of function, and survival by Donabedian;[26] as longevity, physical abnormalities, psychologic abnormalities, physical symptoms, psychologic symptoms, and function by Sanazaro and Williamson;[66] and as death, disease, dissatisfaction, disability, and discomfort by White.[81] Sanazaro and Williamson have also defined a number of process outcomes, listing attitudes toward care, attitudes toward condition, compliance, risks, hospitalization,

and costs as legitimate outcomes of medical care. Williamson has more recently focused on diagnostic outcome (false positive and false negative diagnoses) as the major process outcome in his system of health accounting.[84]

Starfield has proposed a scheme for categorizing the dimensions of health outcome, incorporating seven continua, including resilience, achievement, disease, satisfaction, comfort, activity, and longevity.[72] Resilience encompasses the ability to cope with adversity, and achievement signifies the level of development or accomplishment. Disease represents the classic morbidity category and ranges from not detectable to permanent. Satisfaction and comfort relate to acceptance of one's health state, worry, and distress. Activity encompasses many concepts from previous workers' scales of function, and longevity is a prognostic category from normal life expectancy to death. Starfield rejects administrative outcomes and such measures as utilization and acceptability as being related primarily to process. She points out that patient satisfaction is a legitimate outcome only insofar as it is concerned with a patient's satisfaction with his own health status. She classifies patient satisfaction with health care encounters as a measure of process and satisfaction with health care in general as a measure of structure.

Strict definitions and categorization of outcome dimensions are necessary for communication and to promote coordination in research and developmental activities in quality assurance. However, overemphasis of the process-outcome dichotomy may lead to serious oversimplification in methods. Health care can be viewed as a sequence of clinical functions, including primary prevention, screening, diagnostic evaluation, treatment planning, and ongoing management. Each clinical function can be characterized by its specific objectives, as in Table 13-1. An effective process of health care is a result of timely applica-

TABLE 13-1.   Generic Objectives of the Process of Health Care

	PRIMARY PREVENTION	SCREENING	INITIAL DIAGNOSTIC WORKUP AND PLAN	ONGOING MANAGEMENT
INFORMATION GATHERING	Collect data required to determine if the patient might benefit from preventive therapy.	Collect data required for screening.	Collect data required to: 1. Confirm the diagnosis 2. Determine etiologic factors 3. Baseline pathologic and functional changes 4. Evaluate the prognosis 5. Identify patient factors that may affect treatment (such as allergies)	Collect data required to: 1. Determine new etiologic factors 2. Evaluate current clinical status 3. Evaluate current prognosis 4. Measure the response to treatment 5. Disclose adverse drug reaction 6. Identify spontaneous remission
ASSESSMENT	Determine if preventive therapy is both necessary and appropriate for the patient.	Determine if patient meets criteria for positive screen.	1. Confirm (or reject) diagnosis 2. Establish etiologic factors 3. Diagnose and classify pathologic and functional changes 4. Evaluate the prognosis	1. Establish new etiologic factors 2. Evaluate and classify current clinical status 3. Evaluate current prognosis 4. Determine an acceptable response to treatment (outcome criteria)
TREATMENT PLANNING	Formulate plans for: 1. Preventive measures 2. Follow-up	Formulate plans for: 1. Referral (action to be taken if patient is screened positive) 2. Follow-up (schedule workup if screened positive; schedule re-screening if negative)	Formulate plans for: 1. Initial therapy 2. Patient education 3. Follow-up 4. Referral	Formulate plans for: 1. Maintaining, modifying, or terminating therapy 2. Patient education 3. Diagnostic tests 4. Referral plans 5. Follow-up

tion of each appropriate clinical function in the proper sequence. The tasks within each function should be applied to the proper patients, in the proper sequence, and at appropriate time intervals, and thus effective health care results in the flow of patients from one clinical function to the next.

It is readily apparent from the generic objectives of Table 13-1 that some clinical functions may result in a change in patient health status, but the majority of them will not. However, each clinical function has a definite result, which in many instances is an awareness on the part of the patient or provider of the nature, severity, etiology, or implications of the patients health status. Although this awareness does not directly contribute to a health outcome, it nonetheless improves the probability that the succeeding functions will be applied, moving the patient through the sequence of functions that do result in a health outcome. For example, a positive screening result implies presumptive evidence of disease and as such does not necessarily lead to a health outcome. Yet, an awareness of the positive screen on the part of the provider, patient, or both may improve the probability of subsequent diagnosis and treatment, which in turn may lead to a health outcome.

Another example is the patient who is given a 10-day supply of an oral antibiotic along with education regarding the importance of taking the medication in the prescribed manner. The expected result of the education is compliance on the patient's part. Many investigators will insist that the resulting compliance is not an outcome but rather another element of the process of care, although it clearly is the result of the education and is clearly required to achieve the expected health outcomes. Very few physician activities have a direct effect on health status, and usually patient behavior is the intervening variable. The health education in this example does not achieve a health outcome but may have as its result an awareness on the part of the patient of the importance of filling the prescription and taking the medication, which in turn may result in an improved health status.

It is not to be suggested that the distinction between process and outcome should be abandoned. However, it should be recognized that health care consists of a sequence of clinical functions, which should be applied to appropriate patients, in the correct sequence, and in a timely manner. Each does not have a health outcome as its direct result, but the purpose of health care is to move patients through the sequence to those functions that may realize a direct health benefit.

CHARACTERISTICS OF OUTCOMES

The use of health outcomes in an appraisal of the quality of health care requires an understanding of some of the strengths and weaknesses implicit in outcome appraisal.

Outcome measures are a function of the perspective of the observer. From the medical viewpoint, mortality, morbidity, and functional status are relevant outcomes. Discomfort, anxiety, length of stay, and interruption of life style due to both illness and the prescribed therapy may be the relevant outcomes to the patient. The community perspective may identify unmet health needs, and the health system managers and public administrators may focus on utilization and cost effectiveness as relevant dimensions of the outcome of health care. Varying viewpoints may be found even within the medical perspective: reduction in blood pressure to the physician, change in health attitude to the behavioral scientist, and compliance with suggested well-child care to the home visiting nurse.

The outcome measures most generally available from the medical perspective are mortality and incidence of major complications. However, each is a relatively uncommon event, particularly in an ambulatory care setting, and would require very large study samples to provide meaningful information. As the end results of care, they often occur long after the provision of care that influenced them. Such outcome measures do not provide a timely assessment of current health practices.

Many health outcomes are strongly influenced by factors unrelated to medical care, such as genetic composition, health attitudes and behavior, and the environment. Measures derived from such outcomes are therefore insensitive to the quality of medical care provided and could focus attention on areas of relatively poor outcome that may not be areas of improper or inadequate medical care. However, this weakness could in time become a major strength of outcome appraisal if it serves to diminish the focus on medical care as the major determinant of good health and encourages emphasis on the other factors related to outcome, such as health attitudes, behaviors, and a healthy environment, as noted by Illich.[37]

The timing of observations contributing to outcome measures is critical. If one waits for a stable end point in health status, the resulting information may not contribute to the timely improvement of health care. Although some diseases, such as acute infectious processes, have obvious end points resulting in death or recovery with or without residua, other disease processes develop slowly and may appear to wax and wane. Timing of measurements become even more complex in a multidimensional measure of outcome that may take physiologic, functional, and emotional status into account, where each dimension has its own set of time-critical observation requirements.

When used alone, outcome appraisal does not in itself suggest how to improve health care if it appears to be inadequate. The commonly used outcome measures (mortality and morbidity) when suggesting suboptimal care do not point out specific deficiencies. For example, an unacceptable mortality rate due to hypertension sequelae does not suggest whether improved screening, diagnostic procedures, treatment, follow-up, or patient compliance would more likely reduce the unacceptable outcome.

On the other hand, outcome appraisal used in conjunction with process assessment may lead to conflicting results. In a classic study by Brook, the quality of care was assessed for three chronic conditions using process assessments, outcome assessments, and a combination process-outcome assessment.[7] For a given condition the quality of care varied substantially as a function of the method used. Brook also found that the assessed quality of care varied depending on whether implicit or explicit criteria were used.

Furthermore, several important studies have questioned the relationship between process criteria chosen for study and the corresponding outcome measures. Lindsay and associates studied the outpatient management of acute urinary tract infections and found no statistically significant associations between any of the ten process criteria and the four outcome measures selected for the study.[51] The process criteria had been selected by a committee who chose only those process elements felt to influence outcome directly. In a similar study of hypertension by Nobrega and associates, no substantial correlation existed between explicit process criteria and control of blood pressure.[56]

These studies do not suggest that there is no relationship between the process of health care and the outcomes potentially achieved. Rather, they suggest that process criteria chosen for the study may not always bear a statistical relationship to the outcome criteria chosen. Again, it is important to recognize that very few medical processes lead directly to a change in health status, independent of patient attitudes and behaviors. As depicted in Figure 13-1, medical processes act in conjunction with patient processes to achieve desired health outcomes. It is often sobering to reflect on the relatively small impact of medical processes on health status when they are running counter to prevailing patient attitudes, behaviors, and current health fads. Health education is often used in an attempt to reconcile differences in medical care requirements and patient behaviors, yet far too often this relationship (Figure 13-1) is unilateral. The medical community attempts to educate the patient and change his process of care, but it does not learn from the interchange of needed adjustments in the medical process. Quality assurance activities from the medical perspective will quite legitimately con-

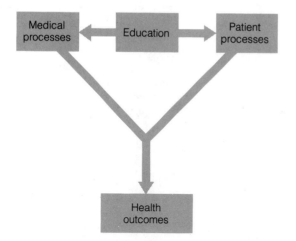

FIGURE 13-1. Relationship of medical and patient processes of care to health outcomes.

tinue to seek process and outcome criteria that seem to be related, such that a change in the level of process performance will result in a change in the observed outcome. However, in so doing, it is well to remember that in a larger context, which one might call the public health perspective, one could add inputs from environmental, genetic, and cultural factors to Figure 13-1 and demonstrate that many desirable health outcomes will not be observed to change dramatically in response to changes in the medical process of care.

Data for many outcome criteria are not routinely available on all members of a recipient population. The patient record, as an obvious source of outcome data, provides outcome measures only for those patients who comply with follow-up visit requests. This would provide a biased sample, because general patient compliance may strongly influence the observed outcome. The cost of collecting high-quality outcome data from an unbiased sample is a significant factor in the use of outcome appraisal.

Nearly any proposed scheme for using outcome measures in quality assurance requires some degree of value judgment. The attainment of optimal outcomes across all criteria selected may be nearly impossible due to the relationship between the outcome criteria themselves. For example, if longevity as an outcome is desired in neoplastic disease, there may well be an associated increase in morbidity due to the side effects of surgical or medical therapy over the extended life of the patient.

MECHANISMS FOR ASSESSING HEALTH STATUS

Physicians have long assessed health status in individual patients as an integral part of routine clinical practice. All physicians specify outcome events that will alert them to the probability of either favorable or adverse health states at a later point in time. In an iterative manner, physicians adjust their therapeutic approach in light of changing health status of their patients. For example, a child with mild anemia might be placed on a therapeutic trial of iron and followed later with a reticulocyte count. If there is an acceptable response, the iron therapy will be continued, with a provisional diagnosis of iron-deficiency anemia and a good expected outcome. If the reticulocyte response is less than acceptable, a more in-depth diagnostic evaluation is undertaken, and a different set of outcomes anticipated.

Assessing the health status of a group of patients, a community, or an entire population, however, requires a different set of cognitive tools. The most comprehensive approach to measuring the health status of a total population involves a complete examination of a sample of that population. Although far too costly for routine use in quality assurance, such an approach was used in England in the 1940s. A similar study has been undertaken more recently in the United States through the

Health Interview Survey, Health Examination Survey, and Health Records Survey. Linder has reported the results of this massive study, which attempts to define the social implications of illness as well as measures of physical and physiologic health status.[50]

In a less costly approach, Sanders constructed a life table of productive man years projected from birth.[67] These modified life tables provide a crude measure of health status but contain very imprecise indicators of well-being and morbidity.

A great deal of work has gone into the development of health status indices. Using data from the U.S. Health Interview Survey, Sullivan constructed an index based on mortality and morbidity, where morbidity consisted of expectation of time free of disability.[75] The Cornell Medical Index is a composite obtained through a self-administered questionnaire.[6] Data elements relating to bodily function, mood, feeling patterns, and frequency of illness are collected and subjected to clinical evaluation. When aggregated, the results form a profile of the target population's health status. The Proxy Measure for Health Status is simpler and is both administered and scored by a nonprofessional.[46] It consists of four data elements—number of days hospitalized, drugs and medication taken, checklist of acute conditions, and a checklist of chronic conditions—and has been validated against independent professional judgment.

Packer and Shellard developed a scale running from death to perfect health and have attached values to occupying given points on the scale.[60] Fanshel and Bush devised a disutility continuum; death and well-being were the two extremes, and weights were assigned to the various states based on economic, behavioral survey, and expert judgments.[30] This method describes the target population's health status at one point in time by aggregating the weighted states across that population.

Many of the health status indices attempt to incorporate specific dimensions of patients' daily functioning. An early effort by Katz and associates produced an index of activities of daily living (ADL), which examines the performance of several functions such as bathing, dressing, and feeding that may be affected by disabling conditions.[41] Ellwood, and Wylie and White developed health status measures using disability as the measure of health.[28,88] Both are administered by professional rehabilitation workers and consist of a checklist of daily routine activities. Although having a great deal of utility in rehabilitation programs, these profiles do not encompass a very broad assessment of health status.

Mushlin has developed a problem status index (PSI) based on frequency and activity of symptoms, anxiety, and activity limitation.[55] Patients respond to a questionnaire at the time of initial contact for a condition and again after 1 month. A combination of disability and distress scales has been described by Rosser and Watts for use with hospitalized patients.[64] Reynolds and associates have also described a function status index (FSI), which has been validated and is considered ready for use in evaluating medical care.[63]

Berdit and Williamson developed a 6-point health status scale for measuring functional limitations.[3] This scale has been used in some quality assessment studies based on Williamson's health accounting system. Kane and associates added restriction of activity as a seventh category of functional status.[40] In use in the family practice clinic at the University of Utah, the scale assesses patient's usual status, status at the initial visit, and status at follow-up.

A comprehensive sickness impact profile (SIP) has been described by Pollard and associates, and Bergner and associates.[62,4] The SIP provides a summary of health status aggregated across 14 categories of functional activity. A patient's SIP is constructed from a self-administered questionnaire dealing with behaviors relevant to each of the 14 categories. A scoring method relies on weighted values placed on each of 235 SIP items. Scores can be calculated for the entire SIP as well as for each of the categories. The categories and selected items of the SIP appear in Table 13-2. The broad range of activities and its sensitivity to minor changes in dysfunction make the SIP particularly appealing for use in a primary care setting.

Very few health status measures view health from the patient's perspective. This, however, is a particularly important viewpoint, because the perceptions of his own health status may well affect the patient's health-related behavior. Brunswick suggests that at some point the assessment of the quality of health care must take into account health status as the individual perceives it.[13] She has devised a measure of health status using four self-reported indicators designed for adolescents. The morbidity indicator includes a checklist of symptoms and illness reported within a given time frame and specific questions regarding vision, weight, accidents, menstrual problems, smoking, and eating behavior. The subjects' attitude is measured in response to the question, "Is your health very good, good, fair, or poor?" Functional limitation is assessed from the individual's response reflecting the extent to which his health had limited his activities in or out of school. Finally, disability is measured from the subject's report of school absence due to health problems.

MEASURING OUTCOMES

Shapiro has pointed out the distinction between direct and indirect approaches to outcome appraisal.[68] The direct approach requires an environment structured carefully to control for variables to be studied, and usually outcome measures are defined and collected prospectively from both control and experimental groups. The direct approach is most useful in health services research to validate hypotheses of the efficacy and effectiveness of elements of the structure and process of health care. It has the advantage of requiring smaller sample sizes, but the requirement of carefully structured environments to control for extraneous variables limits its utility in routine quality assessment.

The indirect approach begins with the examination of outcomes, and where differences are found, a retrospective analysis of the structural and process elements contributing to the difference can be initiated. Since its purpose is to monitor results and modify performance rather than validate hypotheses, the indirect approach has its major utility in quality assurance efforts. Its primary appeal lies in its relative simplicity. It does not require the rigid experimental design of the direct approach, and results can be obtained relatively quickly. Shapiro notes, however, that the indirect approach relies on evidence from the direct approach, and this has been slow in coming.

Brook and associates distinguish between prospective and retrospective outcome studies.[11] The prospective approach is that used by clinicians in the routine management of their patients, whereby diagnostic and therapeutic activities are altered as a function of changes in the patient's health status. When used as a quality assurance tool, the prospective approach may evoke a change in the quality of care for those patients whose care is under study. The retrospective approach, on the other hand, examines the care provided to patients in the past with the purpose of improving the quality of care provided to future patients. In addition to its application within a single delivery system, the retrospective approach is useful in comparative evaluations to support policy decisions on a local, regional, or national level.

Outcomes are commonly measured in one of five ways. An outcome may be expressed as the difference between health status measured at two points in time. This approach has been used by

TABLE 13-2.   Categories and Selected Items of the Sickness Impact Profile*

CATEGORY	ITEMS DESCRIBING BEHAVIORS INVOLVED IN OR RELATED TO	SELECTED ITEMS	SCALE VALUES
SI	Social interaction	I isolate myself as much as I can from the rest of the family.	10.2
		I am going out less to visit people.	4.4
A	Ambulation	I am walking shorter distances or stop to rest often.	4.8
		I do not walk at all.	10.5
SR	Sleep and rest activity	I lie down more often during the day in order to rest.	5.8
		I sit around half-asleep.	8.4
E	Eating	I am eating no food at all, nutrition is taken through tubes or intravenous fluids.	13.3
		I am eating special or different food, for example, soft food, bland diet, low-salt, low-fat foods.	4.3
HM	Household management	I have given up taking care of personal or household business affairs, for example, paying bills, banking, working on budget.	8.4
		I am doing *less* of the regular daily work around the house than I usually do.	4.4
M	Mobility	I stay within one room.	10.6
		I am not going into town.	4.8
BCM	Body care and movement	I am in a restricted position all the time.	12.5
		I dress myself, but do so very slowly.	4.3
C	Communication	I communicate mostly gestures, for example, moving head, pointing, sign language.	10.2
		I often lose control of my voice when I talk, for example, my voice gets louder, starts trembling, changes pitch.	8.3
RP	Recreation and pastimes	I am doing more inactive pastimes instead of my other usual activities.	5.1
		I am going out for entertainment less often.	3.6
AB	Alertness behavior	I sometimes behave as if I were confused or disoriented in place or time, for example, where I am, who is around, directions, what day it is.	11.3
		I have difficulty reasoning and solving problems, for example, making plans, making decisions, learning new things.	8.4
EB	Emotional behavior	I act irritable and impatient with myself, for example, talk badly about myself, swear at myself, blame myself for things that happen.	7.8
		I laugh or cry suddenly.	6.8
W	Work	I often act irritable toward my work associates, for example, snap at them, give sharp answers, criticize easily.	8.0
		I am working shorter hours.	4.3

*From *Sickness Impact Profile Project,* Department of Health Services, University of Washington.

several investigators cited previously. Rosser and Watts measure the change in health status occurring during hospitalization and have found consistent improvement.[64] Mushlin reports measuring health status at the time of initial contact and again after 1 month.[55] Kane and associates derive an outcome measure using health status from three points in time, including usual status, status at the initial visit, and status at follow-up.[40] When outcome is characterized as a change in health status, the problem of timing of the health status measurements becomes critical. A fixed interval between the two measurements may not capture the entire change that will occur or may result in an interval that does not distinguish between optimal or suboptimal care, particularly for acute and self-limiting conditions. Rosser and Watts' approach does not utilize a fixed interval but measures health status change between admission and discharge. The general improvement that they observe may be due in part to a natural improvement in health status or to the tendency to discharge patients only after they have improved. The approach of Kane and associates measures change not only between initial and follow-up visits (presumably not a fixed time interval across various conditions) but also has the potential to examine outcome as a difference between usual health status and health status at follow-up. Although this approach is attractive for such acute conditions as accidents and infectious disease, the determination of usual health status may be difficult for chronic conditions. The problem of timing of the health status measurements may become more complex as the number of dimensions of outcome chosen for study increases. In the multidimensional health status, certain dimensions may change slowly, change rapidly, or continue to wax and wane.

Similarly, the problem of making value judgments appears in outcomes derived from changes in health status in terms of how great a change is desired or acceptable. Presumably if change is measured from patients' usual health status or patients' desired health status, this problem may be reduced somewhat. If a multidimensional profile such as proposed by Starfield is used to assess change in health status, a different problem of value judgment emerges.[72] As noted previously, positive change may be observed in one category (such as longevity) in association with a negative change in another (such as activity). The problem of determining the magnitude of positive change that will offset the negative change is not easily solved.

A second approach to measuring outcomes derives from comparing a single measure of health status with norms or normative criteria. Norms are numerical or statistical measures derived from direct observation,[59] whereas normative criteria are derived from opinions of what constitutes good medical practice.[23,27] Comparison of observed health status with norms presents enormous problems in data collection, particularly for measures other than incidence, prevalence, mortality rates, and so forth that may be readily available. Also, norms may not necessarily reflect ideal or even acceptable health status. Comparison of observed health status with normative criteria, on the other hand, has some obvious advantages in that no costly data collection effort is required to establish them, and issues of timing and value judgments can be managed.[9,86] The work of Brook and associates and Avery and associates utilized a panel of experts to define normative outcome criteria for eight diseases and surgical conditions.[2,9] In addition to dealing with issues of timing and value judgments, the panel identified nonmedical care variables that might affect the outcome measures chosen and suggested methods for controlling them.

A third method of measuring outcomes involves comparison of health status measures in two or more study areas. Thompson and associates used this approach to compare perinatal mortality in two U.S. Air Force hospitals.[76] Applying the tracer methodology, Kessner and associates examined outcomes of health care in five different practice configurations, and Morehead studied outcomes in prepaid and fee-for-service practices.[45,54] Although this approach does not lend itself to assessments of ''good'' or ''bad'' health care, it may be extremely useful in identifying the relative deficiencies in health care within a geographic area or large system of care.

Outcomes for selected patient cohorts can be expressed also as the transition rate from one discrete health state to another. Chen and associates and Bush and associates have devised a method whereby prognosis is expressed as the transitional probability of movement from one point on their health index scale to another.[15,19] The transitions among the health states/functional levels are determined empirically by population monitoring and follow-up studies on specific patient cohorts. In a prospective study, Nutting and associates assessed the effectiveness of direct care by tribal health workers for infant gastroenteritis through the use of transitional rates among five discrete stages of gastroenteritis.[58] This mechanism has also been used to monitor the care provided to groups of patients and to validate a method of prospectively identifying infants at high risk for gastroenteritis.[58]

Finally, population outcomes may be expressed as a proportion of a target population that meets normative outcome criteria during successive iterations of a quality assurance program. Shorr and associates have described an application of this approach in ambulatory care, whereby the local physicians set normative outcome criteria as a proportion of the target population.[70] Two criteria are specified: one as the minimally acceptable level and the other as an exceptional level. Through the use of a computerized health information system the proportion of the target population can be ex-

pressed from two perspectives. The provider-based perspective expresses a given outcome indicator as a proportion of the population utilizing services, whereas the population-based perspective expresses that proportion including the entire beneficiary population in the denominator. Since the latter includes also those patients who have either reduced access to care or who choose not to utilize services, the two perspectives when used in conjunction aid in focusing on the reasons that outcomes may be unacceptable.

USES OF OUTCOME MEASURES

Outcome measures have been found to be useful in three general areas. They have been used extensively to aid in the decision process regarding establishing health policies, setting priorities, and assessing the effectiveness of major health programs. They serve a central role in evaluative research as the primary criteria to validate the efficacy and effectiveness of the processes of health care and the organization of health services. In this regard they have utility as the ultimate criteria against which the value of quality assurance programs themselves should be judged. Finally, outcome measures are finding an increased usage in quality assurance programs either in conjunction with process evaluation or as a screening tool to identify the need for an in-depth investigation of the process of care.

Decision-Making Aid

Much of the work using outcome measures to assess the effectiveness of health care programs has been reported by Bush and his associates. They have described a model to determine the impact of health programs on disease in target population.[16] They have subsequently refined the model and applied it to an analysis of a tuberculin testing program and later to the PKU screening program of New York State.[15,17]

Miller developed and tested three indices of health status using mortality and morbidity to assess the impact of preventive, control, and curative health programs in the Indian Health Service.[52] The first index measures years lost due to premature death, institutionalization, and disability. The second considers the ratio of time that would be lost to those disease cases not known to the health care system to time lost to those known, and the third measures time lost due to premature death and institutionalization. Weaknesses of this method are principally due to the inability to measure precisely some of the model inputs and the assumed causal relationship between health program intervention and change in functional time loss.

Torrance and associates developed a mortality-morbidity index that assigns a utility value to every possible health state as a function of time spent in that state.[78] Effectiveness of health care is expressed as a function of days spent in a given health state, and cost-effectiveness ratios are calculated to assess health care programs in terms yield per dollar cost. The relative weakness of each of these methods is their relatively narrow concept of health and the problems attendant on weighting and assigning values to the health states.

Outcome measures have also been used to assign program priorities. Miller developed the Q-Index to aid program planners in assigning priorities to different disease entities.[52] The model compares the target population with a standard reference population and examines mortality and morbidity (represented by time lost in the hospital or outpatient clinic). The model suggests that diseases resulting in the greatest time loss should receive priority attention. Stewart uses a similar method but takes into account the program cost and the estimated disease vulnerability.[74] The latter is expressed as the likelihood of treatment impact on the disease on a scale of 0 to 10. Stewart's priority formulation is:

$$\frac{MTV}{C}$$

M = magnitude of the disease (mortality/100,000)
T = importance of M on a scale of 0 to 10
V = disease vulnerability on a scale of 0 to 10
C = cost

Chen expands Miller's Q-Index to account for potential improvement in health status, which presumably would follow if a higher priority were placed on that disease.[18] However, the potential improvement is defined as the difference in mortality and morbidity between the target and reference populations.

Each of these methods has shortcomings as measures of outcome for quality assurance. They encompass a relatively narrow concept of health outcome in that they focus on mortality and morbidity statistics. They focus on time loss and place only a socioeconomic value on days hospitalized and time spent in the outpatient clinic. Finally, they attempt to set disease priorities without very precise data on the potential impact that would result from rearranging priorities. However, in the intended role of their developers, they have a value in imbuing the health planning process with some objective rationality. They may have utility in quality assurance in aiding in the identification of tracer conditions and diseases to be examined by virtue of their incidence and system work load.

Finally, outcome measures may be of value in support of policy decisions. They have been used successfully to shed light on issues such as whether the quality of care provided by U.S. medical graduates is significantly better than that provided by foreign medical graduates, how the quality of health care in a health insurance plan compares with that in the medical welfare system, or whether the design of the health care delivery system measurably impacts on the quality of care provided.[45,68,83]

Evaluative Research Tool

Outcome measures are most commonly used to validate the efficacy of specific elements of the process of care. Drugs and surgical procedures are usually subjected to an outcome-oriented assessment in a study comparing them with those currently available or with a placebo. Experimental designs have been used in cancer research to examine the 5- and 10-year survival rates resulting from various chemotherapeutic agents. Unfortunately, many elements of the process of care have not been validated against outcome measures. For example, much of that which is done in the name of prenatal and well-child care is supported by conventional wisdom rather than objective outcome data.

Outcomes also are used frequently to validate the effectiveness of selected processes and delivery strategies in health care. Lewis compared outcomes for patients seen in an experimental nurse clinic and patients receiving care in the medical clinic of a university medical center.[48] Nutting and associates employed health problem staging to assess the effectiveness of tribal health workers utilizing protocols to provide direct patient care in the home.[58]

A major role of health outcome appraisal in quality assurance has been relatively unexplored to date. Virtually no evidence exists that any quality assurance program design will positively affect the health status of patient populations. Outcome appraisals are thus needed to determine which, if any, design approaches to improving the quality of health care do in fact result in an improvement in health status of the recipient population. Shorr, Nutting, and Berg have outlined an approach to outcome assessment of quality assurance programs in which outcomes are expressed as a proportion of the recipient population that meets normative outcome criteria.[70] During successive assessment phases of the quality assurance program, changes in the proportion reflect the impact of the program on the health status of the population. There is an urgent need to develop and apply this type of evaluative approach to PSROs.

Quality Assurance Tool

Although it was not mandated in the original legislation, there has been encouragement to incorporate outcome appraisal in the MCEs under PSRO.[32] The general model that has emerged utilizing outcome assessment in routine quality assurance studies makes use of outcome measures as a screening tool to identify areas of health care that require closer scrutiny. These approaches assume that the logical first step is to identify health care processes in need of improvement by comparing observed health status with normative criteria.

The original work on this method was reported by Williamson and his associates, who have called it health accounting.[84,86] The process begins with a selection of a problem to be studied. Normative criteria are established specifying diagnostic accuracy (unjustified diagnoses and missed diagnoses) and the degree of impairment expected following appropriate medical intervention. Williamson and his associates term these diagnostic outcome and therapeutic outcome, respectively. Outcomes are assessed by a combination of chart review, patient survey, and in many cases, an independent reexamination of the patient by the study team. Where outcome measures are not in compliance with the normative criteria, an in-depth process analysis is initiated and the results presented to the clinicians as part of a continuing education process.

Brook and associates reported a modification of the work of Williamson and his associates in which diagnostic and therapeutic outcomes were assessed by chart review using implicit criteria rather than employing independent reexamination of the patients.[8,10] Outcome data collected included persistence of symptoms, disability, and abnormal physical or laboratory findings.

Similarly, Mushlin and Kane and associates obtained outcome measures without requiring costly reexamination of the patient.[40,55] In the method employed by Kane and associates, the clinician records the patient's usual functional status, status at the initial visit, and status at follow-up. Mushlin determines frequency and activity of symptoms, anxiety, and activity limitation from a patient questionnaire at the time of the initial visit and again after 1 month. Both approaches could be used to trigger an in-depth process analysis when outcomes are found to be inadequate.

The health accounting approach to medical care evaluation and the subsequent modifications of that approach hold a great deal of promise for the use of outcome appraisal. It is conceptually simple and feasible in most practice settings, including evaluation of both inpatient and ambulatory care. As noted by Brook and associates, it has been tested in 23 ambulatory and hospital settings.[9] Although somewhat expensive, particularly if independent patient reexamination is undertaken, it may forego the need to examine many processes of care that are associated with acceptable outcomes. However, health accounting techniques also tend to ignore those aspects of medical care with little or no demonstrable impact on outcome. A comprehensive quality assessment method should examine inappropriate care as well as deficient care. Furthermore, in relatively small target populations using outcome measures of relatively low inci-

dence, the health accounting approach may incorrectly assume adequate care. For example, in a target population of less than 10,000 people, the lack of any cases of rheumatic fever would not necessarily suggest that the management of streptococcal pharyngitis was adequate.

Health accounting is oriented toward identification of medical care deficiencies and feeding these into educational programs. This is its major strength, and as noted by Palmer, it may also be its major shortcoming for application in PSRO.[61] Unlike process evaluations, the nature of the results of health accounting are not readily applicable for use in controlling reimbursement for inadequate or inappropriate health services. Nonetheless, the concept of examining health outcomes to pinpoint areas of process deficiency and subsequent feedback of process information to the providers of health care appears to be a constructive approach to assuring quality of health care. Further experimentation with additional measures of health status in this context is needed.

Other investigators have used outcome measures in conjunction with process measures in study designs in which both are assessed simultaneously. In some of their early work with the tracer methodology, Kessner and associates used measures of both process and outcome to make assessments of the quality of care.[43] Greenfield and associates have utilized simultaneous measurements of process and outcome assessment.[33] Although their goal is to develop process maps that have a strong correlation to patient outcomes and thereby eliminate the need to measure outcome, they nonetheless are currently using both process and outcome appraisal. Shorr and associates also employ simultaneous measures of process and outcome for quality assessment within the Indian Health Service.[70] In their operational quality assurance programs with target populations of under 15,000 persons, they feel that outcome measures alone are not adequately sensitive to the quality of care and particularly to changes in the quality of care. Their experimental program provides performance feedback to the individual provider of care. If only outcome measures were used, the feedback would be less specific with regard to necessary changes in provider behavior and would totally ignore inappropriate care, such as antibiotic therapy for upper respiratory infections. More importantly for those providers of care who are improving their performance, outcome measures alone might not reflect such an improvement, and the opportunity for positive reinforcement could be lost.

IMPLICATIONS FOR PSRO

The implementation of the PSRO program through the BQA represents a sizable investment in dollars and professional manpower. Operational PSROs provide an opportunity to continue experimentation with mechanisms for outcome assessment and to contribute significantly to the body of knowledge relating process of care to outcome. It would be regrettable if this opportunity were to be lost. In view of the state of the art and the need to continue developing and testing innovative approaches to outcome appraisal, the following are offered not as specific suggestions but as issues to consider in the use of outcomes in PSRO.

Outcomes can be viewed from a variety of perspectives, as noted previously. In light of the tendency of physicians to focus on physical and physiologic parameters and the legislative requirement of provider control of PSRO activities, it is unlikely that outcome measures employed in the immediate future will extend beyond measures of morbidity, mortality, and physical/physiologic dysfunction. However, the works of Mushlin, Berdit and Williamson, Pollard and associates, and Kane and associates attempt to extend outcome

measurement to incorporate measures of functional limitation and patients' perceptions of symptoms, anxiety, and dysfunction and deserve more widespread application.[3,40,55,62] Further work should also be done to incorporate and test outcome measures based on patients' perceptions of their own health, such as that reported by Brunswick.[13]

The community perspective is very likely to be ignored in PSRO activities unless an attempt is made to assess the quality of care provided to the entire recipient community. The PSRO legislation requires review of care provided to only those patients who utilize health services payable under Medicare and Medicaid. However, a committee of the Institute of Medicine of the National Academy of Sciences has recommended that quality assurance efforts be directed as well to all persons in the review area, most of whom will not be receiving services during a specific study period.[34] The quality assessment method of Shorr and associates described previous attempts to examine health care from the standpoint of care provided by the system as well as care received by the community.[70] Various types of outcome measures that reflect more than the medical outcomes of one-on-one patient care deserve further exploration if the PSRO is to be more than a mechanism for control of federal expenditures under Titles V, XVIII, and XIX.

An early step in the development of any strategy for assessing the quality of health care is the selection of topics for review. Kessner and associates were some of the first investigators to specify the criteria for selection of health problem topics.[43] More recently, other authors have specified the criteria by which they choose health problem topics. These are summarized in Table 13-3 as compiled by Brook and associates.[9] The comprehensive quality assurance system (CQAS) developed and in use by Rubin in the Kaiser-Permanente system suggests that topics for review should be identified by the providers in an open

TABLE 13-3.   Criteria Used to Select Conditions for Outcomes Measurement and Quality Assessment, Classified by Previous Users*

CRITERION	BROOK (1973)	KESSNER et al. (1973)	LEWIS (1974)	PAYNE et al. (1976)	OPSR†a (1975)	SIBLEY et al. (1975)	WILLIAMSON (IN PREPARATION)
High frequency (prevalence or incidence)	+	+	+	+	+	+	+
Functional impact on patient	+	+		+	+		+
Well-defined; easy to diagnose	+	+	+	+			
Medical care has positive impact on natural history	+	+	+	+	+	+	+
Techniques and impact of treatment are well-defined		+					+
Nonmedical factors affecting natural history are well-defined		+					
Mix of conditions is representative of many specialties and types of service		+		+	+		
High (social) cost					+		
Course not unduly dependent on patient cooperation				+			
Preventive care and/or early detection have positive effect on natural history				+			

*From Brook, R.H., Avery, A., Greenfield, S., et al. 1976. Quality of medical care assessment using outcome measures: An overview of the method, R-2021/1-HEW. Santa Monica, Calif.: Rand Corp.
†aOffice of Professional Standards Review.

format.[65] Rubin stresses that topics selected in this way are not restricted to health problems but may include administrative and logistic issues as well. Such an approach, however, is likely to focus attention on topics that have only an indirect relationship to patient health status. An implicit assumption underlying this approach is that providers of health care know in advance what the major impediments are to quality health care. Several recent studies suggest that providers of health care cannot accurately estimate from their day-to-day experience the level of quality of health care that they are providing.[12,57]

Establishing the outcome criteria provides a number of options. In a general sense outcome measures may be disease or problem specific or may be aggregated across a large number of diseases (such as infant mortality or man days lost from work). Within a given health problem category, one may select only a few outcomes that are particularly relevant or may attempt to measure a large number of outcomes for that health problem. Finally, outcome criteria may be implicit or explicit. The former requires that the review process be performed by a credible professional, whereas with the latter, records may be screened or in some cases completely assessed by a nonprofessional. The decision to use implicit or explicit criteria should not be made lightly, however. As Brook has shown, the results of the assessment may be in part a function of this decision.[7]

The selection of the panel to establish outcome criteria may affect the assessment results. There is some evidence derived from establishing process criteria that internists from different parts of the country and pediatricians from academic centers and community practice will set similar criteria.[36,77] There is very little similar evidence regarding outcome criteria, and in fact, Kane and associates note that practicing physicians may tend to underestimate the degree of disability reported by patients at follow-up.[40] Establishing outcome criteria requires a different set of skills than that needed to set process criteria, because outcomes are usually derived from groups of patients and may be affected by factors other than medical care.

Setting of outcome criteria by the local providers whose care will be evaluated has some obvious advantages. Providers who are assessed against their own criteria are likely to be more responsive to the results. However, if the results fall short of their criteria, they are likely to be more lenient in setting criteria in the future. This may be particularly apparent in criteria set as suggested by Rubin. In the CQAS method a set of criteria is made progressively more lenient until it has 100% acceptance by the local staff. Although this approach ensures local acceptance of the resulting criteria, the effort may be self-defeating in some settings. In the Indian Health Service, Shorr and associates have the local providers specify two levels for each outcome criterion.[70] The minimally acceptable and exceptional levels define the range of expected performance. Results may be expressed either as the proportion of the patient population who meet each criteria level or as the population who meet a given criterion where the proportion itself is set at two levels of performance.

By whatever technique the criteria are established, the final criteria list should bear at least a theoretical relationship to some process of health care that potentially could be changed. Ideally the outcome measures derived from the criteria should be sensitive to changes in the process of care and less sensitive to nonmedical factors. Finally, unacceptable results from the outcome measures should suggest further action. This might include the need to strengthen specific elements of the process of care. In this regard it is most helpful if the outcome measures suggest a distinction between unacceptable provider behavior and unacceptable patient compliance. On the other hand, outcome measures may be used to pinpoint areas of health care in need of in-depth process evaluation, as in the health accounting system.

Another critical consideration is the timing of the outcome measure. Those generally available, such as mortality and sequelae of illness, may occur far after the health care to be assessed. The concept of final outcomes is not terribly useful if results are to be used in a timely manner. Proximate outcomes can be measured while the care episode is in progress or shortly thereafter and are a reasonable proxy for end results if there is a known relationship between the proximate outcome and the end result. Starfield and Scheff used posttreatment hemoglobin levels for anemia, and several investigators have used diastolic blood pressure in hypertension as proxy measures for final outcome.[73] Even with proximate outcome measures, the timing of measurements remains important. The measurement must be made after sufficient time has passed for the medical care to exert its effect but not so long after as to be overshadowed by the natural course of the illness.

Regardless of the types of outcome measures used, some degree of value judgment will be required. The situation becomes more complex when several types of outcomes are assessed simultaneously. For example, an appropriate treatment plan for an asymptomatic hypertensive patient will result in a significant disutility in terms of daily routine and life style to achieve an acceptable diastolic blood pressure. There is virtually no information on the relative values that society or the individual places on longevity versus conformation to a self-determined life style. Furthermore, there is not adequate ongoing research employing techniques such as formal decision analysis to provide guidelines for the trade-offs that will inevitably have to be made. Acton has described techniques for determining society's values in the trade-offs, including the human capital approach and various modifications of a willingness-to-pay approach.[1] At the other end of the spectrum, Bickner has observed that for certain types of value judgments, "we must decide the answer ourselves, somewhat arbitrarily, or we must ask for an answer from higher authority, which will be somewhat arbitrary, or we must seek an answer from the voting, spending, demonstrating, or rioting public, which will also be somewhat arbitrary."[5]

The cost of data collection is likely to be a major consideration in the use of outcome measures in the PSRO. Here the old adage is quite true, "the data you have is not what you want, the data you want is not what you need, and the data you need is not available." The outcome data that are most likely to be available, and hence presumably less expensive to collect, are mortality and incidence of major sequelae. To view outcome in a broader

perspective, such as a patient's functional status, disutility, or satisfaction with his health status, would require acquisition of data not routinely collected. Although several authors have pointed out the need to restructure medical care data systems to support quality assurance activities, this is not likely to occur in the immediate future.[80,87,89] In the short run it is important to consider the cost of data collection for quality assurance against the predicted benefit of that same cost invested back into direct patient care. In the long run, however, it is also necessary to consider the benefits that may accrue from a quality assurance effort based on more meaningful outcome data. These will not be easy decisions to make.

Finally, professional standards review as a specific design decision for assuring the quality of health care is untested. There is virtually no objective evidence to suggest that substantial benefits will result in terms of improved health status of the recipient target populations, and thoughtful arguments as to its potential to do so have been raised.[82] It is of utmost importance, therefore, that the PSRO concept be validated against an improved health outcome, just as one would argue for validation of any other structural or process element of health care. It is very possible that the major immediate application of outcome appraisal in the PSRO program rests in this area. Quality assurance programs may continue to emphasize process assessment due to cost and state-of-the-art considerations, but such programs themselves should be evaluated with outcome measures.

REFERENCES

1. Acton, J.P. 1973. *Evaluating public program to save lives: the case of heart attacks.* R-950-RC. Santa Monica, Calif.: Rand Corp.

2. Avery, A.D., Lelah, T., Soloman, N., et al. 1976. *Quality of medical care assessment using outcome*

measures: eight disease-specific applications. R-2021/2-HEW. Santa Monica, Calif.: Rand Corp.

3. Berdit, M., and Williamson, J.W. 1975. Function limitation scale for measuring health outcomes. In Berg, R.L., editor. *Health status indexes: proceedings of a conference conducted by health services research.* Chicago: Hospital Research and Educational Trust, pp. 59–69.

4. Bergner, M., Bobbitt, R.A., and Pollard, W.E., et al. 1976. The sickness impact profile: validation of a health status measure. *Med. Care* 14:57–67.

5. Bickner, R.E. 1970. *Measurement and indices of health: outcomes conference I and II.* Rockville, Md.: U.S. Department of Health, Education, and Welfare, National Center for Health Services Research and Development.

6. Brodman, K., Erdmann, A.J., Lorge, I., Wolff, H.G., Broadbent, T.H.

7. Brook, R.H. 1973. *Quality of care assessment: a comparison of five methods of peer review.* DHEW Publication No. HRA-74-3100. Rockville, Md.: U.S. Department of Health, Education, and Welfare.

8. Brook, R.H., Appel, F.A., Avery, C., et al. 1971. Effectiveness of inpatient follow-up care. *N. Engl. J. Med.* 285:1509–1513.

9. Brook, R.H., Avery, A.D., Greenfield, S., et al. 1976. *Quality of medical care assessment using outcome measures: an overview of the method.* R-2021/1-HEW. Santa Monica, Calif.: Rand Corp.

10. Brook, R.H., and Stevenson, R.L. 1970. Effectiveness of patient care. *N. Engl. J. Med.* 283:904–907.

11. Brook, R.H., Williams, K.N., and Avery, A.D. 1976. Quality assurance today and tomorrow: forecast for the future. *Ann. Intern. Med.* 85:809–817.

12. Brown, C.R., and Uhl, H.S.M. 1970. Mandating continuing education: sense or nonsense? JAMA, 213:1660–1668.

13. Brunswick, A.F. 1976. Indicators of health status in adolescence. *Int. J. Health Serv.* 6:475–483.

14. Bush, J.W., Blischke, W.L., and Berry, C.C. 1973. *Health indices, outcomes, and quality of care.* No. BHSR 74–49. Rockville, Md.: U.S. Department of Health, Education, and Welfare, Bureau of Health Services Research.

15. Bush, J.W., Chen, M.M., and Patrick, D.L. 1973. *Analysis of the New York state PKU screening program using a health status index.* Report to the New York State Health Planning Commission. New York: The Commission.

16. Bush, J.W., Chen, M.M., and Zaremba, J. 1971. Estimating health program outcomes using a Markov chain equilibrium analysis of disease development. *Am. J. Public Health* 61:2362.

17. Bush, J.W., Fanshel, S., and Chen, M.M. 1972. Analysis of a tuberculin testing program using a health status index. *J. Socio. Econ. Plan.* 6:49–68.

18. Chen, M.K. 1973. The G-Index for Program Priority. *In Health Status Index,* ed. R.E. Berg, Chicago: Hospital Research and Education Trust.

19. Chen, M.M., Bush, J.W., and Patrick, D.L. 1975. Social indicators for health planning and policy analysis. *Policy Sci.* 6:71–89.

20. Codman, E.A. 1914. The product of a hospital. *Surg. Gynecol. Obstet.* 18:491–496.

21. Codman, E.A. 1916. *A study in hospital efficiency: the first five years.* Boston: Thomas Todd Co.

22. Decker, B. 1973. Outcome appraisal of medical care. In Decker, B., and Bonner, P., editors. *PSRO: organization for regional peer review.* Cambridge, Mass.: Ballinger Publishing Co.

23. Decker, B.D., and Bonner, P. 1974. *Criteria in peer review.* Boston: Arthur D. Little Corp.

24. Densen, P.M. 1965. The quality of medical care. *Yale Biol. Med.* 37:523–536.

25. Donabedian, A. 1965. *A guide to medical care administration, vol. 2, medical care appraisal.* New York: American Public Health Association.

26. Donabedian, A. 1966. Evaluating the quality of medical care. *Milbank Mem. Fund Q.* 44 (2):166–206.

27. Donabedian, A. 1969. *A guide to medical care administration, vol. 2, medical care appraisal—quality and utilization.* New York: American Public Health Association.

28. Ellwood, P.M., Jr. 1966. Quantitative measurement of patient care quality. *Hospitals.* 40:42.

29. Esovitz, G.H. 1973. The continuing education of physicians: its relationship to quality of care evaluation. *Med. Clin. North Am.* 57:1135–1147.

30. Fanshel, S., and Bush, J.W. 1970. A health status index and its application to health services outcomes. *Operations Res.* 18:1021.

31. Garratt, A.E. 1973. A comprehensive health care data system. *Computer Med.* 3:9.

32. Goran, M.J., Roberts, J.S., Kellogg, M., et al. 1975. The PSRO hospital review system, *Med. Care* 13(4).

33. Greenfield, S., Nadler, M.A., Morgan, M.T., et al. 1977. The clinical investigation and management of chest pain in an emergency department: quality assessment by criteria mapping. *Med Care* 15:898.

34. Haggerty, R.J. 1974. *Advancing the quality of health care: key issues and fundamental principles.* A policy statement by a committee of the Institute of Medicine. IOM Publication No. 74-04. Washington, D.C.: National Academy of Sciences.

35. Haggerty, R.J. 1976. *Assessing quality in health care: an evaluation.* Institute of Medicine, IOM Publication No. 76-04. Washington, D.C.: National Academy of Sciences.

36. Hare, R.L., and Barnoon, S. 1973. Medical care appraisal and quality assurance in the office practice of internal medicine. *Am. Soc. Intern. Med.*

37. Illich, I. 1976. *Medical nemesis: the exploration of health.* New York: Pantheon Books, Inc.

38. Jacobs, C.M., and Jacobs, N.D. 1974. *The PEP primer: the JCAH performance evaluation procedure for auditing and improving physician care.* Chicago: Quality Review Center, Joint Commission on Accreditation of Hospitals.

39. Johnson, W., and Rosenfeld, L. 1969. Indices of performance in ambulatory care services. *Med. Care* 7:250–260.

40. Kane, R.L., Wolley, F.R., Gardner, H.J., et al. 1976. Measuring outcomes of care in an ambulatory primary care population: a pilot study. *J. Comm. Health* 1:233–240.

41. Katz, S., Ford, A.B., Moskowitz, R.W., et al. 1963. The index of ADL: a standardized measure of biological and psychosocial function. *JAMA.* 185:914–919.

42. Kessner, D.M., and Kalks, C.E. 1973. *Contrasts in health status, vol. 2, A strategy for evaluating health services.* Washington, D.C.: National Academy of Sciences.

43. Kessner, D.M., Kalk, C.E., and Singer, J. 1973. *Assessing health quality: the case for tracers. N. Engl. J. Med.* 288:189–194.

44. Kessner, D.M., Singer, J., Kalk, C.E., and Schlesinger, E.R. 1973. *Contrasts in health status, vol. 1, Infant death: an analysis by maternal risk and health care,* Washington, D.C.: National Academy of Sciences.

45. Kessner, D.M., Snow, C.K., and Singer, J. 1974. *Contrasts in health status, vol. 3, Assessment of medical care for children,* Washington, D.C.: National Academy of Sciences.

46. Kisch, A.I., Covner, J.W., Harris, L.J., and Kline, G. 1969. A new proxy measure for health status, *Health Serv. Res.* 4:223.

47. Last, J.M. 1965. The measurement of medical care in general practice. *Med. J. Aust.* 1:280–282.

48. Lewis, C.E. 1974. The state of the art of quality assurance, 1973. *Med. Care.* 12:799–806.

49. Lewis, C.E., Resnick, B.A., Schmidt, G., et al. 1969. Activities, events, and outcomes in ambulatory patient care. *N. Engl. J. Med.* 280:645–649.

50. Linder, F.E. 1966. The health of the American people, *Sci. Am.* 214:21.

51. Lindsay, M.I., Hermans, P.E., Nobrega, F.T., et al. 1976. Quality of care assessment: evaluating methods of peer review, a study of the outpatient management of acute bacterial cystitis. Rochester, Minn.: Mayo Clinic.

52. Miller, J.E. 1970. An indicator to aid management in assigning program priorities. *Public Health Rep.* 85:725.

53. Miller, J.E. April 1970. Performance indices for community health programs. Presented at the annual meeting of the Operations Research Society of America, Washington, D.C.

54. Morehead, M.A. 1970. Evaluating quality of medical care in the Neighborhood Health Center Program of the Office of Economic Opportunity. *Med. Care* 8:118–131.

55. Mushlin, A.I. 1974. An experimental mechanism for quality assurance in a pre-paid group practice. Proceedings of the Group Health Institute.

Washington, D.C.: Group Health Association of America, Inc., pp. 130–136.

56. Nobrega, F.T., Morrow, G.W., and Smoldt, R.K. 1977. Quality assessment in hypertension: analysis of process and outcome methods. *N. Engl. J. Med.* 296:145–148.

57. Nutting, P.A., and Helmick, E. Provider estimates of quality of health care: comparison with study results. (In preparation.)

58. Nutting, P.A., Shorr, G.I., and Berg, L.E. 1975. Process and outcome measures of tribal health workers in direct patient care. In Flagle, C.D., editor. *Advanced medical systems: issues and challenges.* New York: Stratton Intercontinental Medical Book Corp., pp. 173–190.

59. Nutting, PA.A, Shorr, G.I., and Burkhalter, B.R. Assessing the performance of Medical Care Systems: A Method and Application. *Med. Care* (In press).

60. Office Professional Standards Review. 1974. *PSRO program manual.* U.S. Department of Health Education, and Welfare. Rockville, Md.

61. Packer, A.H., and Shellard, G.D. 1970. Measures of health systems effectiveness. *Operations Res.* 18:1067.

62. Palmer, R.H. 1976. Choice of strategies. In Greene, R., editor. *Assuring quality in medical care: the state of the art.* Cambridge, Mass.: Ballinger Publishing Co.

63. Pollard, W.E., Bobbitt, R.A., Bergner, M., et al. 1976. The sickness impact profile: reliability of a health status measure. *Med. Care* 14:146–155.

64. Reynolds, W.J., Rushing, W.A., and Miles, D.L. 1974. The validation of a function status index. *J. Health Soc. Behav.* 15:271–288.

65. Rosser, R.M., and Watts, V.C. 1972. The measurement of hospital output, *Int. J. Epidemiol.* 1:361–368.

66. Rubin, L. 1975. Comprehensive quality assurance system: the Kaiser-Permanente approach. Alexandria, Va.: American Group Practice Association.

67. Sanazaro, P.J., and Williamson, J.W. 1968. End results of patient care: a provisional classification based on reports by internists. *Med. Care* 6:123–130.

68. Sanders, B.S. 1964. Measuring community health levels. *Am J. Public Health* 54:1063.

69. Shapiro, S. 1967. End-result measurements of quality of medical care. *Milbank Mem. Fund Q.* 45:7–30.

70. Shapiro, S., Williams, J.J., Yerby, A.S., et al. 1967. Patterns of medical use by the indigent under two systems of medical care. *Am. J. Public Health* 57:784–790.

71. Starfield, B. 1973. Health services research: a working model. *N. Engl. J. Med.* 289:132–136.

72. Starfield, B. 1974. Measurement of outcome: a proposed scheme. *Milbank Mem. Fund. Q.* 52:39–50.

73. Starfield, B., and Scheff, D. 1972. Effectiveness of pediatric care: the relationship between process and outcome. *Pediatrics* 49:547–552.

74. Stewart, D. 1968. Planning as an integral and essential part of a national health program. *Med. Care* 6:439.

75. Sullivan, D.F. 1971. A single index of mortality and morbidity. *Public Health Rep.* 86:347.

76. Thompson, J.D., Marguis, D.B., Woodward, R.L., et al. 1968. End-result measurements of the quality of obstetrical care in two U.S. Air Force hospitals. *Med. Care* 6:131–143.

77. Thompson, H.C., and Osborne, C.E. 1976. Quality assurance of ambulatory child health care: opinions of practicing physicians about proposed criteria. *Med. Care* 14:22–31.

78. Torrance, G.W., Thomas, W.H., and Sackett, D.L. 1972. A utility maximization model for evaluation of health care programs. *Health Serv. Res.* 7:118.

79. Vail, D.J. 1961. Strategy in evaluating the effectiveness of community mental health programs. *Public Health Rep.* 76:975–978.

80. Vallbona, C., Quirch, J., Moffett, C.L., et al. 1973. The health illness profile: an essential component of the ambulatory medical record. *Med. Care* 11(suppl.): 117.

81. White, K. L. 1970. Evaluation of medical education and health care. In Lathem, W., Newberry, A., editors. *Community medicine: teaching, research, and health care.* New York: Appleton-Century-Crofts, pp. 241–270.

82. White, K.L. 1974. Caveats for PSRO's, *West. J. Med.* 120:338–343.

83. Williams, K.N., and Brook, R.H., Foreign med-

ical graduates and their effects on the quality of medical care in the United States. R-1698-HEW. Santa Monica, Calif.: Rand Corp.

84. Williamson, J.W. 1971. Evaluating quality of patient care: a strategy relating outcome and process assessment. *JAMA*. 218:564–569.

85. Williamson, J.W., Alexander, M., and Millder, G.E. 1967. Continuing education and patient care research. *JAMA*. 201:938–942.

86. Williamson, J.W., Aronovitch, S., Simonson, L., et al. 1975. Health accounting: an outcome-based system of quality assurance—illustrative application to hypertension. *Bull. N.Y. Acad. Med.* 51:727–738.

87. Wirtschafter, D.D., and Mesel, E. 1976. A strategy for redesigning the medical record for quality assurance. *Med. Care* 14:68–76.

88. Wylie, C.M., and White, B.K. 1961. A measure of disability, *Arch. Environ. Health* 8:834.

89. Zuckerman, A.E., Starfield, B., Hochreiter, C., et al. 1975. Validating the content of pediatric outpatient medical records by means of tape-recording doctor-patient encounters. *Pediatrics* 56:407–411.

14

Medical Care Evaluation Studies

Richard Chamberlin

A primary component of the PSRO program is the activity described in the *PSRO Program Manual* as medical care evaluation studies (MCEs). This chapter relates this component of the program to the PSRO legislation, guidelines, and regulations and places this activity into the context of the current state-of-the-art of quality assessment and quality assurance systems. In so doing, some comments are made about the current limitations of the medical care evaluation process; however, this chapter does not present a thorough analysis of these. Reference to some of the more extensive recent reviews of the subject is made where appropriate.

There are some who have criticized the evolution of the PSRO program on the grounds that the legislation was not followed promptly by the promulgation of specific regulations. In the instance of MCEs, this criticism is unfounded, because it is important to acknowledge from the outset that the fields of quality assessment and assurance are continually evolving. That the PSRO program has the potential to contribute to this science should not be overlooked—an output that could have been hampered by early regulation. The early history of the PSRO program as it applies to the approach taken toward MCEs does, in fact, reflect this evolution.

LEGISLATION

The term "medical care evaluation studies" does not appear in the legislation that created the PSRO program. It is, however, important to relate MCEs to the legislation as it was written to understand how this activity meets the intent of the law. This can perhaps best be done by recalling some direct quotations from the law, highlighting some of the key words and phrases.

Section 1151 of the Title XI of the Social Security Act declares the purpose of professional standards review to be " . . . to *assure,* through the application of *suitable procedures of professional standards review* that services for which payment may be made under the Social Security Act will conform to appropriate professional standards for the provision of *health care . . .*" This purpose is further qualified by adding the words ". . . [to assure] . . . that payment for such services will be made:

(1) Only when, and to the extent, *medically necessary,* as determined in the exercise of *reasonable limits of professional discretion,* and
(2) In the case of services provided by a hospital or other health care facility on an in-patient basis, only when and for such period as such services can not, consistent with *professionally recognized health care stan-*

dards, effectively be provided on an out patient basis or more economically in an in-patient health care facility of a different type, as determined in the exercise of *reasonable limits of professional discretion.*

These quotations from the law are not complete without adding that the legislative language includes a reason for declaring these to be the purpose of professional standards review. That reason is "... In order to promote the effective, efficient, and economical delivery of health care services of *proper quality* for which payment may be made . . . and in the recognition of the interests of patients, the public, practitioners, and providers in *improved* health care services . . ."

Section 1155 of the act further details the specific duties and review functions of each PSRO, and Section 1156 requires that each PSRO ". . . shall apply professionally developed norms of care, diagnosis and treatment based on typical patterns of practice in its regions . . ." while accomplishing the review.

GUIDELINES

The term "medical care evaluation studies" as it relates to the PSRO program first appears in Chapter 1, Section 106 of the *PSRO Program Manual* published in March, 1974—1½ years after the legislation was signed into law. This section says in part: "For review in short stay general hospitals, the PSRO will at a minimum perform (a) admission certification concurrent with the patient's admission, (b) continued stay review, and (c) medical care evaluation studies." The details of each of these component parts of the review system are then described in Chapter 7 of the *PSRO Program Manual.* Here the term "medical care evaluation studies" is first defined in Section 705.3 as follows: "MCES are a type of retrospective medical care review in which in-depth assessment of the quality and/or the nature of the utilization of health care services is made." The objectives of such studies were then stated as:

(a) To assure that health care services are appropriate to the needs of a patient and are of *acceptable quality.*

(b) To assure that health care organization and administration support the timely provision of quality care.

Using the mechanism of draft transmittals and comments thereto, the BQA attempted to further refine the requirement for MCEs in an effort to reflect even more closely the state-of-the-art and to make the PSRO program requirements as nearly compatible with those of other programs and agencies as possible.

On August 20, 1976, the first draft transmittal on the BQA policy for MCEs was circulated. Based on the responses from 60 organizations and individuals and of the NPSRC, the final transmittal on the subject was released on January 25, 1977, almost simultaneously with the publication of the regulations for procedures for review of hospital services in the *Federal Register* also dated January 25, 1977.

The medical care evaluation transmittal defined the term slightly differently than did the *PSRO Program Manual:* "Medical Care Evaluation Studies are a form of health care review in which an indepth assessment is made of the quality of the delivery and organization of health care services." The transmittal also made some slight changes in wording of the purposes of medical care evaluation activity: ". . . to assure that (1) health care services are appropriate to the patient's needs and are of *optimal quality* and (2) health care organization and administration support the timely provision of quality care."

REGULATION

The *Federal Register,* vol. 42, No. 16, Part 3, published on January 25, 1977, contains the notice of proposed rule making that would add a new subpart G of Part 101 of Title 42, Code of Federal Registration. The sections pertinent to MCEs are 101.702(p) (definitions) and 101.710 (describing the specific requirements). The definition of medical care evaluation study is given as ''. . . a process, usually performed retrospectively, in which an in depth assessment of the quality and/or the nature of the utilization of health care services is conducted, corrective action is taken, where indicated, and a subsequent analysis is made of the impact of the corrective action.'' The purposes of MCEs are listed as follows:

(1) Assuring that health care services are appropriate to the patient's needs and are of *appropriate quality*.

(2) Assuring that health care organization and administration of hospitals support the timely provision of quality care;

(3) Focusing on patterns of service which may require modification review efforts as described in . . . (concurrent review);

(4) Identifying changes necessary to improve the quality of care and the effectiveness and efficiency of the utilization of services.''

From 1972 to 1977, during the time that these policy statements were being developed, a number of reports and studies relevant to the general area of the review of medical care were published. Among these were reports of the evaluation of the Experimental Medical Care Review Organization (EMCRO) program,[1] a report by the Institute of Medicine titled *Assessing Quality in Health Care — An Evaluation,*[2] a book by R. Greene,[3] *Assuring Quality in Medical Care,* and a publication of the continued work by Robert Brook.[4,5] The variation in terminology contained in the various policy statements, such as ''acceptable quality'' in place of ''optimal quality'' and ''health care review'' in place of ''medical care review,'' is an example of the difficulty of directing the MCEs component of the PSRO program in such a way as to accommodate the intent of the law to the current developments in this general field of endeavor.

It is also important to understand and acknowledge that in spite of the problems of terminology, it was by the process just described that MCEs became one of the ''suitable procedures of professional standards review'' required by the legislation.

THEORETICAL AND CONCEPTUAL CONSIDERATIONS

Notwithstanding the generally negative reaction of the medical profession to the PSRO legislation as evidence of further intrusion of the federal government into the practice of medicine, a frequent debate stimulated by the legislation was that the intent of the law was focused more on the cost than on the quality of medical care. Although it is clear from the legislative language just reviewed that Congress expressed concerns for both the cost and the quality of medical care, this debate affected the degree to which the medical profession accepted and cooperated with the implementation of MCEs. However, even if it were not for this reaction, it is helpful, if not essential, to have a conceptual framework within which medical care evaluation activity may operate.

The key words and terms contained in the purpose of the PSRO legislation as they relate to MCEs are: improved, quality, and medical (health) care services.

The word ''improved'' implies a change — a change for the better. Thus, since one focus is on change, a method for measuring change is required. The word ''quality'' is difficult to define in any context but is particularly difficult to define in relation to medical or health care services. Nevertheless, a working definition of quality is helpful since these are the items being measured for change.

The Measure

The measuring tool that serves as the basis for MCEs is a process by which the care rendered to patients is compared with explicit criteria or standards. This process, usually conducted retrospectively, has traditionally utilized information contained in the medical records of the patients under review as documentation of the care that was given. A common model of this process is seen in Figure 14-1. This model, developed by Slee, utilized the term "medical audit," because the frame of reference was the medical care rendered by and under the primary control of physicians.[6]

The BQA and the NPSRC wrestled with the terminology to adopt for use in the PSRO program and considered such terms as "patient care evaluation" and "health care evaluation" to reflect a broader focus of review to be consistent with the legislation. The term "medical care evaluation" was adopted primarily because it had been in accepted use longer than other specific terms referring to medical audit type of activity in utilization

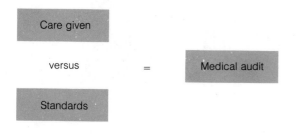

FIGURE 14-1. Measurement of medical care.

review under Medicare.[7] Regardless of the term, the concept represented in Figure 14-1 is the same—a measuring device used to determine whether the objective of improved quality has been attained.

Definition of Quality

Many authors have attempted to define quality as it is used to describe medical or health care. A complete discussion of the various attempts to reach such a definition is beyond the scope of this chapter. Two recent reviews by Decker and Bonner[8] and by Greene[9] are helpful references to study. The important point is that any student of the problem of medical care evaluation would benefit by the exercise of developing a working definition of quality. Without this, the efforts to measure it or changes in it will likely be discouraging in view of the many recognized imperfections in the accepted methodologies available today.

Because the primary initial emphasis of the PSRO review program has been on the short-stay acute general hospital inpatient population, one helpful and practical approach to the definition of quality of medical care has been that of Ralph Reinfrank of the American Society of Internal Medicine. This definition says that quality ". . . includes the correct diagnosis, medical, psychological and social, arrived at by a disciplined and logical process of clinical thinking and judgment, resulting in the application of any or all treatment maneuvers available at that point in time in an effort to restore the patient to an optimum degree of health."[10]

A strong point of this definition is that it speaks to issues with which practicing physicians are comfortable and relate to easily while also being reflective of some of the problems they encounter when they react to some aspects of federal health programs and when they conduct medical care evaluations. They recognize, for instance, that the diagnoses of their patients may involve more than medical factors and contain elements of a psychologic or social nature. They have no problem with the goal of restoring their patients to a maximum degree of health. On the other hand, they are aware of the fact that when they deal with the Medicare program, there are limitations to the reimbursement for services rendered by them when their patients' problems appear to be primarily of a "social" nature. This is discussed further under the concept of medical necessity. Physicians are also aware of the difficulty encountered in conducting medical audit if they attempt to measure that element of care referred to in the definition as ". . . disciplined and logical process of clinical thinking and judgement." Parenthetically, the approach to this aspect of the medical audit problem made by the problem-oriented medical information system developed by Lawrence Weed has been of assistance.[11]

The exercise of deriving a definition of quality, regardless of the specific definition itself, is helpful not only toward an understanding of the medical care evaluation process but also toward placing the cost versus quality equation in proper perspective. The fact that the quality of medical or health care is closely wedded to the cost of such care should become clear. Donabedian has stated this fact:[12]

It is a truism that quantity is a necessary precondition of quality . . . the absence of necessary or appropriate care connotes the absence of quality . . . excessive procedures [quantity] may be harmful, but even when not, they constitute a waste of resources and reduce the availability of services to others who might need them . . . for these reasons wasteful or inappropriate use is an element in the appraisal of quality.

It has been recommended by some authorities on medical care review that review activities focused on quality should be separate and distinct from those whose primary focus is cost. This may have been true when it was applied to the medical audit programs of the past. However, if one does struggle with a working definition of quality as it applies to medical and health care in the PSRO program, the appropriate balance of concerns for both quality and cost can be achieved.

Health Care vs. Medical Care Services

It is important to have a clear concept of health care and medical care services, because these are the services to be measured to determine if they have the attribute of improved quality. One model proposed to apply to medical care is seen in Figure 14-2.[13]

This model describes three conceptual levels of medical practice, one of which is medical care. It is possible to apply this same model to health practice and health care. The first level described represents the large body of fact that has been determined by research in the laboratory, in clinical experiments, and by epidemiologic studies. Medical or health students acquire some of these facts through the process of their education, creating the second conceptual level of practice—medical or

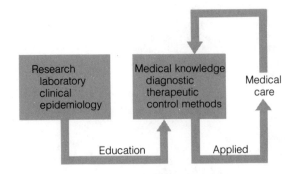

FIGURE 14-2.   Medical practice model.

health knowledge, including that which enables them to make diagnoses, treat disease, or control disease processes. It is through the application of this knowledge that the entities desired to be measured are created—medical or health care.

A critical part of this model is the feedback arrow, which could be labeled "observation," because it is by means of observing a change in a patient—a change hopefully for the better—that practitioners either reinforce or in some other way alter their knowledge base. The model as it was originally displayed was used to show that the focus of the medical audit process was on the second and third levels of this universe, a fact that is helpful to reinforce the thought that medical audit and MCEs are not meant to be research in any sense of the term. This model, particularly its feedback loop, is also helpful in defining the concept of medical necessity.

Medical Necessity

Medical necessity is worthy of consideration as background to MCEs, not so much because of how it relates to measuring and improving quality as because of how it can help one understand the relationship between physicians and the Medicare and Medicaid programs. In its simplest form, the Medicare section of the Social Security Act established as a basis for reimbursement for medical services the principle that those services medically necessary could be reimbursed and those not medically necessary could not. The definition of the term "medically necessary" was not explicitly stated, but the original mechanisms used to determine it were. One mechanism took the form of a statement signed by the practicing physician stating that the services rendered were medically necessary. This statement of physician certification was initially required for all services rendered to a patient as an outpatient, upon admission to a hospital, and

periodically thereafter in cases of continued stay in the hospital. The background of this method is contained in a report of the Senate Finance Committee dated June 30, 1965. "The committee's bill provides that the physician is the key figure in determining utilization of health services and provides that it is a physician who is to decide upon admission to a hospital, order tests, drugs and treatments, and to determine length of stay. For this reason the bill would require that payment could be made only if a physician certifies to the medical necessity of the services furnished."[14] In 1967, the Medicare law was amended to eliminate the requirement for such certification for outpatient services and upon admission. The Senate Finance Committee determined at that time that "Outpatient hospital services and admissions to general hospitals are almost always medically necessary and the requirement for a physician's certification of this fact results in largely unnecessary paperwork."[15]

A second mechanism used to decide medical necessity was contained in the claims review process used by the fiscal intermediaries. Claims were subjected to a screening process involving several levels of complexity and screening parameters. The final level of review required a decision to be made by a physician consultant employed by the intermediary. This physician's decisions were made using a combination of criteria and guidelines developed by the Bureau of Health Insurance and the physician's implicit judgment. All too frequently this decision was contrary to the attending physician's statement of medical necessity, and a constant adversary relationship developed between practicing physicians and the Medicare program.

This background is important, because a careful examination of the definitions and concepts detailed in this section shows a potentially positive relationship between the concept of medical necessity and quality assurance systems such as MCEs. This relationship has been jeopardized by the adversary situation that has evolved as described.

The practicing physician's concept of medical necessity may be approached by examining the definitions of the words. "Medically" is the adverb of medical, which means ". . . of or pertaining to, dealing with the healing art or science of medicine." "Art" is ". . . the skill in performance acquired by experience, study, or observation." "Science" is ". . . knowledge" or "any department of systematized knowledge" or "art or skill." "Necessary" has at least two meanings: (1) ". . . essential to an end or condition," and (2) a legal definition, ". . . requisite for support of an incompetent or dependent in his station in life."[16]

Using these definitions, one is able to construct the following concept. A patient with a problem presenting himself to a physician becomes dependent at that station in life on the knowledge, (science) art, and skill of that particular physician. That physician's knowledge has been acquired by an educational process, and that physician's skill has been acquired by experience, study, and observation. Thus, that physician's services are "of or pertaining to his particular knowledge of and skill and art in applying medicine" and are therefore by definition medically necessary at the time the physician rendered them.

In an attempt to unify these concepts, one might consider Greene's schema describing the complexities involved in assessing and assuring the quality of medical and health care services. This schema is shown in Figure 14-3.[17]

In the diagram the circle A represents what Greene terms conventional medical wisdom, only a small portion of which (represented by the shaded area) is based on empiric evidence. This collection of conventional medical wisdom can be likened to the first two conceptual levels of medi-

cal practice shown in Figure 14-1. As such, the smaller shaded area in Figure 14-3 would be that portion of a practitioner's wisdom affected by his or her observations of patients' responses to the physician's services, which are rendered in various locales represented by the dotted-line box (B) in the diagram. A patient brings to this setting a variety of problems, comprising his status A, and his journey to the physician may be affected by factors such as finances and geography, all of which might well relate to the definition of quality as it applies to the correct diagnosis presented earlier. Also related to the definition of quality in respect to outcome, depicted as Patient status B in Figure 14-3, is the factor of patient compliance. Coloring all of this may be the physician's own belief that his or her services were medically necessary for reasons just described.

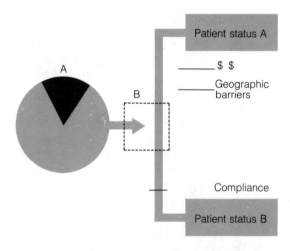

FIGURE 14-3. Complexities of assessing and assuring quality of medical and health care services. (From Green, R. 1976. *Assuring quality in medical care: The state of the art.* Cambridge, Mass.: Ballington Publishing Co., p. 5.)

Summary

The medical care evaluation study portion of the PSRO program presents a number of challenges to its successful implementation, challenges that are based on some complex and as yet unanswered problems in the delivery and evaluation of health care services. That these challenges may be viewed as opportunities for the program to contribute to the fields of quality assessment and assurance is an aspect of PSRO that deserves continual emphasis.

BASIC STEPS OF MCES

The BQA acknowledged from the outset that many different procedures are available for the conduct of MCEs. It was the bureau's position that it should not endorse any specific methodology for the purpose of the PSRO program but rather should identify certain generic characteristics that any medical care evaluation must have to be acceptable as a medical care evaluation for purposes of meeting the PSRO requirements. These generic characteristics are listed, and then certain points are made about each of them. These characteristics are of critical importance, because as is shown, it has been the failure to adhere to these characteristics that has led to many of the criticisms of the medical care evaluation process and to charges of its ineffectiveness.

Generic Characteristics of Medical Care Evaluation[18]

1. To focus on a known or suspected problem area impacting on the quality of health care.
2. To focus on a well-defined topic and to be carried out in accord with objectives explicitly stated in, and specifically developed for, the study.
3. To utilize written criteria against which actual patterns of health care practice are compared.
4. To provide for the collection of data on a sample of patients, the size and composition of which is appropriate to the study topic and objectives.
5. To provide for thorough peer analysis of the reasons for any discrepancies between the written criteria that reflect optimal achievable health care practices and the data collected on actual health care practices to determine whether variations are objectively justifiable or represent problems that require corrective action.
6. To result in specific written recommendations where indicated to improve the quality of care and promote more effective and efficient utilization of facilities and services.
7. To include documentation regarding when, where, and by whom the recommended actions were, in fact, implemented.
8. To include a plan for follow-up evaluation where indicated to determine what changes have occurred as a result of actions recommended in No. 6 to correct specific deficiencies identified by the study.
9. To provide for such a follow-up evaluation where indicated to be completed in a reasonable period of time.
10. To provide for at least periodic reporting of a summary of the quality assurance activity to the governing board of the hospital.

Focus on a Known or Suspected Problem

The famous bank robber Willy Sutton, when asked why he robbed banks, replied, "Because that is where the money is." A frequent criticism of the medical care evaluation process is that a medical staff has done a number of audits and has failed to find any problems. There may be several explanations for this occurrence, but a common one is that the selection of a topic for the study was poorly done. It is important to choose as a topic for any medical care evaluation one in which the professional staff involved in the study suspects a problem might exist in the first place. In addition, it should be a problem area that would be logically expected to have an impact on the quality of care. So often a topic is chosen in the haste to do the required number of MCEs that little thought is given to the possible problem areas to study. Regarding the conceptual working definition of quality, for instance, an element of quality is making the correct diagnosis. One might then ask the question, "Are the diagnoses being made in the hospital validated by the information in the medical record?" A quick survey of some of the commonly made diagnoses in the hospital might show a possible problem area that would warrant a medical care evaluation. Another approach to topic selection would be to identify those areas in which medical intervention is particularly and specifically critical to patient outcome. Still another approach is to focus on areas in which outcomes of care are less than acceptable and choose medical care evaluation topics from these patient populations. An additional important point is that even if a medical care evaluation fails to reveal a problem and documents perfectly acceptable care, that medical care evaluation should not be considered a failure. Topic selection may have been in error in terms of possible problems, but the medical staff should report the MCEs documenting good care just as proudly as it endeavors to correct problems when they are found.

Objectives

Another common area of weakness in the medical care evaluation process as it has been in medical audit is the failure to establish written objectives

for each specific study. This point has not been stressed strongly enough in most of the common audit methods in use, and like the first characteristic, failure to establish objectives often results in what appears to be a failure of the study. The objective should be more specific than the global objective of any medical care evaluation—improving the quality of medical care. The objective should be stated in terms that are as measurable as possible. Examples of such objectives as taken from some specific MCEs are as follows:

Study Topic	Objective
Carcinoma of breast	To determine if pathologically proved cases of breast carcinoma are managed appropriately.
Therapeutic diet orders on discharge	To determine if the physician's order for therapeutic diet orders upon discharge is followed by appropriate dietary instruction to the patient.
Myocardial infarction	To determine if patients with clinically proved myocardial infarction are managed by using the accepted coronary care protocol.

The writing of objectives specific to the particular study enables the staff to truly focus in on the suspected problem area and avoid the collection of data that are not appropriate to the study (see the following section).

Utilization of Written Criteria

A critical point in the medical care evaluation process is the development and adoption of the criteria to be used in the study. The criteria should be as specific as possible and related to the focus and objectives of the study. Decker and Bonner have published an analysis of criteria used in peer review based on the experience of the EMCRO program. This review is particularly helpful, because it studies the problems with criteria in a recent program that was similar to the PSRO program.[19]

The criteria may be arrived at either by the use of normative expressions of accepted practice (empiric criteria) or may be developed by a consensus of the professional staff involved in the study. Here again is an area that has been the cause of alleged failure of the study. Because of the complexities of the care of patients' problems, it is often difficult to arrive at a consensus on a given criterion. The discussion that such a process stimulates is often an educational experience for the group of professionals involved, a fact that should be viewed as a positive spinoff of the medical care evaluation process. In the event that a consensus cannot be accomplished and there is no normative experience available, the particular criterion under consideration should probably not be used in the study. On the other hand, if this is the case and in the judgment of the medical staff the study is still considered important, the focus and objective of the particular study might be changed to a fact-finding study to determine what the practice norm in that particular instance is in the institution. The important points are that the medical care evaluation process should use explicit criteria that are widely discussed by the professional group involved so that the care that was rendered can then be compared with these criteria.

Collection of Data
on Appropriate Sample of Patients

To collect data on an appropriate sample of patients would seem to speak for itself. Experience to date with medical audits has demonstrated techniques of data collection utilizing nonphysician personnel effectively, providing they are given appropriate

instructions. Techniques and formats for the display of the data collected are readily available. Nevertheless, the step of data collection also has some inherent weaknesses that are discussed here and under the next characteristic of peer analysis.

What is the appropriate sample size? An important approach to the answer to this question is to reiterate that MCEs are not research studies and are therefore not bound by the usual constraints of statistical significance. The key is clinical significance, and the sample size then is related to the degree of clinical significance of the particular study. A reasonable but arbitrary rule of thumb might be to attempt to include a minimum of 20 to 30 cases in any medical care evaluation. If this continues to be a problem, as it well might be for small hospitals or in study problems that occur infrequently, the mechanism of an areawide medical care evaluation offers a solution.

Nonavailability of Data

Occasionally a topic is well chosen, and objectives and criteria are well stated, only to find that in retrospective collection attempts some items of data needed are not recorded in the patient records. This may be due to the common problem of lack of documentation of items of medical care on the part of the professional involved in the care of the patient, or it may be due to the fact that perfectly acceptable practice has not required certain elements of care to be recorded. William Jesse has proposed the model in Figure 14-4, which is of help in this instance as well as assisting in approaches to peer analysis.[20]

In this model the critical data elements are collected concurrently, usually by the patient care coordinator while he or she is conducting concurrent admission certification and continued stay review. The data are then analyzed retrospectively in the traditional medical audit fashion.

Concurrent	Concurrent PIPSRO type	Retrospective
Peer analysis		
Retrospective	Collection concurrent analysis retrospective	Traditional medical care evaluation

FIGURE 14-4.   Data collection. PIPSRO stands for Private Initiative in PSRO.[24]

Other limitations of the medical record as a data source are recognized. If the source of data for a particular medical care evaluation is contained in an abstract of the medical record, studies of the reliability of such data have shown significant problem areas of variation from the original record, depending on the type of data element involved.[21] Those conducting MCEs should be aware of these variations and take them into consideration according to the nature of the specific study and the specific data elements required. Also, the medical record frequently does not document the reasoning, or logic, that was involved in making certain clinical decisions. The fully implemented problem-oriented medical information system designed by Weed is an exception to this.[22]

Peer Analysis of Variation

It is perhaps misleading to designate one of these ten essential characteristics of the medical care evaluation process as more important than another, because all of them are felt to have implications for the success or failure of any given study. However, certainly this characteristic is of primary importance with regard to the principles of peer review.

Among the several aspects of this characteristic are consideration of the members of the peer group, the opportunities available in the analysis itself, the interpretation of a variation from a criterion as displayed by the data, including the problem of lack of documentation, and attention to the relationship of this characteristic to the next characteristic of written recommendations.

Although the appropriate peer group obviously should be involved in choosing the topic and establishing the objectives and criteria for any given study, it is at the point of peer analysis of the data that peer review in the true sense of the term is brought to bear in the conduct of MCEs. The many ramifications of the definition of the word "peer" is beyond the scope of this chapter; however, it is important to emphasize that the success of any MCEs may depend on the degree to which a professional staff organizes the team to analyze the data from any given study. This is complicated by a number of factors, including the complexities of subspecialization and the involvement of non-physicians in the delivery of direct services to the patient. An approach to the solution of this problem is to consider carefully the nature of the particular study and the locale in which the study is being conducted. A study that focuses very clearly on care that is primarily medical should be analyzed by physicians having qualifications as close as possible to the type of training and experience considered appropriate for the study population. That this still presents problems in some locales with few physicians and few specialists is further complicated by the recent modification of the "locality rule" defined in the courts during litigation of malpractice cases. In such decisions, the courts have determined that the community standard previously established is now broadened. A PSRO should stand ready to offer technical assistance in the form of appropriate consultants when needed. A discussion of the health care professionals other than physicians follows in a section on multidisciplinary MCEs. The important practical point relating to the effectiveness and credibility of any given study is how the entire professional staff involved views the expertise of the peer group doing the analysis.

The analysis of the data presents one of the opportunities to counteract the potential rigidity of the explicit criteria. This alleged rigidity stems from the limitations of criteria to describe the reality of the variables encountered by physicians in the care of patients. Since the use of criteria in the medical care evaluation process amounts only to a screening mechanism to identify possible problem areas or cases, the members of the peer analysis group have an opportunity to evaluate all of the information in the medical records involved and apply a more flexible decision-making process to arrive at a conclusion that the variation from criteria is or is not medically or clinically justified.

Most existing data display methodologies are helpful in that they lead the reviewers toward making one of two decisions in relation to a variation that does not seem to be otherwise clinically justified. Those decisions are that the variation is due to a problem in knowledge or that it is due to a problem of performance. This is obviously vital in terms of making specific recommendations for appropriate corrective actions. A frequent criticism made by physicians of the medical audit programs has been that they do not have the link to continuing medical education that they were claimed to have. Experience from many audit programs has shown that of the deficiencies in care identified, only about 15% of these were felt to be deficiencies of knowledge, whereas 85% were due to deficiencies of performance. Of the latter only a small percentage involved the performance of the physician.[23] Thus, this step in the analysis is critical, because a continuing education approach to the improvement of deficiencies can be effective only

if it is targeted to the appropriate subject matter and the appropriate professional group.

Documentation in the medical record as it relates to a variation from a criterion is important to mention. When confronted with the problem of documentation, physicians frequently respond, "I take care of patients, not records." There have been studies that do show a correlation between good records and the delivery of good care. Decker and Bonner commented on the medical record in their concept of good quality medical care. "Quality medicine restores health, prevents disability and/or death, improves function and relieves suffering. Such quality outcomes are anticipated from the application of appropriate medical processes since knowledge of the later is ultimately based on controlled clinical experiments. The medical record documents the processes applied and can therefore serve as a source of data for quality audit."[24] As Decker and Bonner point out, however, the logic of the statement may be clear, but the correlation of one part of the statement with the next is less than perfect, particularly when it comes to the medical record.

The answer to the problem of documentation at present must lie with the nature of the specific study under consideration and the relative degree of importance that the particular variation based on lack of documentation has to the overall evaluation of the data from the study. This would seem to be justified by the experience of the Private Initiative in PSRO study. The critical criteria adopted for the seven diagnoses included in the study were divided into several categories, the first two of which were criteria elements particularly prone to the documentation problem. These criteria, which described elements in the present illness and past history of the patient, were found to be subject to poor documentation, and yet in the final analysis of the data this lack of documentation was not correlated with poor outcomes in any significant way.[25]

Specific Written Recommendations

The characteristic of specific written recommendations is the most self-explanatory. A key point is the emphasis that the written recommendations should be specific as to their relationship to improved quality or to their attention toward more effective and efficient utilization of facilities and services. These should be self-evident by the focus of the study and its objectives. In the event that a study revealed care of acceptable quality or utilization, the recommendations still should reflect this fact by recommending continuation of the practice patterns so identified.

Documentation of Implementation of Corrective Action Steps

Medical audits have in the past been weak in the documentation of the implementation of corrective action steps. Problems that have been identified and corrective action steps that have been recommended have not as a rule been followed by a clear statement of the specific accountability of the person or persons who are responsible for the corrective action steps. An example is the case in which the written recommendations indicate the need for a continuing education program designed to correct an identified knowledge deficiency. Who is responsible for the design of such a program to assure that it is appropriate to the specific deficiency? Even in the event that the task will be assigned to a committee, the study report should designate the person responsible for the committee accomplishing its assignment and the time table for its work.

Plan for Follow-up Evaluation

Medical evaluation study is not complete until a follow-up has been accomplished when indicated. This has caused confusion, because the follow-up evaluation is usually and logically at some time in the future—up to 1 year. Does that mean that the medical care evaluation is not considered complete until the follow-up is accomplished? The present policy states that medical care evaluation is considered complete in its first phase at the point when a specific follow-up plan is decided on and documented. The medical care evaluation may then be reported by the hospital, the PSRO, or both. The plan should specify, as in the previous characteristic, who or what group is to be accountable for accomplishing the follow-up, at what time, and in what manner.

Follow-up Evaluation

As previously stated, follow-up evaluation is actual implementation of the follow-up plan as detailed. This may vary in its character from the relatively simple collection of some key data elements related to the deficiency identified to an extensive revision of the criteria requiring in a sense a fairly complete repeat of the entire previous study.

Periodic Reporting of a Summary of Quality Assurance Activities to Governing Board of Hospital

Periodic reporting of a summary of the quality assurance activities to the governing board of the hospital has caused some concern among physicians, even allowing for the recognized and accepted legal doctrine of the ultimate accountability of the governing body for the quality of care in the hospital. The key words here are periodic and summary. The decision as to the timing of the periodic reports and the extensiveness of the summary has been left for the individual hospital professional staffs and boards or the individual PSROs to make.

The ten generic characteristics of an acceptable medical care evaluation are considered to be applicable whether the medical care evaluation is designed and conducted within a hospital to which the medical care evaluation component has been delegated by the local PSRO or whether the activity is conducted by the PSRO in the nondelegated hospitals, even though the corrective action steps may be more difficult to achieve in the latter instance.

In summary, by defining these basic characteristics of MCEs, the Health Standards and Quality Bureau has built on the basic components of the processes of quality assessment and quality assurance as they are understood and have been experienced by those who have attempted to implement such procedures up to and including the early days of the PSRO program. They are intended to incorporate all of the elements required by other agencies, such as those responsible for other government programs, including the most recent utilization review regulations, and such voluntary programs as that of the JCAH, while at the same time not recommending any specific program by name or methodology.

A discussion of the medical care evaluation portion of the PSRO program is not complete without detailing other program elements relating to MCEs, including the number of MCEs required, multidisciplinary MCEs, areawide MCEs, the relationship of MCEs to other PSRO program components, and the evaluation of MCEs.

NUMBER OF MCES REQUIRED

There was confusion in the first years of PSRO implementation in that there seemed to be a conflict between the number of MCEs (audits) required by the program compared with requirements of other agencies, particularly the JCAH. The specific requirement published in the 1974 edition of the *PSRO Program Manual* was that each hospital must complete four studies each year. Following discussions with the JCAH, the PSRO program requirements were made consistent with those of the JCAH and are based on the size of the patient population being treated in the hospitals as follows:

Number of Admissions Per Year	Number of MCEs Required
0–2499	4
2500–4999	6
5000–9999	8
10000–19999	10
More than 20000	12

One must be cautious, however. Experience has shown that the requirements of a certain number of MCEs has often been the only motivation for doing the studies. When this has been the case, one has found not only that the process has been delegated to a single medical staff committee—often to a single individual—but also that the studies are done in batches usually just before a hospital survey. This is contrary to the goal of any quality assessment/assurance system. The intent of these programs is to monitor continuously all care being rendered to all patients all of the time, with the in-depth assessment represented by MCEs to be an ongoing process. This should mean that at any given time any number of studies are in some stage of implementation. The Commission on Hospital and Professional Activities has devised a simple but effective schedule that can be of help. With the use of this schedule, a number of study topics are chosen, and assignment of specific time frames for each of the steps of the medical care evaluation (audit) process for each study is set forth.[26] By this method a delegated hospital or a PSRO in the non-delegated hospitals, knowing the number of studies required, can more efficiently meet the number requirements while distributing the actual work throughout the year.

MULTIDISCIPLINARY MCES

As discussed previously, one reason for choosing the term "medical care evaluation studies" instead of "medical audit" to describe this component of the PSRO program has been to guide the program toward the intent of the law—to promote the effective, efficient, and economical delivery of health care services of proper quality, recognizing the interests of patients, the public, practitioners, and providers in improved health care services. Medical audit alone in the sense that it has usually focused primarily on the care rendered by physicians can clearly be only one approach to meeting this intent. With the recognition that involvement of health professionals other than physicians has been sporadic before implementation of the PSRO program and that the outcome of hospitalization is generally dependent on care rendered by more than one health care discipline, the policy of the PSRO program has been strongly to encourage more participation of members of all health care professions in the medical care evaluation process.

The most logical guide to this involvement is the nature of the particular medical care evaluation being planned. An analysis of the suspected problem area under study should indicate which disciplines are active in patient care involved in the problem area. The appropriate individual professionals from each such discipline should then be assembled to participate in each step of the medical care evaluation design, including writing of objectives, formulation of criteria, analysis of data, writing of recommendations for corrective action, and follow-up.

This involvement may well identify a specific problem in the delivery of a service that is under the direct control of a professional group other than physicians and could then lead to an in-depth assessment of that problem area by that discipline alone, such as a physical therapy audit by physical therapists or a nursing audit by nurses. A unified concept of patient care by a variety of health professionals working as colleagues would suggest that the multidisciplinary approach to MCEs is likely to have more impact on patient care, however.

AREAWIDE MCES

Areawide MCEs have been mentioned thus far only as a mechanism by which smaller hospitals might participate in the medical care evaluation process by combining the data on their patients with those of other small institutions to have a patient population in some disease categories large enough to conduct a meaningful medical care evaluation. This is an important potential benefit of an areawide medical care evaluation, but it is not the most significant one. In comments based on the experience of the Private Initiative in PSRO, Paul Sanazaro has noted that the PSROs are the only organizational structures that can conduct such areawide studies of health care services and be entrusted with the confidentiality of the data involved. Because a PSRO is also required to conduct profile analysis (such profiles being constructed from data relating to the entire spectrum of health care services in its area, including patients, practitioners, and institutions [ambulatory, hospital, and long-term care facilities]), it is in a position to identify problems in the health care delivery system that are generic to any or all groups or institutions. Using these data, areawide MCEs having the same basic characteristics of any MCE described earlier may be designed, the focus of which transcends any single group or institution. By this mechanism, a major role of the PSRO in quality assurance is to raise the results of care in all settings to acceptable levels.

The effectiveness of the areawide medical care evaluation approach is dependent on the same basic principle that would determine the effectiveness of any medical care evaluation. That principle is the need for involvement of all appropriate individuals in the conduct of the medical care evaluation. In the case of areawide MCEs, this requires participation of representatives of all hospitals involved in the study at all stages of implementation. In addition, it may be of some importance to recognize that participation in an areawide study on the part of an institution qualifies that institution for meeting the number requirement of that particular institution, just as if the institution had conducted a study of its own.

Relationship of MCEs to Other PSRO Program Elements

Although the PSRO program has been presented as consisting of three main components, concurrent review, MCEs, and profile analysis, it should be considered an integrated review system in which each component part is interdependent. This is best seen in the medical care evaluation component, a fact that argues strongly for the quality orientation of the entire program. Several areas of interdependence and integration are discussed using the generic characteristic of MCEs as a guide.

Topic selection and objectives for MCEs are clearly related to concurrent review and profile analysis. If a hospital PSRO team is working smoothly, whether in a delegated or nondelegated hospital setting, the patient care coordinator and physician advisor frequently may identify problem areas that require further study, as with a medical care evaluation. If communication between members of the concurrent review team breaks down, the analysis of profiles constructed from data gathered from the concurrent review process may allow the PSRO itself to identify the same problem areas leading to a medical care evaluation.

Selection of criteria may also relate to the concurrent review process. In some instances this relationship may be in both directions. Depending on the nature of a specific medical care evaluation, some of the criteria used in concurrent review in that subject area may be used as such or modified for use in the medical care evaluation. A result of a medical care evaluation might be a recommendation to change the criteria used in subsequent concurrent review. In other words, both concurrent review and the medical care evaluation process may be used as a method of validating criteria.

A previous section has already described how concurrent review may be used as a mechanism for gathering data for a planned retrospective medical care evaluation. The data base already incorporated in the profile construction may well contain some data that would be useful in some MCEs.

Because a medical care evaluation process results in written recommendations, every segment of the PSRO program may be affected by these. There may be a recommendation to change a criterion in use for concurrent review, or it is possible to use the medical care evaluation process in the decision to drop a given diagnostic category from concurrent review entirely, as in focused (waived) review. There may be a recommendation affecting the data base used to build profiles, and there may even be a recommendation in respect to a topic area for a subsequent new medical care evaluation.

The follow-up plan and follow-up itself may be related to profile analysis in that the data needed for a follow-up may already be contained in the profile data base, and follow-up could then consist of simply monitoring changes in the profile over time. Concurrent review may be the method of follow-up, particularly of short-term problems where the PSRO is interested in fairly immediate feedback on the results of corrective action steps taken.

Thus, the interrelationships that exist among the component parts of the PSRO program are easily emphasized using the medical care evaluation component as a hub.

EVALUATION OF MCES

The medical care evaluation component of the PSRO program is subject to evaluation of its effectiveness at several different levels and in several different ways. There is evaluation of the individual MCEs at the hospital level, PSRO level, or both. An evaluation is conducted of the individual studies as well as the aggregate of all studies at the national level. Finally, the entire PSRO program is being evaluated. The individual MCEs may be evaluated by reviewing the process of doing the study, that is, were all ten characteristics present and satisfactorily performed, and may be evaluated by the impact the medical care evaluation had on the quality of care or the utilization of health care services.

Evaluation of the MCEs at the hospital or PSRO level occurs at several different times, the first of which is at the time a hospital is being considered for delegation status. Early experience would indicate that the importance of this level of evaluation should not be overlooked. It should include a review of the evidence available in the hospital that there is sufficient experience and commitment to the audit process on the part of the professional staff to conduct a meaningful program. This should include evidence that the hospital will provide the staff with the necessary support resources.

The next time frame for evaluation is at the time a study is complete for the purposes of initial reporting, that is, up to and including a documented plan for follow-up. At this stage, the PSRO Program Management Information System has required that a medical care evaluation be rated on a 3-point scale of poor, good, and excellent for reporting purposes. There have been no criteria or guidelines provided to allow for a uniform approach to these ratings. PSROs have developed a variety of evaluation approaches toward their own MCEs, most of which have been essentially an evaluation of the process.

A third time frame for evaluation of MCEs at the local level is at the time of PSRO monitoring of delegated hospitals or at the time of site assessment visits to the PSRO from the Health Standards and Quality Bureau. Techniques for the local monitoring efforts are continually being refined, but again, the monitoring devoted to the MCEs has generally been attentive only to the numbers required and to process evaluation.

Because there is a lack of published reports detailing the specific approaches taken toward MCEs evaluation by the individual PSROs, the remainder of this section describes the approach being developed to evaluate the studies as they are submitted to the Health Standards and Quality Bureau. The initial reports of this work were released in September of 1977 and were based on almost 3000 MCEs submitted between 1975 and June 1, 1977.[28] It should be emphasized that these approaches are continually evolving, yet the information contained in the report is helpful to an understanding of the problem of evaluation.

The evaluation report recalls the goals of the medical care evaluation component of the review program as stated earlier in this chapter and, with these in mind, defined the goals of medical care evaluation as: to demonstrate the efficiency of the MCEs program in (a) the mechanics (process) of conducting MCEs, (b) the effect of the MCEs on the behavior of the health system, and (c) the effect of the MCEs on patient health status.

The report first displays the studies submitted in such a way as to establish some early normative data that allowed an assessment of the compliance with the MCEs, numerical requirement. Additional interesting findings included:

1. Of the 305 topic areas included in the universe of medical care evaluations studied, those in the medical and surgical areas were about equal at 45% of the total, with the remaining 9% being topics of an administrative or miscellaneous nature.

2. The 20 most commonly audited topics comprised about 46% of the total number of audits, but data from the most recent reporting quarter indicated that this distribution was changing toward a wider diversification of topics being studied.

Following the development of a system that rated the medical care evaluation topic categories according to their relative likelihood of containing MCEs having a high impact, a sample of specific studies was chosen for an in-depth analysis. Each of these studies had been completed through the reaudit stage, and all pertinent material, including criteria used, action steps taken to correct deficiencies, and follow-up specifics, were studied. Each medical care evaluation was evaluated by a five-member team using a weighted scoring system that was applied to both process and outcome elements. Process was studied by looking at two of the ten medical care evaluation characteristics considered most essential, namely, topic selection and action steps planned. Outcome was studied by looking at implementation of recommended actions and corrections of types of deficiencies.

An outline of the approach taken to the evaluation is as follows:

I. Process evaluation
  A. Topic selection; factors considered in rating
    1. Topic-specific factors
      a. Prevalence of disease/problem/ procedure
        (1) Size of patient population directly or potentially affected
        (2) Size of provider population affected
      b. Potential benefits achievable by optimal or by reasonable care
        (1) Degree of agreement by physicians on therapeutic approach
          (a) Indications for treatment
          (b) Modes of therapy
          (c) Likelihood treatment will reduce morbidity and mortality
      c. Direct economic impact of the disease or problem
    2. Situation-specific factors
      a. Importance of results or experience with concurrent review or profile analysis
      b. Patient-generated complaints, litigation, or both
      c. Other (including locally perceived problem)
  B. The degree to which follow-up of action steps accomplished
    1. Action required, action carried out, follow-up done
    2. Action required, action carried out, no follow-up audit done
    3. Action required, no action carried out
    4. No action required
II. Outcome: health system performance
  A. Elements considered in scoring for the sample of studies chosen for evaluation
    1. Whether deficiencies were found

2. Percentage and types of deficiencies removed on reaudit
3. Percentage of recommended actions implemented
4. Other
   a. Further problem areas identified
   b. Educational programs developed
   c. System changes suggested
III. Outcome: intermediate patient outcomes
   A. Studies with high-impact scores in respect to systems performance then evaluated
      1. Outcome specific criteria
         a. If present, what effect on intermediate patient outcome
         b. If absent, extrapolation made from nature and number of deficiencies removed to determine effect on intermediate patient outcome

Although a relatively small number of MCEs were eligible for the entire evaluation process, because many PSROs had not completed an entire cycle of the medical care evaluation (that is, through restudy), a number of important preliminary findings resulted from the evaluation effort. First, MCEs can be effective both in elucidating problem areas relating to the medical care process and to intermediate patient outcome and in eliminating these problem areas. Second, in terms of eliminating these problem areas (specifically in those studies in which the process was considered well done), more than half of all deficiencies identified were, in fact, eliminated on follow-up study.

It cannot be emphasized too strongly that the evaluation methodology described has studied proximate patient outcomes only. The evaluation methodology is expected to undergo revision, and the efforts at design of long-term evaluation are continuing.

SUMMARY

This chapter has described the component of the PSRO program known as medical care evaluation studies. It has attempted to relate this component to the legislation and regulations as well as to the current state-of-the-art of quality assessment and quality assurance both in conceptual and pragmatic frameworks.

Three conclusions cannot be overemphasized. The first and most important of these is that many critical hypotheses on which all quality assurance systems, including MCEs, are based remain to be tested with the degree of exactness and objectivity that the application of the scientific method requires. The health care professional community must place a high priority on efforts to solve these problems as an integral part of improved health care.

The second conclusion is that by the inclusion of MCEs as an integral part of the PSRO review system, the federal government is now in a position to have an influence on the further development of quality assurance mechanisms, certainly as they will be applied in programs designed to finance health care in all federal programs.

Thus, the third conclusion, one that was reached by the Management Committee of Private Initiate in PSRO, must be supported, that is, "PSROs are necessary as a professionally controlled mechanism of quality assurance interposed between third party purchasers of services and providers (physicians and hospitals) on the one side and patients on the other . . . PSROs are potentially the best mechanisms so far devised to protect the medical interests of all patients."[29]

REFERENCES

1. Decker, B., and Bonner, P. 1974. *Criteria in peer review.* Cambridge, Mass.: Arthur D. Little, Inc.

2. Institute of Medicine. 1976. *Assessing quality in health care: an evaluation*. Washington, D.C.: National Academy of Sciences.

3. Greene, R. 1976. *Assuring quality in medical care: the state of the art*. Cambridge, Mass.: Ballington Publishing Co.

4. Brook, R.H. 1973. *Quality of care assessment: a comparison of five methods of peer review*. DHEW publication No. HRA 74-3100. Washington, D.C.: U.S. Department of Health, Education, and Welfare.

5. Brook, R.H., Williams, K.N., and Avery, A.D. 1976. Quality assurance today and tomorrow: forecast for the future. *Ann. Intern. Med.* 85:809–817.

6. Slee, V.N. 1966. *The medical audit*. Ann Arbor, Mich.: Commission on Professional and Hospital Activities.

7. Goldberg, G.A., Needleman, J., and Weinstein, S.L. 1972. Medical care evaluation studies, a utilization review requirement. *J.A.M.A.* 220:383–387.

8. Decker, B., Bonner, P., 1974. *Criteria in peer review*. Cambridge, Mass.: Arthur D. Little, Inc. pp. 11–15.

9. Greene, R. 1976. *Assuring quality in medical care*. Cambridge, Mass.: Ballington Publishing Co., pp. 13–14.

10. American Society of Internal Medicine. 1972. *Task force on assessment by performance*. Preliminary report to the Board of Trustees. San Francisco: The Society.

11. Weed, L.L. 1969. *Medical records, medical education, and patient care: the problem-oriented record as a basic tool*. Cleveland: Case Western Reserve University Press.

12. Donabedian, A. 1969. *A guide to medical care administration, vol. 2, Medical care appraisal: quality and utilization*. American Public Health Association.

13. Slee, V.N. 1966. *The medical audit*. Ann Arbor, Mich.: Commission on Professional and Hospital Activities.

14. *Congressional record*. June 30, 1965. Eighty-ninth Congress. First Session. Senate Finance Committee Report No. 404, part 1, vol. 2, p. 46.

15. *Congressional record*. Nov. 14, 1967. Eighty-ninth Congress. First Session. Senate Finance Committee Report No. 744, vol. 2, p. 64.

16. *Webster's collegiate dictionary*. 6th ed. 1979. Springfield, Mass.: G & C Merriam Co.

17. Greene, R. 1976. *Assuring quality in medical care: the state of the art*. Cambridge, Mass.: Ballington Publishing Co., p. 5.

18. U.S. Department of Health, Education, and Welfare. Jan. 25, 1977. *Policy on medical care evaluation (MCE) studies*. PSRO Transmittal No. 43. Washington, D.C.: Bureau of Quality Assurance, Health Services Administration.

19. Decker, B., and Bonner, P. 1974. *Criteria in peer review*. Cambridge, Mass.: Arthur D. Little, Inc., pp. 31–101.

20. Jessee, W.F. 1977. Personal communication.

21. Institute of Medicine. Feb. 1977. *Reliability of hospital discharge abstracts*. Report of a study. Washington, D.C.: National Academy of Sciences.

22. Tufo, H.M., Eddy, W.M., Van Busen, H.C., et al. 1973. Audit in a practice group. In Walker, H.K., Hurst, J.W., and Woody, M.F., editors. *Applying the problem-oriented system*. New York: Med Comm Press, pp. 29–41.

23. Tufo, H. M., Bouchard, R.E., Rubin, A.S., et al. 1977. Problem-oriented approach to practice. II. Development of the system through audit and implication. *J.A.M.A.* 238:502–505.

24. Decker, B., and Bonner, P. 1974. *Criteria in peer review*. Cambridge, Mass.: Arthur D. Little, Inc., pp. 90–91.

25. *Private initiative in PSRO*. Nov. 1977. Management Committee Final Report. Calif.: The Committee., p. 145.

26. Commission on Professional and Hospital Activities. April 1975. *When and how to do a medical audit study*. Workshop of American College of Physicians, Fifty-sixth Annual Session. San Francisco, Calif.: The Commission.

27. Sanazaro, P.J. 1977. The PSRO program: start of a new chapter? N. Engl. J. Med. 296:936–938.

28. U.S. Department of Health, Education, and Welfare. Sept. 2, 1977. *MCE evaluation report*. Washington, D.C.: Health Care Financing Administration, Bureau of Health Standards and Quality.

29. Sanazaro, P.J. 1977. The PSRO program: start of a new chapter? *N. Engl. J. Med.* 296:936–938.

15

Criteria for the Determination of the Quality of Care

Claude Welch

Critical assessment of patient care always has been important but will assume even greater significance in future years. Third parties will demand that quality controls be required as a condition for the provision of financial payments. Such controls theoretically could be effected by each individual practitioner, but this is not practical; members of the medical profession must review care provided by their colleagues and must assume the burden of the extensive peer review that is involved. Such peer review can be exerted at all levels of patient care—in the home, office, hospital, or in various posthospital facilities, such as nursing homes. The amount of effort that could be expended on this purpose could be enormous and, if carried to an extreme, mean that the time and the cost devoted to medical care could rise explosively.

At the present time some basic concepts and methods for such review have been established. It will remain for the future to decide whether these efforts have actually produced improvement in medical care and to determine the influence such procedures will have on the costs to the public.

The enormity of the task can be illustrated by the fact that there are somewhere between 15 and 20 million operations performed in hospitals in the United States and that there are a few billion contacts made between physicians and patients in var-

ious locations in the course of a year. It is no wonder that this situation invites dismay, and by the same token it becomes apparent that it will be necessary to select a small segment of the entire medical care industry to determine the applicability and efficacy of any system that is devised.

It is for this reason that criteria for care have been developed in particular for one of the most crucial parts of the system—the short-stay general hospitals. It is in this segment that the greatest costs of medical care are generated. The PSROs, the present organization of hospital staffs, the influence of the JCAH, and the recent authorization of investigations by various third-party payors have combined to make this milieu the site of the most intensive development.

To determine whether care has been provided that is of a given quality, certain standards must be established. Furthermore, various criteria must be outlined by which it may be determined whether these standards have been met. It is clear, therefore, that the development of criteria to determine the quality of care becomes a very critical feature in any review system. The purpose of this chapter is to sketch briefly the historical developments and then consider in detail the efforts of the combined AMA/specialty society/DHEW contribution to the solution of the problem.

DEFINITIONS

The definition of the terms applicable to this chapter is of great practical importance. Some of the terms used most frequently are defined in detail, because they are important in the later discussion.

norms Numerical or statistical measures of usual observed performance of medical care.

standards Professionally developed expressions of the range of acceptable variations from a norm or criterion.

criteria Predetermined elements against which aspects of the quality of medical service may be compared and that are developed by professionals relying on professional expertise and on the professional literature.

admission certification In some systems certification for admission requires that certain predetermined criteria for admission be met.

length of stay (LOS) Entire length of stay in the hospital or, in certain instances, the preoperative or postoperative stay.

concurrent continued-stay review Review of a patient's progress while in the hospital to determine whether indicated procedures are carried out, in proper sequence, and in a minimum time range.

retrospective review Review of the record after the patient has left the hospital.

screening criteria Criteria employed to screen out the bulk of patients' records in which care apparently has been adequate and will not require review but will serve to pinpoint certain records in which the care must be examined more carefully to determine whether it has been adequate.

utilization review Comprehensive review of all procedures carried out, equipment used, and personnel involved in individual cases and the determination of whether they were appropriate.

claims review Lists of procedures identified for payment either by the patient or the third-party payor.

medical care evaluation studies (MCEs) Studies based on previously determined standards and criteria, studies designed to determine whether the care has been adequate and to correct any difficulties.

HISTORICAL SUMMARY

Early systems to review medical care in hospitals were produced by individuals, EMCROs, and foundations. Some of these review systems were essentially made for claims review and served as monitors to various third-party payors as to whether reimbursement was indicated for such services. Some were very extensive, such as those developed by the San Joaquin County Foundation for Medical Care, in which monitoring was extended to individual patients, prescription of drugs, and pharmacists. Generally, long lists of applicable procedures compatible with the care given to individuals with definite diagnoses were made.

The AMA/HEW criteria, on the other hand, departed from this system. They represent attempts to avoid such long lists and to identify relatively few items that can serve to identify the presence or absence of good care. A somewhat similar system was developed independently by the New York Chapter of the College of Surgeons in which "predictors" of surgical care were identified, and by them the adequacy of care could be determined in a retrospective fashion.

Some valuable lessons have already been secured from the application of these systems. For example, it has been generally accepted that the inclusion of long lists of all potentially applicable procedures in any given situation is inflationary and may have medicolegal connotations. Two focal points of interest have been obvious throughout this whole development; third-party payors are interested almost entirely in cost control, whereas physicians must emphasize quality first and cost second. Recently it has become apparent that collection of such data is important not only from the point of view of the individual physician and patient but also because the data can be used to provide solid evidence that can focus on such problems as unnecessary surgery.

AMA PROJECT

Prior to the passage of the Bennett Amendment to PL 92-603, the development of some type of standards for medical care throughout the country was a prime subject for consideration by the Interspecialty Council of the American Medical Association. It was decided after considerable debate that this specific organization could serve as a catalyst to devise some standards that could serve as models that could be elaborated by individual states and hospitals. The exact method by which this could be done was far from clear at the outset; however, the passage of PL 92-603 spurred the AMA into a sustained effort to produce some document that would be of great aid to the developing PSROs and to individual hospital staffs throughout the country. The effort led to a large grant from DHEW and to a collaborative effort that involved 38 specialty societies. A large committee comprised of representatives from each of these societies was formed and named the Project Policy Committee. An executive committee of seven persons, known as the Project Steering Committee, acted to meet with a third committee, known as the Technical Advisory Committee, appointed by HEW. The last committee was composed of men whose competence in this field had been demonstrated by past experience. The combined efforts led to numerous meetings of the committees and the final publication of a document in June 1976 entitled *AMA*

*Sample Criteria for Short-Stay Hospital Review.** During this period of approximately 4 years, numerous questions of policy were considered. Those of major importance are described in the following pages. Because the whole field of peer review is still in a dynamic state, the reasons for the decisions that were made must be recorded.

Practical Questions

The first decision made was to limit the development of criteria to diseases encountered in short-stay general hospitals. It was recognized that a large amount of important medical care is delivered in offices; this is particularly true of pediatric patients and in certain other specialties such as psychiatry. However, in most instances development of methods by which review of such care can be carried out for office practice is in an elementary phase and poses many more practical difficulties than concentration on hospital patients.

When hospital patients are considered, if independent review is carried out on all of them, essentially all medical care and decisions will be duplicated. This would lead to an enormous waste of time, because it is very clear that the great majority of procedures would be approved by an independent reviewer. Hence, it is necessary either to select a random sample of patients for review, or if some special problem is encountered, to focus sharply on it with review of all pertinent records.

Peer review can be carried out only by physicians. Undoubtedly screening will be conducted even more frequently in the future by nurses or clerks, who will attempt to perform the preliminary review functions. It must be emphasized strongly that the purpose of such employees is to select records that may indicate a deviation from the ac-

*The readers should obtain a copy of this publication to follow the remaining discussion. It can be obtained free of charge from the AMA.

cepted standard; the determination then of proper or improper procedures must be made on an individual basis by physician peers.

The cost of such a review is an important feature. It may vary from $5 to $15 per admission. Much of this expenditure is due to physicians' time. It is therefore imperative that nurses, clerks, and computers be employed as much as possible for screening procedures. This will identify the relatively few records that will require review by physicians.

The ultimate purpose of the review is to identify substandard procedures and to correct them. Corrective action will be primarily directed toward education of physicians. Although sanctions are provided for repeated deviations, it is not expected that they will be used frequently.

This brief overview is supplemented by a detailed discussion of the major features of the project.

Scope of the Criteria

Screening criteria will be of greatest value when they are developed for diseases that are encountered in a hospital. If a disease is infrequent, it is possible that all such admissions could require individual physician review. To develop screening criteria for such cases would be more difficult than this examination of each record.

In accordance with this principle, each specialty society was asked to consider the diagnoses that accounted for 75% of the admissions to hospitals in that specialty. Data obtained from the Commission on Professional and Hospital Activities were used as a basis. By this method, approximately 300 common diagnoses were obtained. In some instances as diverticular disease of the colon, for example, both physicians and surgeons would be involved so that separate criteria sets could appear from each involved specialty group. This then in-

volved a coordination of viewpoints. At times final decisions had to be made by the Project Steering Committee.

Inasmuch as each separate criteria sheet had been prepared by an individual society, these societies were indicated on each sheet to identify the actual authors in each instance.

It is recognized that in certain institutions other diagnoses not covered in this manual may be encountered frequently; therefore, the individual hospital or PSRO will wish to develop screening criteria for these diagnoses. Additional criteria sets are suggested on the bases of (1) the greater local frequency of certain diagnoses or problems, (2) the degree to which local health status could be improved by appropriate identification and treatment of certain local medical problems, and (3) local evidence indicating possible inappropriate utilization of services or delivery of substandard health care.

In the final document, approximately 300 diseases are included, representing 75% of admissions. In contrast, the remaining 25% would include about 4000 different diagnoses. This indicates the impracticality of any attempt to make an extensive development of criteria to cover all cases.

Development of the Format

The major decision in the development of any criteria set is the construction of a format that is followed in each individual instance. Some of the philosophy of possible formats was previously discussed. It should be reemphasized here that the decision was made to limit the format to relatively few elements. Too extensive a review leads to serious practical problems involving the use of a great deal of time and the production of a great deal of data that will probably be of little use. It was decided that answers to approximately 30 questions should be sufficient to provide an indication as to whether or not care of high quality was being obtained; such a method should probably identify at least 95% of the problems and would be a relatively simple task. On the other hand, it was recognized that when MCEs are carried out, it would be necessary for the reviewer to expand on such criteria to obtain answers to specific questions.

The format may be understood better by the example in the boxed material on p. 147. The critical questions include the title, admission review, continued-stay review, validation of diagnosis and reasons for admission, the critical diagnostic and therapeutic services, the discharge status, and complications. The maximum number of entries required is 40. Comments are made about each of these items, but for a full discussion of the method of application, the AMA/HEW manual should be consulted.

Diagnoses and Problems

Patients may be admitted to a hospital because of a definite diagnosis or because of a specific problem that usually will be resolved during the hospital stay so that a definite diagnosis can be applied before discharge. Thus, many patients will enter with a basic problem, such as severe headache, and be discharged with a specific diagnosis, such as brain tumor. In some instances, a definite cause of the symptom cannot be established. In such an instance, the discharge diagnosis would read, "headache, severe, cause undetermined."

In any such compendium, it is necessary to employ some system of identification. The two codes that are used most frequently in hospitals are the *International Classification of Diseases Adapted*, eighth edition (ICDA-8) and the *Hospital Adaptation of International Classification of Diseases*, second edition (H-ICDA). For that reason, each diagnosis is coded for these two systems.

Ready access is provided by cross indexing. Inasmuch as nearly all of the criteria are developed on the basis of diagnoses, it is possible then to develop methods of comparison with other series of statistics. In particular, the figures on length of stay (LOS) can be obtained for H-ICDA from the Commission on Professional and Hospital Activities. When admission is made on the basis of a problem, it is assumed that a working diagnosis should be established relatively briefly after admission to the hospital and that use of a criteria set for this new diagnosis would then be required to establish a new and definite LOS.

Admission Review

The purpose of admission review in the format is to establish the reasons that a patient is admitted to a short-stay hospital rather than to some other type of health facility and to assign an initial length of stay.

At the outset a list of diagnoses or problems that will justify admission to a short-stay acute-care hospital without any further qualifications should be established. Unfortunately, because of the lack of availability of beds, such a policy may have to be modified from time to time. For example, under optimal conditions all patients with the diagnosis of malignant disease should be admitted without delay. However, if there is a shortage of beds, such conditions as acute abdomen, shock, or severe trauma with suspected visceral injury will have to take preference. With other diagnoses, such as burns, it will be necessary to specify certain types that should be admitted immediately, for example, any third-degree burn or any second-degree burn that involves the face, head, neck, or genitalia, or the hand and foot, or if over 15% of the body is involved. A sample list of these diseases that demand immediate admission has been compiled by the various specialty societies.

SAMPLE CRITERIA FOR SCREENING PATIENT CARE*

Diverticular disease of colon

I. Admission review
   A. Reason for admission
      1. Obstruction, perforation, or abscess
      2. Fistula formation
      3. Fever, hemorrhage, pain, or mass
      4. Scheduled for operation
   B. Initial length of stay assignment (see explanation on p. 149)
II. Continued-stay review
   A. Reasons for extending the initial length of stay
      1. Fever (over 100 F, or 37.7 C), hemorrhage
      2. Wound infection, obstruction, or perforation
      3. Atelectasis, pulmonary emboli, or pneumonitis
      4. Urinary obstruction, infection, or both
   B. Extended length of stay assignment (see explanation on p. 149)
III. Validations of:
   A. Diagnosis (only one required)
      1. Positive barium enema
      2. Positive pathology report or operative findings
   B. Reasons for admission
      1. Radiologic evidence of perforation, abscess, fistula, obstruction, or bleeding site
      2. Failure to respond to medical treatment
      3. Recurrent diverticulitis
IV. Critical diagnostic and therapeutic services
   A. Digital rectal examination and sigmoidoscopy
   B. Antibiotics in acute diverticulitis with complications
   C. Surgical consultation for complications
   D. Radiologic examination of the abdomen to include barium enema except in acute diverticulitis with free perforation and peritonitis
V. Discharge status
   A. Alive
   B. Ambulatory
   C. Bowels functioning
   D. Clinically stable and improving
   E. Documentation of follow-up plan
VI. Complications
   A. Primary disease and treatment-specific complications
      1. Obstruction, perforation
      2. Urinary infection, obstruction, or both
      3. Hemorrhage
      4. Pneumonitis, atelectasis, or emboli
      5. Sepsis (temperature over 100 F, or 37.7 C, for 4 days)
   B. Non-specific indicators
      1. Any extension of initial length of stay assignment
      2. Second operation
      3. Transfusions in absence of overt bleeding or operation

*Adapted from material developed by the American College of Gastroenterology/American Gastroenterological Association/American Society for Gastrointestinal Endoscopy, American College of Surgeons, and American Society of Colon and Rectal Surgeons, with modification by the Project Steering and Technical Advisory Committees.

These sample criteria are for screening patient care for subsequent physician review only and do not constitute standards of care.

Diagnoses Requiring
Immediate Admission

Abdominal tumors, pediatric age group
Abortion, spontaneous (inevitable or incomplete)
Abortion, spontaneous (threatened)
Acidosis, diabetic
Amniotic membranes, premature rupture
Anemia, sickle cell (crisis only)
Aneurysm (dissecting or ruptured, thoracic, abdominal, cerebral)
Appendicitis
Arthritis, septic
Brain abscess
Breast, carcinoma
Cerebral hemorrhage
Cervix, carcinoma
Colon and rectum, malignant neoplasm
Coma—stupor
Diabetes, juvenile, uncontrolled
Drug overdose
Encephalocele
Encephalopathy (toxic-metabolic)
Endocarditis, infectious
Endometrium, malignant neoplasm
Endotoxic shock
Esophageal atresia and tracheoesophageal fistula, pediatric age group
Esophagus, chemical injury, acute
Foreign body, intraocular or intraorbital
Fracture of base of skull
Fracture of hip, femoral neck, or intertrochanteric
Fracture, open (compound)
Fracture, skull vault
Fracture of vertebrae, cervical/dorsal/lumbar, acute-traumatic
Gastrointestinal hemorrhage
Hemorrhage, traumatic, into vitreous, eye
Hyphema, traumatic (hemorrhage into anterior chamber)
Intestinal obstruction
Intussusception, pediatric age group
Jaundice, obstructive, in infancy
Meningitis, bacterial, fungal, tuberculous
Meningitis, viral
Myocardial infarction, acute
Omphalocele or gastroschisis, pediatric age group
Osteomyelitis, acute
Pancreatitis, acute
Pericarditis, acute
Poisoning, acute
Pregnancy, bleeding in latter half

Pregnancy, ectopic
Pregnancy, preeclampsia or eclampsia
Pulmonary edema, acute
Pulmonary embolism, acute
Pyloric stenosis, congenital, hypertrophic
Renal colic
Respiratory distress of newborn
Retention of urine, acute
Septicemia
Shock, acute
Shunt complications, ventricular or cerebrospinal fluid
Spinal cord injury or paralysis
Status asthmaticus
Status epilepticus
Stomach, malignant neoplasm
Stroke, acute or impending
Suicide or suicidal (attempt, risk, or tendency)
Torsion, spermatic cord
Tracheal or bronchial foreign body
Tumors, central nervous system
Wound, open, of orbit
Wound, perforating, of eyeball

In addition to the list of diagnoses for which immediate hospitalization is indicated, other diagnoses or problems will justify hospitalization. For example, a suspicion of acute myocardial infarction would be sufficient. A problem that could require hospitalization would be abdominal pain; however, it is obvious that not every patient with abdominal pain should be admitted to a hospital, so that some modifier would be necessary. In this instance, for example, abdominal pain with a physical finding suggestive of an acute abdomen would be sufficient.

A certain number of diagnostic or therapeutic procedures other than surgery will also justify hospitalization. For example, cardiac catheterization should be performed on hospitalized patients. Colonoscopy can usually be carried out as an outpatient procedure but in certain instances in old or poor risk patients should be done as a hospital procedure.

Many of these admissions will be for surgical operations that theoretically should be carried out with a minimum of delay in the hospital. This means that before admission adequate diagnostic work should have been carried out to establish the diagnosis. For example, if a patient is believed to have gallbladder disease, an admission should not be scheduled for question of gallbladder disease when cholecystograms have not been taken before entry. On the other hand, if cholecystograms have confirmed the diagnosis of gallstones, the statement under the reasons for admission would be "scheduled for operation."

At the time of admission, an initial LOS assignment is made. This will depend primarily on the admitting or working diagnosis but will require adjustment in the presence of secondary or concomitant diagnoses.

The LOS assignment is a very sensitive consideration. Comparison with statistical data gathered from the Professional Activities Study of the Commission on Professional and Hospital Activities must be used as guides. In these data it is quite interesting to note the varying LOS assignments in various sections of the country. For some reason that is not entirely clear, discharges have occurred more rapidly in the West than they have in the East. Such factors as availability of home or extended care facilities are very important. On the other hand, there is an impression that much of the hospital stay is decided on the basis of tradition and that shorter lengths of stay are completely compatible with good care.

In individual instances because of other concomitant diagnoses, lengths of stay may be extended considerably, but an average figure covering a large number of cases should show no significant difference from the collected data of the Professional Activities Study.

Continued-stay Review

The continued-stay review will include five or fewer reasons for extending an initial LOS and then will also include revision of the LOS that is justified under these circumstances. The entries in this element will include the most common reasons, such as complications of therapy that have arisen, which indicate that continued care in the hospital is indicated for a patient with this particular diagnosis or problem.

In some instances it may be necessary to list one particular sign or symptom that will indicate the requirement for extending the LOS. For example, continued fever, either after an operative procedure or in a patient with pneumonia who has been properly treated with antibiotics, could be given an extended LOS merely on the basis of this continued symptom.

In certain instances there will be a shift in the diagnosis so that a new protocol must be established. This is particularly true when the patient is admitted for a certain problem, but a definite diagnosis can be made within the course of the next 2 or 3 days. The extended LOS is then made on the basis of this new diagnosis.

Validations

Validations must be made of both the diagnosis and the reasons for admission.* In both instances five or fewer entries will be used.

Validation of the diagnosis is designed to specify the few pieces of documented, easily retrievable data that will validate the diagnosis. Preferably this should be objective, and for this reason, laboratory data provide the most solid evidence. If that is not available, as in some instances of back pain, physical findings will serve as the second most satisfactory evidence. Finally, if both of them are lacking, items abstracted from the history or

---

*Validation of discharge diagnosis must be made on record review after discharge; however, under certain circumstances, validation of admitting diagnosis could be done as a task of concurrent review.

from the course of the patient in the hospital will be required. Thus, severe back pain may continue to be present despite negative physical findings.

Validations of the reasons for admission must consider each of the indications for admission previously listed. Here the evidence that will validate each reason for admission listed under the admission review on p. 146 should be included.

Admittedly this is a somewhat difficult entry. For example, if the reason for admission is to perform a herniorrhaphy, it is conceivable that one might ask whether a herniorrhaphy is indicated in this particular instance. The general consensus among surgeons is that herniorrhaphy is wise in every case of inguinal hernia regardless of age. Some family physicians might dispute this claim. It should not be expected that individual records will include a full description of the pros and cons of hernia repair. The criteria set on inguinal hernia indicates that the reason for admission is validated if the presence of a groin hernia or history of inguinal bulge, or hydrocele, on physical examination is obtained.

Critical Diagnostic and Therapeutic Services

Critical diagnostic and therapeutic services are a very important part of the review. The selection of five or fewer questions that will decide whether adequate care has been given is a very difficult task. These few key services should have a very critical relationship, so that either their presence or absence is sufficient to justify review of a record by a physician. This should answer the question whether these services should be provided in an acute-care hospital. They may emphasize that care should be provided in a special unit of the hospital, for example, in the respiratory care unit. Such an entry could be essential in the determination of the diagnosis or in the selection of therapy.

To determine whether or not these services are

critical, a benchmark of either 100% or 0% is selected. It could be inferred that this means that some procedures should be done every time and that others should never be done. However, this interpretation is not correct. The correct interpretation is that if the benchmark is 100% and a procedure has not been done, this item should be reviewed by a physician; if the benchmark is 0% but this procedure has been done, again there should be a physician's review. There may be exceptions to every rule. For example, it might be considered that every physical examination should include a rectal examination. Such a benchmark would be 100% for all physical examinations. However, in the presence of any acute myocardial infarct, this could be a very dangerous procedure and should be omitted. Benchmarks of 0% are less common. As an example, however, the use of antibiotic therapy following an operation on a carpal tunnel syndrome could be an indication that the procedure was not performed in the proper fashion.

A feature that may make interpretation of this entry more difficult is the fact that many physicians will have ordered certain diagnostic tests before the patient's entry into the hospital. Consequently, these notations would be present in the office records but not in the patient's hospital records. It is desirable that such material be available in the hospital record, but it must be recognized that there are many instances in which this will not be done, and if cases are brought up for review on this basis, the physician should have an opportunity to present the material he or she has obtained before admission to the hospital.

In some instances it will be found that there are local variations from the entries in this section of the AMA criteria. For example, in the AMA criteria on cholecystitis and cholelithiasis, an EKG is regarded as 100% necessary in patients over 40 years of age. It may be found in local areas in retrospective review that only 50% of patients over

40 have had this done. This should invite a critical review and assessment of the procedures in the local area. It is possible that in some instances the AMA criteria will be too strict, but in general I believe that they will be found to be correct.

It would be possible to extend the list of critical diagnostic and therapeutic services enormously were it not for the fact that routine services should not be included in this list. For example, a history, physical examination, complete blood cell count, and urine examination are considered part of the routine treatment of all hospitalized patients; therefore, they are not included in this protocol.

Discharge Status

Five or fewer entries again are required under discharge status. The point of these particular entries is to select the few key indicators easily retrievable from the record indicating that the patient has received the maximum benefit from hospitalization. The goals that should be attained during hospitalization also can be included.

In most instances it will be found that one of the key entries will be that the patient has survived hospital care. If one of the entries therefore is "alive," it will mean that the records of all patients who died will be reviewed by physicians. In general terms this is correct. It is conceivable, however, that if there were, for example, a large number of deaths from metastatic cancer, it would not be deemed necessary by local groups that all such records be reviewed. However, I believe that this is in all cases essentially necessary and that there will be few times in which a death should not be reviewed by the physician.

In certain instances the goals to be sought during hospitalization are important to specify. For example, the patient who has received a colostomy should have been instructed in the care of the stoma before he leaves the hospital.

Complications

Two particular sections are included in complications. The first section is the complications referable to the primary disease or to the treatment. Any list of the innumerable complications that might follow an operative procedure would be undesirable. The point of these entries is to find five or fewer that occur reasonably frequently that have a significant effect on morbidity and mortality and are potentially preventable.

The second section consists of the nonspecific indicators, and again these are restricted to five or fewer entries. Listed in this area are such items as a transfusion after an inguinal herniorrhaphy, a second operation after appendectomy, the use of antibiotics for clean orthopedic operations, or the transfer to surgery of a patient with congestive heart failure.

VALUE OF QUALITY CARE CRITERIA

The final test of any criteria developed for the care of patients will reside in the determination as to whether better care has resulted from their application. Obviously this will be a very difficult matter to assess. For example, the mere knowledge that such criteria have been developed will influence many physicians to examine their practices and institute improvements. Furthermore, with the changes that are occurring every day in the practice of medicine, it is impossible to ascribe improvement to one particular factor.

Published data that indicate the influence of the development of criteria of medical care are very few. Hopefully, the passage of time will lead to the establishment of some studies that will indicate their value. Attention should be called to two reports that would indicate the value of such procedures.

Dyck and associates have conducted a study on hysterectomies in Saskatchewan and the effect of the establishment of criteria on the reduction of the number of unjustified procedures. It was noted that in 1971 there were 86.4% more hysterectomies carried out than in 1964. In 1972 the College of Physicians and Surgeons of Saskatchewan established a committee that carried out a number of studies. They established accepted criteria that would justify a hysterectomy, that is, malignant and premalignant lesions of the female reproductive tract, endometriosis, adenomyosis, leiomyomas with a uterine weight of 200 gm or more, salpingitis and oophoritis, hysterectomy associated with pregnancy, benign ovarian neoplasms, cervical dysplasia, hyperplasia of the endometrium, dysfunctional uterine bleeding, and pelvic congestion syndrome. Any hysterectomy carried out for one or more of the accepted indications was categorized as justified, and all other hysterectomies were categorized as unjustified. After publicity and education, the annual number of hysterectomies in Saskatchewan in 1975 returned to the figure that it was in 1964. The number of unjustified hysterectomies dropped from 23.7% at the time of first review in 1973 to 7.8% in 1974.

A second important study was completed by Emerson in New York State. The medical society of the state of New York and the Brooklyn–Long Island Chapter of the American College of Surgeons established ''surgical criteria predictors'' for the common surgical diseases in the year 1973.

These predictors included material that could be obtained on retrospective review and included significant details of the history, physical examination, laboratory data, indications for surgery, preoperative preparation, operative description, postoperative course, criteria for discharge, and average length of postoperative stay. If a numerical value is assigned to each one of these items, a final score card can be reached on each individual patient. A level of standard performance can then be set and the conformance to the standards judged. By the use of these predictors and their application to such common operations as cholecystectomy, appendectomy, and hysterectomy, Emerson concluded that only about 1% of operative procedures performed in the hospitals reviewed could be classed as unnecessary.

THE FUTURE

The future development of criteria is impossible to predict. Without question, any that are used today will require modification. The increased emphasis on ambulatory care will require extension to such facilities; office practice will be subjected to greater scrutiny. Reduction in the number of short-stay hospital beds can have a profound effect. It is obvious that further revisions and extensions of the protocols discussed in this chapter will continue. The prospects are that their use will increase with the passage of time.

16

Data Requirements

Philip Walker

Data policy for support of the PSRO has evolved in the same general method as the rest of the PSRO program, with the basic pattern being taken from existing models. Prior to PL 92-603, a few electronic data processing (EDP) firms were providing processing support to review organizations. Also in existence were a number of abstracting services performing data collection for individual hospitals.

A number of alternatives were considered by the BQA prior to a data policy. These alternatives included consideration of the following:

1. Federal, nationwide processing of all data; this was briefly considered and found not to be feasible.

2. Regional federal processing with the department contracting for services of processing and automation; this alternative was explored to a considerable extent and finally ruled out in that many PSROs then operating already had contracts and were resistant to submitting all review data to a federal processor.

3. Individual PSROs subcontracting for EDP services through competitive bid; this option eventually developed into policy; however, it necessitated that BQA develop guidelines for the PSROs to follow and meet in the subcontract process.

Since the decision was made as to what alternatives were to be used to support data processing, the evolution of an efficient, effective system has been evolving as new needs are identified. Currently, a number of different approaches are being used throughout the program. Selection of the processors has been a result principally of competitive bid. The federal office has developed its own data system, and as previously stated, all the uses of an EDP system in the PSROs have not yet been identified.

FEDERAL GUIDELINES GOVERNING EDP IN THE PSRO PROGRAM

The first of the guidelines affecting data processing was released in May 1975 as *Provisional Policies for PSRO Data Routing and Processing,* with the first revision in September of the same year. The latest modification is dated February 1977, and was released as PSRO Transmittal No. 45. These contain the requirements for services as well as constraints.

Much of the content has changed over this time period, although two items have withstood the test of time. First, the recommendation that PSROs consider existing systems; specifically, those that have used or are using federal or state funds or nongovernmental hospital discharge abstract service organizations already collecting data in the PSRO's geographical area. The second item that has remained is the 75¢ per abstract maximum limit that a PSRO may spend for processing.

The following points are addressed in the latest (February 1977) policy. Most reflect considerations that an organization must debate in determining a method of data collection to be used in any activity.

1. What are the organization's data needs? In other words, why are the data being collected? To what use will the data be put? Is the volume of data such that automation is required?

2. Once the need has been determined and delineated, one must determine if these data are already being collected by asking, "Will our needs duplicate data already being collected?"

3. If duplication is evident, an organization must determine if duplication is necessary. That is, can whoever is currently collecting the data provide the data to you in a form that is acceptable and in a manner that will meet requirements with validity and reliability?

The federal provisional policy addresses each of these questions in a manner that allows each organization to obtain the answers in its own way but at the same time provides the reinforcement required to assure that answers are obtained. After the answers have been obtained, a further decision is possible as to which method to use. Generally speaking, there are three alternatives: (1) to use an already existing system, (2) to incorporate parts of an already existing system, and (3) to bid competitively for the development of a "new" system. Models of these three alternatives are discussed in a later section of the chapter.

Regardless of which option is selected, the PSRO data system must provide the organization with some specific results:

1. Provision of the PHDDS to the BQA in the specified format and content prescribed by the bureau.

2. Capability of profiling activities of patients, practitioners, and providers as specified by DHEW and the local organization.

3. Capability of assisting in the management and monitoring of the local review process.

4. Capability of meeting the PSRO management information system's needs.

5. Capability of assuring confidentiality of data processed.

6. If so desired, capability of supporting MCEs.

If it is found that any of the three alternatives available in processing meet all of the six stated capabilities, the PSRO may consider utilizing that option, providing it does not cost more than 75¢ per abstract.

Other federal constraints include the need for the organization to utilize the competitive bid method of acquiring a subcontractor unless justification is documented showing clear evidence in terms of efficiencies and economics of subcontracting to a sole source. This is a federal requirement but legally a protective measure for the PSRO.

FEDERAL DATA PROCESSING

Because the BQA requires each PSRO to provide the PHDDS in machine readable form to the DHEW, a portion of this chapter is allocated to that function.

PL 92-603 Section 1155 (f) (1) (B) authorizes the secretary to establish federal reporting requirements for the PSROs. Under this authority, an automated data system has been developed with the stated goal of providing "feedback to plan, operate, monitor, and assess the PSRO program at local and national levels."*

It is expected that this federal system will enable the BQA to:

1. Allow PSROs to assess their local activities.
2. Monitor PSRO operations.
3. Support comparative self-assessment among PSROs.
4. Identify technical assistance needs of PSROs.
5. Provide summary information about PSRO activity and costs to respond to the DHEW, congressional, and Office of Management and Budget (OMB) inquiries.

Obviously, this is a large undertaking and has not been completed, although progressive activity is taking place at the federal level. Part of this activity appears duplicative; however, it may prove justified if the resulting information is useful in meeting the other expectations both at the federal and state levels. Figure 16-1 illustrates the federal PSRO EDP system.

For the data to be useful outside the BQA, the definition of data elements must be very solid, and each PSRO must be interpreting and utilizing the definition in exactly the same fashion. The volume of data being acquired will help adjust this if all interpretations are not the same; however, the exact extent is still in question.

*From U.S. Department of Health, Education, and Welfare. 1977. *Overview of Professional Standards Review Organization management information system.* Health Services Administration, Bureau of Quality Assurance (undated draft).

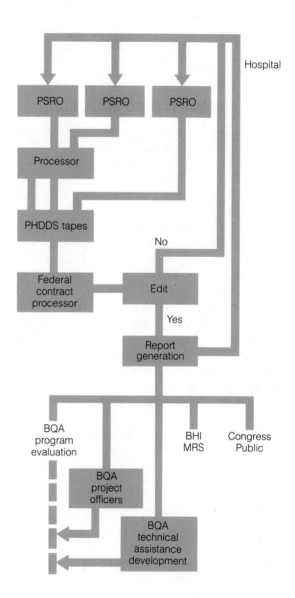

FIGURE 16-1. Federal PSRO EPD system.

The final note as to the utility of the data is that the requester must know the specific purposes for which the data collection took place. This must not only include the PHDDS definitions but more generally the purpose of the PSRO itself.

COMPETITIVE BID PROCESS

Unless a sole source subcontract is approved by the BQA, each PSRO must select a processor through a competitive bid process. The BQA must approve each step of the process, and for purposes of discussion, it is assumed that approval is requested and granted.

The first step in the process has already been addressed—that of determining data needs and justifying any data elements above and beyond the PHDDS. This task is usually completed as part of the development of the local data policy and plan. Also included in the plan are the results of what method of collection and data flow will work in the PSRO area.

Most pertinent is the assessment of whether the PSRO will be allowed by the community to develop a new data collection instrument or whether each hospital will insist on using one with which it is familiar.

After each of these questions is answered, the competitive bid process may begin. The basis for the process is the request for proposal.

Request for Proposal

The request for proposal (RFP) may be considered the technical specifications book and the informational presentation of how to make a bid. The RFP must include:

1. The requesting organization's name, address, and so forth.

2. The officer's name to whom questions may be addressed.

3. The criteria that will be used in evaluating the proposals.

4. Format requirements.

5. The deadline for response.

6. If desired, the organization's option to select either the lowest priced or the best technical system.

7. The right of the organization to refuse all bids.

8. Sociodemographic, geographic, and other volumetric data concerning the area.

9. The specific type of bid that will be considered: (a) one proposal addressing both collection and reporting, or (b) the option for the respondent to bid on either the collection or the reporting function.

10. Statement as to method of contracting.

11. Statement as to maximum dollar amount to be considered.

12. Technical attachments including: (a) data elements to be used, (b) PHDDS tape specifications, (c) edit expectations, (d) report expectations, (e) local data policy, (f) description of how system will work, and (g) minimum confidentiality requirements.

13. Performance expectations, including time of implementation, performance time limits, and penalties.

14. If available, proposed contract.

The researching of the content and the writing of the RFP is an important function in acquiring a data processor. If the RFP is loose, nonspecific, speaking to the general rather than the specific, the responses will be nonspecific and loose.

The contracting process is not a time to be learning; it should be the end product of a research and learning experience. Researching the content of the RFP should be an intensive process with involvement of both pertinent staff and representatives of the organization's membership. The process should not be measured in days of preparation but in months, with the end product (the RFP) a total description of the expected data system that has been justified, by component, to the satisfaction of the board of directors and the BQA.

The Process

First, once the RFP has been written, approved by the board, and printed, notice of its availability must be published and, if desired, copies sent to major known processors. Publication should be run for at least three consecutive days in a prominent paper that has distribution throughout the PSRO area. Another method is to have the notice printed in the *Commerce Business Daily.*

The notice must include instructions as to how to request a copy, deadline for request, and the purpose of the contract.

Second, on receipt of the request, the PSRO must respond in a timely manner, and it is advantageous to reiterate a few of the points contained in a cover letter including: (1) any request for a letter of intent to bid, (2) deadline for receipt, (3) contact person, (4) availability of additional data, and (5) when the contract selection will take place.

Third, during this time the PSRO must select key people to review the proposals. These should include key staff and physician representation, and in some cases, an outside consultant is more than justified. The RFP has the evaluation criteria listed, and from this staff should develop evaluation work sheets that can be used during the selection process to document the evaluation.

Fourth, on receipt of proposals, each one will be evaluated following the criteria for evaluation. Questions should also be noted and request for answers distributed to the appropriate offerer.

Fifth, the final selection, based on the indepen-

dent evaluators, should be made by the board of directors, and minutes should be kept of that meeting.

Sixth, the contract is negotiated.

THREE BASIC MODELS

Utilization of an Existing System

Figure 16-2 is a schema of a system utilizing an already existing system. This method of obtaining PSRO-EDP support has been used only infrequently to date and has been the result of sole source contracts in all cases. This discussion does not address any one specific system but some general observations.

The purposes of selecting and exclusively using an already existing data system are multiple. Principally, it hypothetically is already in place in a major portion of the hospitals in the PSRO area, and only the cost of collecting additional data elements would be defined as "new costs" in those hospitals, whereas the total per-abstract costs would be incurred only in those hospitals not on the system.

Because the system was already in place, time savings would be realized from the time of contract award to the time of data report generation.

Negotiation of additional data elements and reports must be negotiated between the PSRO and the processor; however, it must be remembered that the system was in place in the community and was developed for purposes other than the PSRO. This may cause the PSRO to reassess its need for certain data and for perceived data coding conventions.

Hence, it can be expected that the PSRO may have to forego some of its proposed data elements, coding conventions, or both to conform to a previously designed system that can be expected to

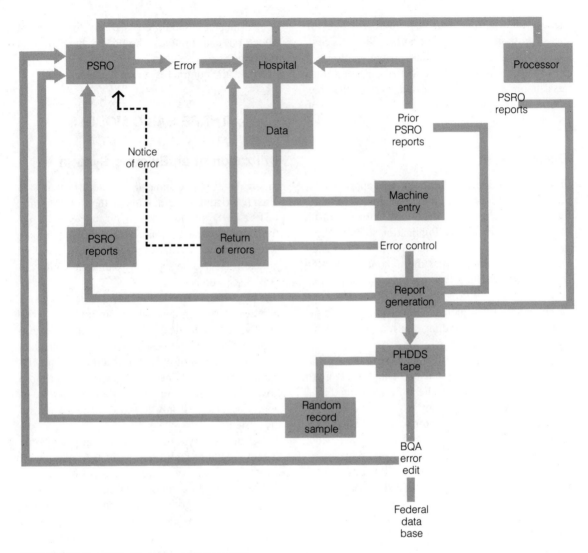

FIGURE 16-2.   Utilization of existing system.

have been implemented for reasons other than PSRO.

Data collection can be expected already to be in place and a prime contract already in existence. This will usually be between the hospital and the collector. The PSRO must actively delineate and define responsibility of data flow control and introduce methods of determining data accuracy.

This task is important in that concerning PSRO data, it is ultimately the PSRO that must stand accountable for the data's quality.

Use of Already Existing Collector and a Different PSRO-Selected Report Processor

Figure 16-3 illustrates the option of using already existing collectors and a different PSRO-selected report processor, which is found more often than the first option of using an already existing system. The major reason is that there is often more than one established collector in any given PSRO area. Utilizing this process is very similar to that of the first option, with the addition of needing to select a report processor that will receive machine readable data from collectors, edit the data, and aggregate them into a consolidated data base from which the PSRO reports may be generated.

The same caution may be observed using this method as in using an existing system.

PSRO Contracting Separately for Both Collection and Processing

In theory, the system of PSRO contracting separately for both collection and processing may duplicate an existing system; however, it is designed, developed, and installed to meet the specific needs of the PSRO. The PSRO has total control over the data from point of collection through report generation, thus providing for direct access to any problems in the system and enabling it to take direct corrective action. With the use of this option, the PSRO is in control of the data. (See Figure 16-4.)

FUTURE

It is still quite early to determine if any one of the discussed options is better than the other two, and

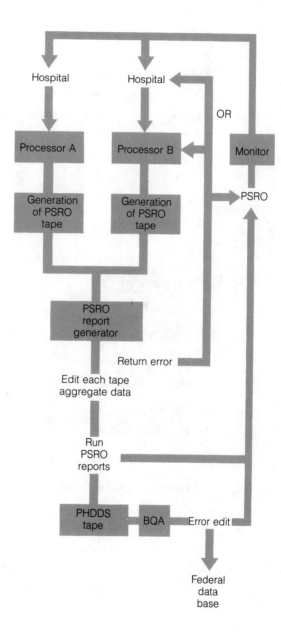

FIGURE 16-3. Use of already existing collector and different PSRO selected report processor.

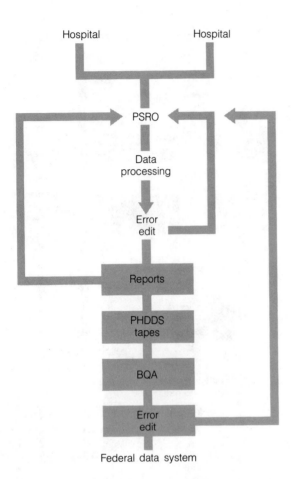

FIGURE 16-4. PSRO control of data.

it may be that none have the opportunity to do so. All of the basic needs of a PSRO-EDP system are not yet identified. As the PSRO evolves in maturity, the focus of the PSRO review also changes. Medical care evaluation, focused review, and monitoring require a level of data analysis that is described as a new need. Questions arising as the PSROs address these relatively new topics require more than the aggregate statistics currently available, leading to a need for personal interaction with the system and access to the total data base. We would hope that this need will be met by easily accessible reports that will be designed to meet these needs and the introduction of automated statistical packages that may assess all the data.

17

Deficiencies of the Health Data System in Quality Assurance and Utilization Review

Robert Barnes
Bruce L. Hulbert

The following discussion describes some of the experiences of the Health Care Review Center, a Seattle-based resource group in the field of quality assurance. During the past 5 years, the staff of the center has worked with over 20 hospitals throughout the state of Washington to assist them in developing programs to review the quality of patient care. These hospitals have varied in size from 25 beds to a 600-bed urban medical center. In addition, the Health Care Review Center helped develop the plan for the Washington State PSRO and recently completed a contract with the BQA, to train nurses and medical records administrators to coordinate and manage health care review programs in community hospitals throughout the Northwest.

This chapter addresses the utilization review decisions made in hospitals and the basic problems that exist regarding the information needed to make those decisions. What follow are some of the actual experiences of the Health Care Review Center in both urban and rural hospitals in the state of Washington.

Two basic problems exist regarding quality-of-care data in hospital settings. First, data generated in the hospital to describe the quality of care and proper utilization of facilities can be characterized as fragmented, often invalid and mismanaged, and therefore, frequently not used. Second, there is lack of incentive by the medical staff to utilize the data properly to identify patient care problems. To underscore why these problems exist and, in turn, how they might be solved, it would be helpful to briefly describe the hospital environment, including its structure and function.

The hospital's primary objective is to provide high-quality care to the acutely ill patient. Services are rendered both by paid employees and a visiting staff of physicians. The legal responsibility for the hospital rests with its governing body, and it, in turn, delegates to an executive officer the task of implementing policy. The third leg to this unique organizational arrangement is the organized medical staff. It is accountable to the governing board, but because each member of the medical staff is licensed to practice medicine, the members of the board have tended to accept their decisions regarding patient care services as final. Furthermore, it must be remembered that each of the long list of hospital committees, including clinical departments, is chaired by a busy volunteer physician whose top priority is his or her own practice, not the hospital. Neither the physician nor the trustee is a trained manager of hospital services and problems. Hospital administrators find themselves in the awkward and sometimes unenviable position of attempting to maintain a balance between these two groups. They must keep the hospital occupancy rate up and therefore must avoid alienating the medical staff. There is an excess of hospital beds in many communities, thus physicians might easily move to other hospitals if they are pressured too much by the one they are attending. Hospital administrators must attempt to meet all the regulations of federal and state governments and insurance intermediaries regarding proper utilization of facilities and quality of care. They are highly dependent on their voluntary, busy medical staff to generate the data required to show that these regulations are being met. Incomplete medical records are a constant block to evaluation of care.

The federal requirement (PL 92-603) that physicians review the cost and quality of care means they have to do certain things that are difficult for them. Traditionally, physicians focus their attention on the care of individual patients. They are most comfortable at the bedside or in their offices examining patients. They are not trained in data management or interpretation or in solving patterns of patient care problems. In general, they solve problems on an individual basis—one patient at a time.

In many hospitals, one or more physicians are interested and knowledgeable about quality of care issues, but this expertise does not extend to the rest of the staff.

Furthermore hospitals do not have a plan to coordinate and manage all of the data they collect. When one considers the variety and multiple sources of data, it is understandable why a plan is needed. The following is a list of some of the kinds of data most community hospitals collect regarding the quality of care, proper use of facilities, and costs.

1. Justification for admission to hospital
2. Length of stay
3. Reason for continued and prolonged stay
4. Total number of patient days
5. Daily census
6. Medical care evaluation studies
7. Mortality review
8. Tissue review
9. Review of use of blood
10. Review of drugs
11. Review of cancer
12. Data regarding infection
13. Running list of surgical procedures, time in surgery, names of member of surgical teams, and so forth
14. Monthly reports from standing committees and clinical departments to executive committee and board of directors: (a) clinical departments (medicine, surgery obstetrics, pediatrics), (b) clinical committees (coronary care unit, intensive care unit, emergency room, respiratory unit), (c) pharmacy and therapeutic committee, and (d) credentials and privileges committee
15. Nursing service, including nurse audits

It is readily apparent from this list that a plan is needed to manage and coordinate the flow of patient care data. However, our experience throughout the state of Washington, in large urban hospitals as well as isolated rural hospitals, reveals the absence of such a plan.

INVALID DATA

To further complicate the problem, the data that are collected describing quality of care may not be valid. An example of this problem is the way mortality is reviewed, which commonly results in misleading information. The review of deaths is one source of information that is available in every hospital for decision making regarding quality of care. In many hospitals the mortality review committee meets quarterly to review a large stack of "death charts." Each member of the committee is assigned a certain number of charts to review before the meeting with the instruction to briefly summarize any case that seems to be a problem. Since every physician has a large number of charts to review, they usually ask only one question, "Was the death justified?" If the patient had a serious disease, such as metastatic cancer, the physician can look at the final diagnosis and justify the death. Surgeons, for example, may skip over an in-depth evaluation of medical complications, such as diabetes, heart disease, or pulmonary infection. Physicians also recognize that the chart does not tell all, and if they did not personally take care of the patient, they cannot be too critical. A physician usually does not have time to discuss the case with the attending physician or to ask for medical evaluation of a surgical case. Therefore, mortality review does not usually provide accurate and meaningful information.

FRAGMENTED DATA

Prevention and control of hospital infections is a high-priority activity, and yet the data collected from multiple sources are often fragmented and poorly coordinated. Data regarding infection may come from the following sources: (1) bacteriology laboratory; (2) hospital epidemiologist; (3) infectious disease committee; (4) medical audit, retrospective; or (5) utilization review, concurrent.

In a recent study at one community hospital, a retrospective review of the complications of emergency colon surgery showed a postoperative wound infection rate of 42%. The audit required a positive wound culture to confirm the diagnosis. In spite of this unacceptably high rate of infection, none of the sources that usually generate data regarding infections had reported the problem to the

chief of surgery or the hospital executive committee. Postoperative wound infections increase the length of hospital stay and thus escalate the costs. A fragmented data system plus poor management failed to identify the problem in a timely fashion and correct it.

DATA NOT COMPARABLE BETWEEN INSTITUTIONS

Under current PSRO requirement, where criteria are adopted locally, the data emanating from MCEs are not comparable between institutions. For example, two hospitals in Seattle recently conducted MCEs in compliance with PSRO regulations. Both hospitals sought to document the incidence of postoperative infections in colon surgery. Hospital A asked how many cases had a positive wound culture, and hospital B simply asked if an infection was documented in the progress note. Hospital A had an infection rate of 23%, whereas hospital B had a rate of 4%. These outcomes are not comparable, because the question asked at hospital B did not identify all infections that actually occurred. It identified only those that were documented in the progress note. This underscores the fact that hospitals auditing the same subject ask different questions, use different criteria, and therefore arrive at different conclusions.

In summary, hospitals collect a great deal of information. It is often fragmented, sometimes invalid, and poorly managed, which makes it difficult for the leadership within the institutions to make proper decisions.

THE NATURE OF UTILIZATION REVIEW

Utilization review (UR) in a hospital setting is an evaluation program designed to assess the medical necessity and appropriateness of care for each Medicare/Medicaid patient beginning with admission and continuing throughout hospitalization.

Agencies such as PSRO, insurance intermediaries, and state governments require data from hospitals regarding proper utilization of facilities and quality of patient care. Examples of such data are claim forms submitted by the hospital to bill for services rendered, uniform hospital discharge abstracts, a document mandated under the PSRO program, and MCEs required by both the PSRO and JCAH. To generate the data within the hospitals for outside agencies regarding utilization review, three main activities are done: justification for admission to the hospital, continued-stay review, and medical care evaluation studies.

Justification for Admission to the Hospital

No one can be denied admission to the hospital. The initial review by the review coordinator must be completed by the end of 48 hours, at which time the necessity for hospitalization is either justified using criteria approved by the medical staff and a review date is assigned, or the coordinator must call a physician advisor to approve further hospitalization.

Continued-stay Review

A review is required for any patient staying beyond the length of stay that was assigned on admission for his problem, diagnosis, or procedure. The staff agrees on criteria that warrant an extension of the assigned length of stay. There are three problems with length of stay and continued-stay review data: First, the length of stay data are obtained from a regional book that has tables developed from past experience. Often length of stay for a particular diagnosis or procedure is not applicable for the hospital in question. Usually it is too long; therefore, the length of stay may have no meaning in monitoring proper use of the facility. Second, the

problem regarding the data describing justification for continued stay is that usually the question is not asked whether the complication could have been prevented. If the patient's complications resulted in death, his chart would be reviewed by the mortality committee. As already described, such review may result in invalid data. Third, the admissions and continued-stay review data are not comparable between institutions. The utilization review nurse screening admissions and continued stay often must make decisions on a subjective basis, and the criteria adopted by the staff for the nurse's use are local, not regional.

Medical Care Evaluation Studies

A further question on continued-stay review is whether a complication is inherent in the disease itself or is a result of the hospital treatment. It is common not to ask this question, and therefore documentation of the quality of care is incomplete.

The 1974 *PSRO Program Manual* defines medical care evaluation studies (MCEs) as retrospective, short-term, in-depth studies that assess the quality, nature, or both, of the utilization of medical care. Since they are detailed studies, they review only a sample of cases or selected data from all cases in a given period of time. Charts that do not meet adopted criteria can be assessed individually. The latter constitutes peer review. The focus is on patterns of care. They stress the outcome of care versus the process of care, and when a problem is identified, they stress the need for corrective action both for patterns of care and for individual patients.

MCEs have a number of limitations. They often are not focused on known or suspected patient care problems. A great deal of analysis may reveal "no problem." The outcome of the audit may document "no problem" when, in fact, there were problems. This may be because the criteria adopted were incorrect or exceptions were made for every case that did not fit the criteria. They are time consuming and therefore expensive. They may overlook or not get at existing problems. Finally, they do not attempt to measure the "art of medicine."

The greatest limitation of MCEs is their dependence on the medical records of patients, written by the provider of care. Records vary greatly in quality. They may contain almost no data or such an abundance of poorly organized data that an exhausting effort is required to read through them. Because it is extremely time consuming to review charts in depth, a variety of medical record personnel have been trained to abstract data and display them for rapid review by a physician or nurse group. A major problem is the inaccuracy introduced by the abstracting process. The most comprehensive abstracting service is the Professional Activity Service (PAS) of the Commission on Professional and Hospital Activities, whose computer contains over 70 million abstracts from 1700 hospitals. It is from these data that regional lengths of stay have been determined.

LACK OF INCENTIVE TO SOLVE PROBLEMS

Most physicians do not have as a high priority the development of an effective patient review process within the community hospital. They give lip service to such a program but do not wish to be their "brothers' keepers." They have no financial investment in the institutions, and often when sanctions need to be imposed on a fellow physician, they may say, "But by the grace of God, there go I." Physicians usually support each other as colleagues and do not desire to threaten each other through a federally mandated monitoring system. In the fee-for-service system, consultations are of economic importance to the specialist. If the specialist becomes an aggressive quality assurance

person, he or she may lose referrals. If hospital privileges are restricted, the administrator is distressed if the census drops. It is difficult to restrict privileges in a rural hospital where the services of one physician may account for up to 50% of the admissions. The great majority of individual physicians wish to provide high-quality care. However, each physician has little incentive to be accountable for the entire profession and is most amenable to change through continuing education rather than through "police action." Furthermore the physician feels that the poor performers are already known and that an extensive medical audit system to identify them is not necessary.

● ● ●

The limitations inherent in MCEs, admissions, and continued-stay review result in inadequate and incomplete descriptions of the quality of patient care and the proper use of facilities. New methods of generating and managing data are needed.

SOLUTIONS

It is difficult to envision an ideal data system that supports utilization and peer review. Many variables, both human and technical, enhance the possibility of fragmentation and error. One principle must be stressed; the further removed one gets from the patient and the bedside, the greater the likelihood that the data will not be valid. The ideal quality assurance system would focus on the service currently rendered, and suboptimal care would be corrected immediately. The following suggestions may help to solve some of the problems described by taking into account the present state-of-the-art and economic restrictions.

Hospital Data Management Plan

The development of a plan to manage data has many implications. It implies that roles and responsibilities for reviewing patient care and correcting identified problems are understood by each person at every accountability level from the board of governors down to each committee. It means that as data describing patient care are generated, they are displayed appropriately and in a timely fashion so that responsible hospital leaders can make appropriate decisions. It also means that there is a feedback system that documents the effectiveness of the program.

The following items list the elements of a hospital data management plan:

1. A member of the organized medical staff must be given responsibility and authority to develop and implement the program, such as chief of health care review. That individual must have staff support, including a health care review coordinator and secretary.

2. All data from the variety of hospital sources must be funneled through his or her office for assessment, coordination, and dispatch to the appropriate person or committee. This might be called the office of quality assurance.

3. A master display of all data and their management must be kept. This requires documentation of data usage at all levels in the accountability system.

4. Chairmen of committees, chiefs of service and staff, and members of the board of directors receive data regularly on quality of care and utilization of facilities. Their monthly meetings are planned around accurate data.

Alternatives to Medical Care Evaluation Studies

The limitations of MCEs, which suggest serious deficiencies in the quality assurance system if too much emphasis is placed on these studies, have been described. It must be emphasized that the key to a successful hospital program is the development of valid data from a variety of hospital sources. Other sources of data that can be utilized regularly are mortality review and "nonspecific indicators," concurrent review, and drug review.

The use of nonspecific indicators is a part of the review process whereby a list of key questions is applied to each chart concurrently to seek out potential or possible patient care problems that might not be detected otherwise. Some of these key questions might be:

1. Did the patient die?
2. Did the patient stay in the hospital 1 day?
3. Did the patient stay in the hospital longer than those in the ninetieth percentile category?
4. Was only 1 unit of blood given?
5. Did the patient receive an antibiotic without a diagnosis of an infection, or no fever, or culture?
6. Did the patient return to surgery during the same admission?
7. Did the patient return to the hospital within 2 weeks after discharge?
8. Did tissue review justify the surgery?
9. Did tissue review show a postoperative diagnosis consistent with the preoperative diagnosis?

There are other nonspecific indicators; these questions are just examples. At the time of discharge, these charts are tagged by the record room person, and in turn they are sent to the appropriate committee for peer review. Occasionally the review of such charts will identify a drug needing review.

Concurrent review of known problems focuses on these problems and corrects them as they occur. Problems identified by the use of nonspecific indicators, utilization review, or MCEs can be reviewed on a daily basis. The principle can be applied to monitoring a single physician, disease, or procedure.

Drug interactions and inappropriate use constitute a major hazard to the patients. A plan to review drugs has a high priority in improving the quality of care and reducing costs. Prescription and daily drug profiles are a source of accurate readily available data. This review process could be worked into the overall hospital data management plan.

Development of Data Comparable Between Institutions

Local review and local decisions are the indispensable conditions of a program acceptable to most physicians. Such decisions are likely to advocate local exceptions to regional or national criteria; however, a compromise is needed. The procedures, problems, and diagnoses that lend themselves to review by national criteria need to be identified. A consortium of hospitals could then adopt the same criteria for these subjects, and comparisons of outcomes of care could be made on a regional basis.

Cost Containment

Cost containment is one of the high priorities in health care planning. Appropriate and valid data from hospital utilization review are essential to making decisions about costs. It has already been stated that use of drug profiles and prescription data has a high probability of decreasing costs. Other areas that warrant more appropriate data are:

1. Continued-stay review. These data do not reflect preventable complications that, if iden-

tified, would be valuable both in evaluating quality of care and identifying reasons for unusual costs.

2. Review of ancillary services. Very few data are available on the appropriate use of x-ray, laboratory, and other hospital services. Data, along with valid criteria, could determine whether or not there is overutilization.

3. Review of level of care. More data are needed justifying the use of various levels of care in the hospital, such as the intensive care unit or coronary care unit. Data showing unnecessary use of these facilities could be used to reduce costs.

4. Use of cost figures as "nonspecific indicators." Charts that fall into the upper 10% of costs could be tagged for local review. This method would identify both high-cost physicians and high-cost procedures and diagnoses. If the cost figure were a regional one, data would be comparable across institutions.

How to Increase Incentive to Improve Quality and Cost of Care

Physicians are busy, and their time with patients is being reduced constantly by increasing loads of paperwork required by endless regulations. They will continue to resist solving hospital patient care problems as the time required erodes into practice and personal life. To obtain cooperation and support, some of the following ideas need to be developed or reinforced:

1. Link quality assurance data closely to continuing education. More research and pilot studies need to be funded to determine how best to do this.

2. Adopt a data management plan as outlined previously.

3. Supply instruction and financial support to voluntary committee chairmen and chiefs of service so that they may accomplish their jobs.

4. Develop a quality assurance/continuing education program unique for small, isolated rural hospitals.

5. Supply hospitals with part-time or full-time (depending on the size) physicians as directors of the programs to take the load off voluntary physicians. These physicians need special training in management, generation and use of data, communications and problem identification, and problem solving. Medical schools or schools of public health need to develop a curriculum to train such physicians.

6. Train nurses and record room administrators to coordinate and manage these programs while being accountable to the physician director.

SUMMARY

The data that are generated within hospitals to describe the proper use of facilities and quality of care reflect the evolving state-of-the-art. The data are often inadequate, sometimes not valid, usually fragmented rather than coordinated, and frequently poorly utilized. The hospital environment that reflects the attitudes of voluntary physicians was described to show its effect on data generation and validity. The lack of a coordinated data management plan was emphasized. Examples were given as to why data are invalid and why they are not comparable across institutions. The limitations of MCEs, the major method of documenting quality of care, were listed. Finally, following a description of some of the problems with the data generated, suggestions were made to improve these deficiencies.

18

PSROs and HMOs— Problems and Opportunities

James Roberts

Currently, there are approximately 700,000 Medicare and Medicaid beneficiaries enrolled in health maintenance organizations (HMOs). This represents 1.5% of the Medicare and Medicaid population and 11% of the 6,041,000 members in the 185 HMOs in the United States.

As with all other Medicare and Medicaid beneficiaries, PSROs are responsible for assuring that institutional health care services provided to Medicare and Medicaid HMO members are medically necessary, appropriate, and of recognized quality. Although the PSRO legislation and HMO regulations briefly address the relationship between PSROs and HMOs, no substantive policy statements or guidelines have yet been issued from either program to further define this important interface. This chapter outlines relevant legislative provisions, describes the genesis and basic structure of HMOs, highlights important efforts of HMOs in quality assurance and utilization control, discusses several policy issues concerning the HMO-PSRO relationship, and emphasizes the opportunity presented to HMOs and PSROs by an effective joint working relationship.

LEGISLATIVE DEFINITIONS OF THE PSRO-HMO INTERFACE

The PSRO legislation makes no differentiation between those Medicare and Medicaid beneficiaries enrolled and those not enrolled in HMOs and thus mandates an interface between PSROs and HMOs. This interface is specifically addressed in Section 1155 (e) (1) of the PSRO legislation, which requires PSROs to "utilize the services of, and accept the findings of, the review committees of a hospital or *other operating health care facility or organization. . . .*"[1] which proves it can effectively conduct mandated review (emphasis added). The report of the Senate's Committee on Finance further clarifies this point as follows:

A PSRO would be required to acknowledge and accept for its purposes, review activities of other medical facilities and organizations, including those internal review activities of comprehensive prepaid group practice programs such as the Kaiser Health Plans and the Health Insurance Plan (HIP) of New York to the extent such review activities were effective.*

Thus, the PSRO is responsible for review of institutional care provided to Medicare beneficiaries and Medicaid recipients who are HMO members. This responsibility must be exercised by the use (called "delegation" in the PSRO program) of HMO review programs where proved effective. PL 92-222, the Health Maintenance Organization Act

*From U.S. Senate. Sept. 1972. *Reports of the Committee on Finance*. Report 92–1230, p. 262.

of 1973, makes no direct reference to PSROs. As a basic requirement for federal qualification, however, the HMO must:

have organizational arrangements, established in accordance with regulations of the secretary, for an ongoing quality assurance program for its health services which program (A) stresses health outcomes and (B) provides review by physicians and other health professionals of the process followed in the provision of health services.*

Subsequent regulations add requirements that the HMO's quality assurance program include (1) systematic data collection, analysis, and feedback, (2) institution of corrective changes, and most important for this discussion, (3) a requirement that the HMO's review program be designed in a manner that allows it to be approved for delegation by the PSRO.[2]

No additional clarifying guidance has been issued, but HMOs seeking federal qualification are expected to have identifiable quality assurance programs. Also, in the process of continuing regulation of qualified plans, close attention is likely to be paid to the group's quality assurance program. Even in the absence of federal qualification, many states have or are considering enactment of HMO enabling legislation that includes requirements for creation of quality assurance programs in HMOs.[3] In short, quality assurance is becoming a fact of life for HMO practitioners.

It is important to recognize that although PSROs were expected to control utilization, the HMO legislation contains no requirements for the development of formal programs of utilization review. The HMO requirements previously noted concern quality assurance rather than utilization

review activities. The HMO's quality assurance efforts will be similar to the medical care evaluation study activities of the PSRO. Utilization review by PSROs (as represented by concurrent review of hospital care) is not mandated by HMO legislation. Yet, HMOs have a basic incentive to control utilization and have established formal and informal programs to do so. Therefore, although the quality assurance interface will be relatively easy to understand and implement, the utilization review interface may not. This important point is discussed in more detail later.

HEALTH MAINTENANCE ORGANIZATIONS—TYPES, CURRENT STATUS, AND QUALITY ASSURANCE ACTIVITIES

An HMO's size, age, organizational arrangements, and relationship to hospitals are factors defining the nature of its quality assurance and utilization control programs. An understanding of these variations will help PSROs determine the nature of the relationship they can establish with HMOs in their area.

The term "health maintenance organization" is a relatively new one. It was coined by Paul Ellwood, a principle architect of plans that resulted in the federal initiative to develop comprehensive prepaid health plans. Although the term is new, and some feel misleading, the history of prepaid comprehensive care is a long one.

There are two basic types of HMOs—the prepaid group practice (PPGP) and the independent practice association (IPA). The features common to both are that (1) a *defined, comprehensive health care benefit* package is provided to (2) a *defined member population* by (3) a *defined group of*

---

*From *Health maintenance organizations*. 1973. Public Law 92-222, Title XIII, Section 1301 (c) (8).

health practitioners for (4) a *predetermined, pre-paid* premium. The basic differences between the two are that IPA physicians practice in their *own offices usually* on a *fee-for-service* basis, whereas PPGP practitioners are located in *one or a few centers* and receive *salaries.*

Prepaid group practice was pioneered by Sidney Garfield in the early 1930s when he provided health services on a prepaid basis under contract to construction companies building an aqueduct to California.[4] His efforts grew to become the Kaiser-Permanente Medical Care Program, which currently enrolls approximately one of every 70 U.S. residents. Practitioners in PPGP plans are employed either directly by the HMO (the *staff model*) or by an independent partnership or corporation of physicians, which, in turn, contracts with the HMO to provide services (the *group model*). Therefore, a PSRO dealing with the PPGP may be dealing with the medical portion of the HMO itself or with an independent medical group that is organizationally separate from the HMO.

IPA plans began in the 1950s with the creation of the San Joaquin County Foundation for Medical Care in Stockton, California.[5] Created in response to the threat of a Kaiser-Permanente group forming in the area, the foundation developed and marketed a comprehensive health insurance program, the enrollees of which received care from physicians in fee-for-service practice. In this case, the physician organization marketed and serviced the insurance plan and represented the participating physicians. Some of the subsequent IPAs have separated the insurance corporation and physician organization.

The success that these pioneering efforts have had in attracting membership and controlling costs coupled with concern over the tremendous explosion in health care expenditures has resulted in increased federal and state interest in fostering the development of HMOs. At the federal level, this interest culminated in enactment of PL 92-222, the Health Maintenance Organization Act of 1973.

The legislation sought to stimulate the creation of HMOs by requiring employers to offer those plans that meet extensive legal, financial, organizational, and benefits requirements ("qualified plans") to their employees. In addition, federal grants and loans became available for feasibility studies, planning, initial construction, and early operations. The early phase of this accelerated interest in HMOs has faltered, but there has been a slow steady growth in the number of such plans and in their enrolled population. A survey done by the Blue Cross Association, DHEW, the National Association of Blue Shield Plans and Inter-Study shows that as of June 1976, there were 185 HMOs enrolling 6,041,000 members, or 3% of the population. Sixty-two percent of the members are in PPGPs. Seventy percent of the members are in plans with over 100,000 members. Sixty-four percent of the members are in the West, and 50% of the total are in California.[6] Since the enactment of PL 92-222, 36 organizations have become federally qualified. Recent statements from the Carter administration health officials make it clear that the climate for the continued federal stimulation of HMO development is favorable.[7]

Many studies have documented the fact that HMOs of either the group practice or IPA type reduce the utilization of inpatient hospital services.[8-11] Reasons for this reduction include (1) the incentives for HMO physicians to utilize appropriately those high-cost inpatient and other services and (2) the existence of funds to provide necessary services in the appropriate yet least expensive setting (such as ambulatory surgery). These basic program incentives and legislative requirements have fostered the development of utilization control and quality assurance efforts in most HMOs. Highlights of some of those programs follow.

HMO UTILIZATION AND QUALITY REVIEW ACTIVITIES

HMOs have been actively involved in quality assurance and utilization review activities for some time. Quality assurance has often taken the form of formal medical auditing, whereas utilization control, particularly in prepaid group practices, has often been less formal.

Quality Assurance

There are numerous examples in the quality assurance literature of research projects and descriptive reports of quality assurance programs based in prepaid practices.[12-17] This abundance of activity is evidence not only of the importance that such practices place on delivering high-quality care but also of the fact that a common medical record, an identifiable and well-defined provider and patient population, and the availability of staff support make organized programs of formal quality assurance relatively easier to conduct in an organized practice compared with a review of care provided in geographically separated practices lacking central organization.

This interest in quality assurance is illustrated by a survey of HMOs conducted by the Health Services Research and Development Center of The Johns Hopkins University.[18] In this study, 30 prepaid group practices of varying sizes and ages were surveyed. Of these, 50% had quality-of-care review programs of their own for hospital care. Another 20% had participated in the review of quality of inpatient services in conjunction with the hospitals to which they admitted their members. Also, 21 out of the 30 surveyed plans had ongoing quality assurance of ambulatory care or were developing such programs.

Another excellent detailed study of a number of ambulatory care quality assurance projects has been published, in which program descriptions are given for the quality assurance activities of 27 ambulatory care practices, including eight prepaid practices and several foundations for medical care.[19] These descriptions illustrate the wide variation in HMO quality assurance programs. An excellent bibliography is also provided.

The American Group Practice Association (AGPA) has assumed responsibility for the development and operation of an accreditation program for ambulatory health care.[20] Using a criteria-based survey program, AGPA surveyors review the operations of an ambulatory care center for accreditation purposes.

One of the most important of the AGPA survey criteria concerns medical audit. This criterion states, ''The organization must provide demonstration of an active, organized peer-based audit procedure for assuring the quality of medical care.'' Further discussion of this criterion, provided in an interim accreditation manual, makes it clear that the association expects an organization to have an audit committee that meets frequently and conducts review using predetermined objective criteria. The importance that the association places on formal quality assurance is illustrated by the fact that failure to meet this medical audit criterion is grounds for denial of accreditation.

Utilization Control

The Johns Hopkins survey previously cited also showed that 18 of the 30 plans surveyed had their own formal review procedures, whereas six more participated with their hospitals. These review efforts took several forms but generally concentrated on the appropriateness of admissions and lengths of stay. All four of the IPA plans had formal mechanisms for review of the utilization of hospital services. Despite this demonstration of a significant level of development of *formal utilization control activities* in HMOs, many feel that the most effective mechanisms of control, particularly in the group practice HMOs, are much more informal. Included in these informal mechanisms are peer discussions of effective alternatives to the use of high-cost services, systemwide interest in and support of economies in medical care practices, the lack of financial incentives to use high-cost services, the lack of financial barriers to the use of ambulatory and home care services, and interest in the prevention and early detection of disease. Although informal, these factors are felt to have contributed significantly to the consistent record of HMOs reducing utilization of high-cost, especially inpatient, services. An illuminating discussion of these informal mechanisms appears in the first volume of an ongoing series of reports of conferences sponsored by the Medical Directors Division of Group Health Association of America.[11]

POLICY ISSUES IN THE RELATIONSHIP BETWEEN PSROs AND HMOs

There is essentially a complete void of policy specifically addressing the relationship between PSROs and HMOs. The major areas requiring policy development are (1) delegation of review from PSROs to HMOs, (2) the delegation process, (3) the impact of review on payment, and (4) the relationship between federal, state, and the JCAH approval of an HMO's quality assurance program and PSRO delegation.

Delegation of Review from PSROs to HMOs

The previously discussed federal HMO qualification requirements will result in the performance by qualified HMOs of MCEs that are very likely to meet the requirements for delegation from a PSRO.

There are important differences, however, in the manner in which PSROs and HMOs control utilization. The HMO represents a *system of health care* that closely integrates patients and providers in a program with comprehensive benefits and defined dollar resources. Comprehensive prepaid benefits give the physician open options to utilize the services that are both least expensive and necessary to meet patient needs. Assuring the appropriate utilization of services is a day-to-day activity of each member of the HMO staff. This consistent, ongoing attention to utilization control is often, but not always, supplemented by formal utilization control programs of the type utilized by PSROs. In addition, the HMO through its budgeting process makes decisions that affect utilization. For example, an HMO may decide that the volume of surgery justifies investment in an ambulatory surgical capability to reduce the use of in-hospital surgical services.

This integrated approach to resource allocation is possible because the HMO has control over both its system of care and of financing and can, within the limits of patient satisfaction and quality control, modify the system to make it more efficient. This is an important contrast to the PSRO program that was designed to meet a narrow objective—the assurance that payment is made only when institutional services are necessary and appropriate and of acceptable quality. Whereas the HMO is an integrated system whose existence depends on each component participating in rational resource utilization, the PSRO is a review body detached organizationally from the financing and delivery of Medicare and Medicaid services. The HMO closely links delivery, financing, and resource allocation, but the PSRO does not and cannot.

In short, HMOs are at financial risk for services rendered, and PSROs are not. Whether lack of risk will be a positive or negative factor in PSRO effectiveness is conjectural. From the HMO's perspective, however, the PSRO's lack of a share in their risk will compel HMOs to continue to conduct their own review and control efforts.

The authors of the PSRO legislation recognized that HMOs did have effective utilization and quality control programs and provided in Section 1155 (e)(1) that the PSRO must allow an HMO ("other operating health care organization") to conduct review when the PSRO found it to be effective. Guidelines and regulations to help implement such delegation have not been issued. Policy discussions, however, have centered on the apparent difference between HMOs that operate their own hospitals and those that utilize the community's hospitals. In the former, delegation to the *hospital committee* follows the procedures established for PSRO delegation to any other hospital. In the latter, the approach to take to fulfill the legislative requirements is not as apparent. There is a concern about the effects of fragmenting review between the hospital or the PSRO for non-HMO patients and the HMO for its patients. If it occurred, such fragmentation could disrupt channels of reporting and increase PSRO program costs by unnecessary duplication of review and support staff.

Several points should be remembered, however. First, hospitals have become accustomed to dealing with several payment sources. Because hospitalization of an HMO member must be approved by the HMO, hospitals have established mechanisms whereby HMO patients are identified on admission, and assurances of authorization for the admission are quickly secured. As a result of this close communication between HMOs, HMO physicians, and the hospitals, it would be simple to identify patients admitted by an HMO that has received delegation and to exclude these from concurrent review by the hospital or the PSRO. Second, recent PSRO regulations encourage the "focusing" of concurrent review.[21] They call for the differentiation of hospital admissions into those requiring and those not requiring review. These regulations will stimulate the development of more sophisticated concurrent review capable of quickly identifying hospitalizations requiring varying levels of review. Even though as currently written they contemplate the development of approaches in which certain diagnoses, problems, services, or physicians may not need review, it is reasonable to extend this concept to allow consideration of HMO admissions for exclusion from review. Such exclusion could occur either by virtue of an HMO having received delegation or in the absence of delegation, because HMO hospitalizations have consistently been appropriate and necessary.

These two factors—available mechanisms that allow a hospital to quickly identify HMO admissions and regulations encouraging the development of targeted concurrent review—increase the feasibility of delegating concurrent review to those HMOs with effective hospitalization control programs, even if the HMO does not operate its own hospital.

A second concern raised by the legislative requirement to delegate review to HMOs, even when they do not operate their own hospital, is that this could lead to unnecessary duplication of review staff and thus to increased review costs. It is important to remember, however, that HMO review programs generally pertain to all members of their population, not just to Medicare or Medicaid members. Therefore, the costs that would need to be covered under delegation are only those allocated to review of the Medicare and Medicaid portion of the HMO's population.

A final concern is that of reporting requirements, both at the local PSRO level and those required of the PSROs by the DHEW. Current requirements are based on a concurrent review system oriented to the fee-for-service system of care. They may not be appropriate either for some HMO review programs or for those programs developed in response to the need to focus concurrent review. For example, HMO programs and many programs of focused review may not include preadmission or concurrent review and approval and, therefore, do not fit well within a reporting system that is based on these forms of hospital utilization review. In light of this need to recognize HMO and focused review programs, current reporting requirements must be reviewed and modified. Reporting requirements that concentrate on the outcome of review (such as admissions per 1000, bed days per 1000, average length of stay, or resource utilization during admission) rather than the process of review must be developed and tested.

Process of Delegation and Monitoring

In the preceding discussion, a case has been made that delegation to HMOs is required by law and is feasible. Yet, the requirement to delegate to a hospital, HMO, or any other organization has proved difficult to implement both from a program policy and an individual PSRO perspective.

There are two principle reasons for this difficulty. First, PSROs generally are wholly new organizations that have often been created in the face of active or passive resistance from local physicians or that have been co-opted by those interested in retaining the status quo. In both situations the organized medical staffs of local hospitals have been able effectively to resist outside PSRO review

by seeking and receiving delegation. PSROs have been reluctant to deny delegation except in those instances where it is obvious to all that review is either not being done or is clearly ineffective.

The second difficulty with the delegation provision is that methods readily to determine the effectiveness of review are lacking. Baseline data rarely exist. It is often impossible to reconstruct from medical charts whether an admission was necessary or whether discharge was unnecessarily delayed, thus making it difficult truly to measure effectiveness. Once delegation occurs, it is equally difficult to monitor performance and identify when change is necessary.

Despite these problems, HMOs and hospitals have the right to seek delegation, and PSROs are obligated to review such requests objectively and determine if delegation to the HMO is warranted.

In considering a request for delegation from an HMO, the PSRO should recognize the basic differences between HMOs and hospitals. HMOs have basic incentives to utilize hospitals appropriately, whereas hospitals have an incentive to keep beds full. Furthermore, HMOs can provide certain services either on an outpatient or inpatient basis without financial jeopardy to the patient, but physicians in fee-for-service practice often provide such services on an inpatient basis because insurance will cover it only as an inpatient. In addition, the response of some practitioners to the fee-for-service financial incentives results in unnecessary hospital utilization not present in the HMO, which lacks such incentives. These differences translate to a hospital review system that on the fee-for-service side must be most concerned with over-utilization. Given the lack of a centralized organizational focus for fee-for-service practice, the review program will need to be organized and formal. The concurrent review system described in current PSRO guidelines and proposed regulations is such a formal structured system.

In contrast to this, the HMO system is more organized. This, plus the previously noted incentives, have often resulted in the creation of less formal and less structured review programs. Often they are retrospective rather than prospective or concurrent. In contrast to review of each individual admission, the HMO's system may consist of initial screening of aggregate figures, such as admission rates and lengths of stay, followed by specific review of apparent problem areas. In concert, incentives and such review have resulted in consistent reduction of hospital bed utilization.

A PSRO must recognize these basic differences as it establishes methods and criteria for the review of delegation requests. In the case of an HMO, I suggest that the PSRO be concerned with:

    1. Does a review program, albeit informal, exist?

    2. Does the program address potential underutilization?

    3. Is the HMO program effective?

Existence of Program

The HMO's review may be relatively informal and unstructured, but a program must exist if delegation is to occur. There are a number of pertinent questions. First, are reports on utilization produced and reviewed? Second, is there evidence that review decisions are formally conveyed to medical group members? Third, are problem areas specifically addressed, and is there an assessment of the impact of attempted changes? Fourth, is there a mechanism in place to assure that Medicare or Medicaid funds are not to be expended for unapproved hospitalizations? Fifth, when the review is retrospective, do plans that call for prospective or concurrent review in situations where retrospective review determines unnecessary admissions have

occurred exist, or have they been implemented? The latter two questions require elaboration.

An HMO with good hospitalization statistics should not be required to implement prospective or concurrent review to receive delegation. Neither need there be mechanisms to recover program funds for unnecessary admissions discovered retrospectively if the HMO has a plan by which prospective and concurrent review can quickly be implemented when it is apparent that unnecessary hospitalizations are occurring. Such an approach will assure both the least disruption to an effective review program and the appropriate use of Medicare and Medicaid funds.

Underutilization of Services

Despite conceptual and practical arguments against an HMO's underutilizing the hospital, the potential exists, and the HMO's review program should address this problem. For example, the HMO might set criteria and review the health status at the time of admission for patients with diagnoses or problems frequently requiring hospitalization. This staging approach, as advocated by Gonella, holds promise for the detection of underutilization of the hospital.[22] Also, an HMO's review of the outcomes of outpatient substitutions for inpatient care (such as ambulatory surgery and home health care) would indicate its concern for identifying and dealing with underutilization.

Effectiveness of Review Program

The most important consideration in the delegation decision is the level of effectiveness of the HMO's review program. Yet, as with the PSRO's consideration of a hospital's request for delegation, this is the most difficult question to answer. There is simply no measure that can be taken that will prove or disprove the effectiveness of review. Despite this, the HMO often has population-based data on hospital utilization by payment source that hospitals do not have. This may include such measures as admission rates and bed-day utilization per 1000 enrollees. Such data can be compared with national and sometimes regional data and indicate the effectiveness of the HMO's efforts to control hospital utilization. Although it may not be possible directly to link reduced hospital utilization to the HMO's review program, such figures are useful indicators of the effectiveness of the HMO's overall efforts at utilization control. The existence of data showing reduced hospital utilization is a strong argument that delegation should occur, but the reverse is not true. The absence of any data (which will also be absent when a PSRO is reviewing a hospital for delegation) or the absence of substantial differences between the HMO's data and that of the nation or region do not constitute a reason to deny delegation, just as it has not constituted a reason to deny a hospital's delegation request. In such instances, the PSRO must rely on analysis of the HMO's review program and, as previously noted, its attention to underutilization. In short, the PSRO cannot make delegation more difficult for an HMO to secure, but it may have the unusual opportunity to review data that will provide strong rationale in favor of delegation.

Impact of Review on Payment

Another area lacking clarity is the impact of review decisions by PSROs on payment for the hospitalization of an HMO member. Where a capitation contract exists between an HMO and a Medicaid agency (for Medicare, there is only one such agreement—an experimental one), the HMO rather than the Medicaid agency or Medicare is the party directly responsible for hospital reimbursement. In the absence of delegation to the HMO, PSRO or hospital review personnel could determine that an HMO admission is inappropriate. How would such a decision affect use of Medicare and Medicaid funds? The PSRO legislation prohibits payment for admissions or continued stays that are denied by a PSRO or its delegate. This prohibition holds true without regard to the existence of a capitation agreement with an HMO. Thus, where an admission or continued stay is denied, the PSRO would notify the hospital, the patient, the HMO, and the Medicaid agency that payment could not be made for the admission. In such instances, the HMO would be prohibited from utilizing Medicaid capitation funds to reimburse for expenses incurred beyond the point of the denial and allowable grace period. That is, the review decision would be binding in this instance as in all others.

Where delegation has been given an HMO, admission of the patient would guarantee payment. In this case, as in all others where the PSRO has delegated review, the PSRO would be responsible for monitoring and periodically evaluating the HMO's performance to assure that review continues to be effective but would not overturn individual review decisions of the HMO.

As noted previously, federally qualified HMOs must as a fundamental requirement of initial and continued qualification have an ongoing quality assurance program. Site visits preceding the qualification determination include a review of the HMO's quality assurance program. However, the site visit teams have few absolute rules that guide them. Those that do exist come directly from the sections of the HMO law and regulations previously cited; therefore, a wide variety of programs can and do exist in qualified HMOs.

Many states have HMO enabling legislation under which organizations have received state HMO certification that affords them some of the advantages of federal qualification (such as dual choice) without many of the stringent requirements of the federal legislation. Many of those state statutes contain provisions that require an HMO to conduct ongoing quality assurance. Although there is no exhaustive analysis of the quality assurance provisions of state HMO laws, it is safe to assume that they vary widely.

Also, the AGPA requirements for quality assurance in ambulatory care centers are quite general, again allowing wide variation across accredited programs.

Adding these requirements from a variety of certifying and accrediting organizations to those of the PSRO program has and will continue to put HMOs in the position of trying to build quality assurance programs that respond to differing rules and guidelines. Without better coordination, the HMO will continue to face multiple site visits, varying reporting requirements, and differing forms of ongoing monitoring. At best, this will be confusing; at worst, it will be destructive to the effectiveness of the HMO's quality assurance efforts. With coordinated requirements, however, the HMO will be stimulated to conduct ongoing effective quality assurance.

Deemed Status

Therefore, it is important that those responsible for developing and implementing federal HMO, PSRO, and if possible, state HMO quality assurance requirements jointly develop mutually acceptable rules and guidelines. With such common understanding, a JCAH-accredited HMO could be deemed to meet federal and state HMO qualification requirements and PSRO delegation requirements. In the same manner, an HMO that has received PSRO delegation could be considered to have met JCAH quality assurance requirements. Recent discussions between the DHEW and the JCAH have resulted in close agreement on the major features of a *hospital quality assurance program* that would be acceptable to both the PSROs and the JCAH. The agreement is not as yet firm enough to consider providing "deemed status" for hospitals, but the agreement is so substantial that such a possibility exists. This dialogue must continue and should include a review of PSRO, HMO, and AGPA requirements for quality assurance of ambulatory care. To explore the feasibility of a common approach, I suggest the creation of a task force of the DHEW, JCAH, AGPA, federal HMO, state HMO, and individuals in PSROs and HMOs to discuss current requirements and programs with the objective of developing initial drafts of common guidelines. These could be tested in JCAH accredited, federally qualified HMOs in areas with progressive PSROs. Such an approach would be a breath of fresh air to an HMO field that is feeling overregulated by organizations and agencies that have vague but differing requirements for quality assurance.

OPPORTUNITY FOR MEANINGFUL COLLABORATION

Their concern for maximizing the return on premium dollars for their members has prompted HMOs to devise numerous mechanisms of utilization and quality control. This experience, coupled with the advantages of a defined system (unit medical records, defined population, and so forth), makes the HMO an ideal locus for testing varying mechanisms for utilization and quality control. Yet, obstacles often exist. HMOs have virtually always developed in the face of vigorous opposition from organized medicine at the community and hospital level. Fears of direct competition and less tangible concern over the development of "socialized medicine" have strained the relationship between HMO and non-HMO physicians.

As a result of statutory prohibitions against the payment of dues and against requirements for membership in other organizations, PSROs will not be an organizational component of organized medicine. Yet, the PSROs have been and will continue to be dominated by fee-for service physicians, many of whom hold deep concerns about the development of HMOs. Although statutory provisions that require delegation to HMOs will probably prevent discrimination against HMO practice by the PSROs, all parties should avoid this defensive posture and work for a relationship between PSROs and HMOs that will take advantage of the strengths of each organization.

For example, PSROs will for the first time in most communities obtain data that reflect community health care practice. This information can be of great interest to HMOs for planning purposes as well as for use in their quality assurance and research activities. Community data on the incidence of particular forms of inpatient surgery could indicate, for example, the feasibility of joint development by HMO and fee-for-service physicians of an ambulatory surgical center. Also, HMOs represent a resource to the PSRO concerning methods of utilization and quality control. For example, as PSROs attempt to focus concurrent review, they may find the experience of HMOs helpful. PSROs and hospitals could study the informal mechanisms of communication utilized by HMOs and adopt those that might assist in rationalizing utilization of expensive services. HMOs could also be used as test sites for new mechanisms of utilization control and quality assurance of interest to the PSRO.

In short, the relationship between PSROs and HMOs can be viewed as constructive for both parties. If this occurs, HMOs need not hide behind the delegation provision of the PSRO legislation, and PSROs need not feel compelled to perpetuate ongoing philosophic and practical divisions between the prepaid and fee-for-service practice models. Just as an open constructive relationship between hospitals and the PSROs will work to the benefit of

both, such a relationship will also work between PSROs and HMOs.

HMOs and PSROs are here to stay. They are becoming and will increasingly become a part of each other's lives. By each contributing to the success of the other, both organizations will benefit as will the populations they serve.

REFERENCES

1. *Professional standards review.* Oct. 1972. Public Law 92-603. Title XI, Part B, Section 1155 (e) (1).

2. *Federal register.* Oct. 18, 1974. 39 FR 37308, Section 110. 118(j).

3. *New York state HMO law.* 1976. Section 14 of the Laws of 1976.

4. Somers, A.R., editor. 1971. *The Kaiser-Permanente medical care plan; a symposium.* New York: The Commonwealth Fund, p. 17.

5. Egdahl, R.H. 1973. Foundations for medical care. *N. Engl. J. Med.* 288:491-498.

6. *National HMO Survey.* Aug. 1977. Washington, D.C.: Cooperative Effort of Group Health Association of America, American Association of Foundations for Medical Care, Blue Cross Association, and Health Insurance Association of America. Group Health Association of America.

7. Champion, H.B. Sept. 1977. *Group Health News.* vol. XVIII, No. 9. Excerpts from speech before the Group Health Institute.

8. Riedel, D.C., Walden, D.C., Singsen, A.G., et al. 1975. *Federal employees health benefits program utilization study.* DHEW Publication No. (HRA) 75-3125. Washington, D.C.: U.S. Department of Health, Education, and Welfare.

9. Gaus, D.R., Cooper, B.S., and Hirschman, C.G. 1976. Contrasts in HMO and fee-for-service performance. *Soc. Security Bull.* 39:3.

10. Wersinger, R.P., Roghmann, K., Gavett, J.W., et al. 1976. Inpatient hospital utilization in three prepaid comprehensive health care plans compared with a regular Blue Cross plan. *Med. Care* 14:721-732.

11. Dorsey, J.L., editor. 1976. How a group practice maintains its own health in a troubled economy. *Pro-*

ceedings of the Medical Directors Educational Conference. vol. I, No. 1. Washington, D.C.: Group Health Association of America, Inc.

12. Rubin, L. 1975. *Comprehensive quality assurance system. The Kaiser-Permanente approach.* Alexandria, Va.: American Group Practice Association.

13. Barr, D.M., and Gaus, C.R. 1973. A population-based approach to quality assessment in health maintenance organizations. *Med. Care* 11:523.

14. Gilson, B.S., Gilson, J.S., Bergner, M., et al. 1973. The sickness impact profile: development of an outcome approach to health care. *Am. J. Public Health* 65:1304.

15. Shroeder, S.A., and Donaldson, M.S. 1976. The feasibility of an outcome approach to quality assurance: a report from one HMO. *Med. Care* 14:49.

16. Shapiro, S. Nov. 1966. End result measurement of quality of medical care. *Conference on Appraisal of Quality and Utilization of Services.* Washington, D.C.: Program Area Committee on Medical Care Administration, American Public Health Association.

17. Mushlin, A.I., Appel, F.A., and Barr, D.M. Quality assurance in primary care: a strategy based on outcome assessment. (In press.)

18. Shapiro, S., Steinwachs, D.M., Skinner, E.A., et al. Jan. 1976. *Survey of quality assurance and utilization review mechanisms in prepaid group practice plans and medical care foundations.* Baltimore: Health Services Research and Development Center. The Johns Hopkins Medical Institutions.

19. Ryland, M.A., White, N.H., Giebink, G.A., et al. 1976. *Ambulatory care quality assurance project.* La Jolla, Calif.: Health Care Management Systems, Inc.

20. Accreditation Council for Ambulatory Health Care. 1976. *Interim accreditation manual for ambulatory health care.* Chicago: Joint Commission on Accreditation of Hospitals.

21. *Federal register.* Jan. 25, 1977. vol. 42, No. 16, Section 101.705, p. 4629.

22. Gonella, J.S., Louis, D.Z., and McCord, J.J. 1976. The staging concept—an approach to the assessment of outcome of ambulatory care. *Med. Care* 14:13-21.

BIBLIOGRAPHY

Health maintenance organizations. 1973. Public Law 93-222, Title XIII, Section 1301 (c) (8).

Professional standards review. Oct. 1972. Public Law 92-603, Title XI, Part B, Section 1155 (e) (1).

U.S. Senate. Sept. 1972. Reports of the Committee on Finance. Report 92-1230, p. 262.

19

Confidentiality Issues in the PSRO Program

Lois S. Eberhard

From the inception of the PSRO program, the confidentiality of PSRO data and information has been recognized as a complex and sensitive topic. PSROs are dependent on data to carry out their duties and functions. Documenting findings and communicating decisions are integral parts of the PSROs' primary responsibility to assure that federally funded health care is medically necessary, is at the appropriate level of care, and meets professional standards. Possession of these data and information, much of it sensitive or personal, creates a need to physically protect the information and to disclose it in a responsible manner. Thus, in defining the scope of confidentiality, one must consider acquisition of information, security (or physical protection) of information, and disclosure (or use) of information.

Although not categorized in these terms, the PSRO statute addresses each of these components of confidentiality. In the statute, PSROs are given access to medical records and other sources of information necessary for them to carry out review. Those who provide information for PSROs are excused from any liability for providing the information to PSROs. Security of information is addressed directly in terms of the need for coding the identification of individuals and indirectly by the emphasis placed on the disclosure of information. That disclosure of information was of particular concern to the Congress is evident by the devotion

of an entire section (Section 1166) of the statute entitled *Prohibition Against Disclosure of PSRO Information*. Under this section, PSRO data (or information) are to be held in confidence and not disclosed except for the purposes of the PSRO statute, for health planning and fraud or abuse purposes, or through federal regulations that must assure the adequate protection of the rights and interests of patients, health care practitioners, or providers of health care. Persons who violate this section of the statute may be subject to criminal penalties. Patient records are specifically protected from subpoena or discovery proceedings in a civil action. The overall prohibition against disclosure, coupled with a clear message that information should be disclosed for special purposes, has been the basis for many of the issues surrounding the confidentiality of PSRO information.

Based on this view of the components of confidentiality, the statutory requirements and limitations affecting confidentiality could be examined. The PSRO statute is threaded with language affecting confidentiality. In addition to the section specifically addressing the need for confidentiality, other sections impact on this topic. The purposes of the statute must be understood to determine the internal and external (to the PSRO) uses of information intended by the Congress. Requirements related to the PSRO duties and functions (such as profile analysis, examination of institutional and physician office records as source documents for the conduct of PSRO review, and the publication and dissemination of the types and kinds of cases selected for particular attention) have confidentiality implications. The responsibilities of the secretary of Health, Education, and Welfare to assure relevant data collection and maintenance of PSRO records, as well as the assessment of PSROs to assure adequate performance, also affect the confidentiality of PSRO information. From the statutory references, a number of overall objectives related to the confidentiality of PSRO information evolved. The objectives are protection of the privacy of individuals, assurance of the viability of the peer review concept and process, sharing of information with other users of health data, and assurance of PSRO and PSRO program accountability. These objectives involve both the need to protect information and at the same time the need to disclose information in a responsible manner.

In the early implementation stages of the PSRO program, the need for some specific guidance to PSROs on confidentiality of information was evident. The potential risk of criminal penalties for unauthorized disclosure prompted action. Efforts to build data systems with adequate security measures and concerns about how much information would or should be shared contributed to the development of federal policies on the confidentiality of PSRO information. These policies were limited in scope in that they addressed only information resulting from the review process and reflected the early stages of PSRO development. Over time, as knowledge and sophistication have increased, the various aspects and components of confidentiality have become more clearly defined.

Based on the view of the confidentiality of PSRO information as a comprehensive system encompassing the acquisition and generation of information, the maintenance of the security of the information, and the use of information (including disclosure for use by others), the issues that emerge are numerous. These issues tend to have legal, technical, and social dimensions, creating complexity and defying easy solutions. Legal problems surface when the PSRO statute or some other statute dictates a particular course of action. Technical problems arise when the most desirable approach is proscribed because it is not feasible. Social problems involve value judgments and frequently choices based on a democratic approach. The issues themselves are often interrelated and interdependent, presenting further complications. The objectives gleaned from the statute provide the basis and framework for developing policies on confidentiality. However, the issues related to the confidentiality of PSRO information arise in those circumstances where these objectives conflict or overlap. Most of the issues concern the disclosure of information, and certainly this is the area of greatest sensitivity. Issues related to the acquisition and security of information tend to be legal and technical in nature. Though often complex, these latter types of issues are usually more easily resolved.

In the following discussion of major issues, no attempt is made to rank the issues in importance. Neither are the issues discussed limited to those of direct concern to PSROs, although ultimately they have a direct impact on each PSRO.

DEFINITION OF CONFIDENTIAL INFORMATION

PSROs acquire and generate a great deal of information ranging in sensitivity from newspaper articles to detailed clinical information on individual patients. The exceptionally broad language of the PSRO statute declares that all information acquired by PSROs shall be held in confidence and not disclosed except for certain purposes. In the case of types of information to be disclosed for health planning and fraud or abuse purposes, the statute is quite specific. For the other two purposes—as necessary for statutory purposes and as the secretary shall provide through regulation to assure the rights and interests of patients, practitioners, or providers of health care—the statute is not specific. Classifying information as confidential and nonconfidential information is helpful in deciding how to meet these latter purposes. It is relatively easy to decide that a newspaper article should be nonconfidential and that clinical information on patients should be confidential. The difficulty begins when information is viewed by some people as nonsensitive and by others as sensitive. The problem is further compounded when viewed in the context of the usefulness of the information for other than PSRO purposes. Finding the balance on both the sensitivity factor and the "need to know" factor is the basis for many of the other issues affecting the confidentiality of PSRO information.

PROTECTION OF THE PRIVACY OF INDIVIDUALS

There is widespread agreement that the right to privacy of patients is of utmost concern. The PSRO statute protects patient records in the possession of a PSRO, a Statewide Professional Standards Review Council, or the NPSRC from subpoena or discovery proceedings in a civil action. The statute further requires that the identity of patients on PSRO reports must be in coded form.

The right to privacy of physicians and other health care practitioners is less generally accepted. On this issue, all four of the confidentiality objectives are involved. The privacy of practitioners as individual persons should be protected. The viability of peer review is seriously affected if practitioners feel threatened by the disclosure of their individual information or their judgments of their

peers, and consequently, they are reluctant to participate in the PSRO. Certainly availability of information on individual practitioners for purposes such as licensing and fraud or abuse investigations would improve the capability of these agencies to carry out their responsibilities. Arguments have been made that information on individual physicians should be available to the public for marketplace decisions and to assure that PSROs are not tolerating harmful or inadequate performance by health care practitioners. Because of widely divergent views on this issue both inside and outside the PSRO environment it is not likely to be fully resolved for some time to come.

DISCLOSURE OF INFORMATION ON INSTITUTIONS

The statute provides for the secretary of DHEW to recognize the rights and interests of institutions as well as those of patients and practitioners. Institutions and organizations, however, are not generally accorded the same rights to privacy as individuals. Nevertheless, the disclosure of certain information on institutions, particularly MCEs (medical audits), seriously erodes the peer review concept. Since PSROs are predicated on this concept, their viability is directly dependent on a healthy peer review system. The need to protect MCEs from disclosure must be weighed against the benefit that might be gained if the findings of the studies were shared.

ACQUISITION OF RECORDS FROM OTHER SOURCES

In some instances, PSROs have had difficulty gaining access to patient medical records and other source records necessary for PSROs to carry out their responsibilities. The problem occasionally arises with a delegated hospital but is more likely to arise when a physician or institution does not have patient consent to disclose the records for purposes such as review. At that point, questions of liability for unauthorized disclosure are raised. The PSRO statute authorizes the PSROs to examine records of federal beneficiaries and excuses the source from liability. But MCEs, for example, are more effective if carried out on all patients, regardless of funding source. This issue is a good example of the interrelationship of the legal, technical, and social aspects of confidentiality. It is a legal question from the point of view of the PSRO's authority to acquire records to carry out its responsibilities versus patient consent. It is a technical problem when the difficulties of acquiring patient consent are examined. It becomes a social problem when the patient's rights to privacy versus society's responsibility to assure the adequacy of health care are considered.

REDISCLOSURE OF PSRO INFORMATION

PSROs share information for a variety of purposes, such as program monitoring, the payment of claims, health planning, and fraud or abuse. The recipients of this information generally have their own rules on disclosure of information. For example, monitors and claims payors are generally subject to federal or state freedom of information statutes; Health Systems Agencies must, under their statute, make all information public. Redisclosure of PSRO information by recipients becomes an issue for two reasons. First, the unauthorized disclosure of PSRO information, regardless of who is the discloser, is subject to the criminal penalties of the PSRO statute. Second, confidential information disclosed to an agency that must make information public negates the confidentiality of the information. It is highly likely that PSRO disclosure rules and recipients' disclosure rules are different,

creating an untenable situation. In some cases the problem can be solved by limiting the types of information disclosed. In other cases it is necessary to recognize the conflicting requirements for disclosure and establish rules that apply to PSRO information regardless of its locale. The Congress took this latter approach with PSRO information disclosed for fraud or abuse purposes by placing statutory limitations on the circumstances of its redisclosure.

GOVERNMENT ACCESS TO PSRO INFORMATION

Government access to PSRO information has many facets. Unlimited access to PSRO information by the federal government is often viewed as a threat to PSRO autonomy and independence. There is genuine concern that PSRO information in the hands of the federal and state governments will be misused or, at least, misunderstood. On the other hand, the PSRO program managers have a responsibility to assure the adequate performance of the PSROs, and the federal and state governments are charged with the proper expenditure of program funds.

It can also be argued that information from the PSROs should be disclosed to assist governments in their broad responsibilities to improve the health care and services provided to all citizens. The use of the Medicare provider number (a numbering system used by the Medicare program to identify individual institutions) illustrates the interplay of these various facets and the difficult decisions required to resolve the issue.

Viewed from a privacy of individuals standpoint, it is not readily apparent that the use of a known institutional identifier may be a potential problem. However, it is possible that if the identity of an institution is known, the identity of a health care practitioner can be deduced. For example, if there is only one obstetric-gynecology practitioner in a small hospital, he or she may be implicitly identified by an examination of the diagnoses for that hospital. (It should be noted that this problem is not limited to government access but to any disclosure that includes this information.)

To continue with the illustration, the PSRO, not the government, is responsible for the performance of the institution. Government intervention could jeopardize the PSRO's authority in this area. However, governments have a strong and responsible role in monitoring PSROs' performance and expenditures. Information on known institutions improves the effectiveness of this monitoring.

Finally, the use of a known hospital identifier permits the linkage of PSRO-acquired information with other information (claims payment, for example). This capability extends the government's ability to examine and improve programs affecting the delivery and financing of health care.

Ultimately, these specific issues and others that affect the confidentiality of PSRO information will be addressed in federal regulations. The regulatory process provides an opportunity for all viewpoints to be considered and for experience and expertise to be effectively utilized. As new issues arise, and they no doubt will as the PSROs refine review responsibilities and expand or modify their information requirements, the confidentiality of PSRO information will need to be reexamined in response to the changing environment.

20

Quality Assurance–Continuing Education in a Community Hospital

Robert H. Barnes
Bruce L. Hulbert
JoAnn G. Roberts

The staff of The Doctors' Hospital in Seattle, Washington completed its first audit on hypertension in 1971. Six years later, it completed its sixtieth audit on the use of cephalosporins. During that time the staff has vacillated between a mood of support and rejection of the program. Questions have been asked: "Was the effort really worth it? What evidence do we have that patient care was improved? Wasn't traditional continuing education much easier than that linked to audit?" If audit had not been mandated by law, the hospital executive committee might have voted to abandon medical audit—too much energy required, too much money, too little payoff!

What was the problem? There were many reasons; perhaps the most basic one was that Congress passed a law mandating a monitoring system for cost control and quality assurance when the state-of-the-art was in its infancy. At The Doctors' Hospital we were in the frustrating position of implementing a program by trial and error. We had no experience in managing a hospitalwide quality assurance program. Education related to needs assessment required expertise that was generally not available.

The director of medical education was given a great deal of responsibility with little authority. A departmentalized audit program was developed with the chiefs of service responsible for completing the audits and correcting problems. Like other voluntary chiefs, they were not trained in quality assessment or educational methodology. The director of medical education also was learning the process. Expectations between clinical departments and the medical board were not clear, and the responsibilities of each concerning quality assurance were not defined.

This scenario is not unique. The staffs of many hospitals have had similar experiences and feelings. The purpose of this chapter is to describe a program called Quality Assurance–Continuing Education (QACE) developed to meet the requirements for continuing medical education for Category I relicensure, as well as those of the JCAH and the PSRO. QACE represents our attempt to build on the lessons learned during the past 6 years. In drafting the QACE program, we were particularly anxious to develop a program that was comprehensive and well managed. Furthermore, we wanted those who participated in it to feel that it was worthwhile. We endeavored to instill a spirit of trust and credibility rather than a threatening atmosphere. It was intended that this program would be linked closely to current patient care problems and to continuing education. Finally, we hoped the program ultimately would become valued by each participant and not be perceived as an unnecessary job to be done to meet external requirements.

LESSONS LEARNED

Physicians and nurses have been frustrated with the inordinate amount of time spent conducting audit studies without receiving the feedback that patients were benefited or that they themselves became better professionals. They have expressed anger at the neglect of time-honored, traditional approaches to the review of care such as clinical-pathological conferences (CPCs), mortality, and individual chart reviews. In analyzing these feelings and our experiences, we have concluded that retrospective audits, process, outcome, or combinations, are limited in their ability to measure quality of care. Even as the experience with audit accumulates and the skills and tools improve, audit has limited ability to define problems in patient care. There is a need for other approaches, including direct observation, concurrent monitoring of drugs and procedures, mortality review, and individual chart review. The first lesson seems clear; a comprehensive quality assurance program requires the documentation and use of data from multiple hospital sources. Furthermore, the closer the review process is linked to current patients, the more effective it is likely to become.

Second, we learned that if we are to use data from multiple sources, we need a hospital data management plan. Most hospitals do not have such a plan, and data are therefore fragmented, often duplicated, and not coordinated for maximum use.

Third, we learned that when voluntary physicians are confronted with information that identifies problems in suboptimal care, they do not know what their options are in solving the problem. When a course of action is decided on, they may not know how to implement the action or may be so uncomfortable with it they avoid the action.

Finally, we learned that we need to redefine the term "continuing education" for the practicing physician and link the new definition to quality assurance. The traditional image of continuing education being limited to the passive transfer of information from the expert to the learner in a formal setting has successfully blocked the realization that problem identification and problem solving represent an alternative mode of learning. Ideally, we would eliminate the labels utilization review and audit, which can produce negative feelings. Instead, we would emphasize that the staff review patient care in a variety of ways, each method being a potential learning experience. Because we decided to emphasize this approach, we called the program QACE—Quality Assurance–Continuing Education.

Taking these lessons into account, we developed a unified program with four parts:

I. Problem identification—a review process encompassing four sources of data
   A. Retrospective audits
   B. Concurrent audits
      1. Utilization review (UR)
      2. Concurrent review of known problems
      3. Infectious disease
   C. Mortality review
   D. Drug review

II. Problem solution—options for corrective action
III. Hospital data management plan
IV. Linking of quality assurance and continuing education

Selection of Sources of Data

Many sources of information in the hospital can form the basis of a comprehensive quality review program. There are so many, in fact, that one has to be selective and choose those sources that are most likely to be valid and will yield the greatest payoff in describing patient care. At The Doctors' Hospital, a 183-bed community hospital, we listed the following possible sources of data:

1. Justification for admission to hospital
2. Length of stay
3. Reason for continued and prolonged stay
4. Total number of patient days
5. Daily census
6. Medical care evaluation studies (MCEs)
7. Mortality review
8. Tissue review
9. Review of use of blood
10. Review of drugs
11. Review of cancer
12. Data regarding infection
13. Running list of surgical procedures, time in surgery, names of members of surgical teams, and so forth
14. Monthly reports from standing committees and clinical departments to executive committee and board of directors:
    a. Clinical departments—medicine, surgery, obstetrics, pediatrics, and so forth
    b. Clinical committees—coronary care unit, intensive care unit, emergency room, respiratory unit, and so forth
    c. Pharmacy and therapeutic committee
    d. Credentials and privileges committee
15. Nursing service, including nurse audits

We felt it was not possible to utilize all of these sources; however, over a period of time using the data we did select, we felt we could build a comprehensive program. As we gain experience managing data from several major sources, we will include others. As mentioned, we initially selected retrospective and concurrent audits as two sources of data, along with mortality and drug reviews.

In reviewing our past experiences at The Doctors' Hospital, we believed that mortality review was inefficient and ineffective and that a new method needed to be developed. Previously there had been no systematic plan to monitor the daily use of drugs. There was also a general consensus among the members of the utilization review committee that their activities had not contributed much to either the quality of patient care or to the proper use of the hospital. A new approach to accomplish their objectives was needed. Therefore, a new approach to mortality and UR was instituted, and a drug review program was developed. A brief description of each follows.

Mortality Review

An analysis of the previous method showed that in the Department of Medicine a mortality committee reviewed the deaths quarterly, which meant that a large stack of charts accumulated in the record room. On a crisis basis several days before a monthly clinical committee meeting, two or three physicians waded through the pile, asking only one question, "Was death justified?" Usually out of this large pile, several questionable cases were presented at the committee meeting. When the minutes of these meetings were reviewed, it was difficult to find any specific action taken or, if an action was recommended, that it was implemented. The surgical committee reviewed deaths monthly, but there was little evidence that any concrete action resulted from the review. Most physicians interviewed who had served on the mortality review committee felt it was not a worthwhile procedure.

The new approach highlights the use of a clinical staff nurse who screens all deaths within 24 hours using questions developed by the staff. These questions not only ask if death was justified but further inquire about the quality of dying. (See the boxed material on p. 190).

The procedure can be summarized as follows:

1. If the nurse has a question concerning the quality of care, a physician advisor is called to review the case. If a surgical patient died for nonsurgical reasons, the physician advisor is instructed to call in the appropriate specialist for further review.

2. If the physician advisor feels there is a problem in quality of care, the case is referred to the quality assurance–continuing education committee for review and recommendation.

3. If the QACE committee agrees that there is a problem, the case is referred to the appropriate clinical service.

4. The action taken by the clinical chief and his committee is reported both to the executive committee and to the QACE committee.

Utilization Review

In the past, the UR committee had listened to a statistical report from the UR nurse on the number of Medicare and Medicaid admissions, the number of reviews by physician advisors, and information regarding lengths of stay according to the fiftieth, seventy-fifth, and ninetieth percentiles. Occasionally, there was a chart to be reviewed when the insurance intermediary questioned a claim. The consensus was that the meeting was seldom worthwhile. The goal of the committee to assure optimal patient care and efficient utilization of the hospital facilities was not being achieved. To address this goal, the committee decided to review a representative sample of charts each month where the length of stay was either greater than the ninetieth percentile or was a short stay of 1 or 2 days. The ninetieth percentile was selected because of the potentially high payoff in identifying patient care problems. The long-stay patients generally have the most severe problems and complications. The short-stay patients were selected because they are usually not reviewed by the UR coordinator. There is a large volume of them, and such charts provide an opportunity to evaluate possible underutilization of the facilities or inappropriate admissions.

A chart is assigned to each member of the UR committee, who summarizes it and identifies problems. Where criteria are available from previous audits, they are used. Otherwise the review is subjective, and a final opinion is dependent on consensus of the group. The committee identifies problems but does not attempt to solve them.

Problems identified by the UR committee most often reflect the care provided by one physician for one patient. This information is sent to the chief of service for action by his committee. If the UR committee feels the problem involves more than one physician, a memo is sent to the QACE committee, recommending it as a topic for in-depth review.

An example of this involved a patient who developed convulsions while on aminophylline therapy. The drug dosage had not been monitored with blood levels. The committee felt that failure to monitor the use of aminophylline was a common problem and referred the topic to QACE for an

SCREENING PROCEDURE
FOR
DEATH REVIEW

LOS_____Chart No._____

Questions	Comments
1. Was patient's condition on *admission* such that death was anticipated? Examples: severe heart disease or failure, COPD with lung failure, renal failure, advanced cancer. 2. Did a complication related to treatment develop, resulting in death? Examples: hemorrhage secondary to use of antibiotics, drug reaction leading to renal shutdown, infection following surgery (peritonitis), death associated with anesthesia. 3. Did the patient die during or within 48 hours after surgery? 4. If the patient was terminally ill on admission, was hospitalization justified? 5. In your opinion, was treatment excessive? Examples: use of blood, antibiotics, cortisone, consultants for each body system. 6. Was pain controlled? Did the physician order prn medication in a hopeless case with severe pain, or was medication given in anticipation of pain? 7. Did the primary condition plus secondary diagnoses justify death? 8. In your opinion, what was the factor(s) that caused death (may not be necessarily disease oriented)? 9. Based on your evaluation, would you recommend further review of this death?	

audit study in addition to sending a memo to the chief of the medical service.

Drug Utilization Review

It is not the purpose of this chapter to describe in detail how to review drugs in a community hospital. We are developing such a program and linking it to the comprehensive QACE program as a crucial source of information. The pharmacy will collect data by documenting daily patient drug profiles, including an adverse reaction detection and prevention program. Both the clinical pharmacist and the pharmacy and therapeutic committee will review these data to identify problems in drug usage. Similar to the UR committee, problems identified involving one physician are referred to the proper clinical service for action, and topics for further in-depth audit study are referred to the QACE committee.

Retrospective Audits

The QACE committee is now responsible for completing the required number of audits. In the past The Doctors' Hospital had a departmental program. The executive committee decided to shift the responsibility for completing all the audits to one central group representing each clinical department and the nursing staff. The change was made to improve the quality of the audits and to reduce the time required to complete them.

To emphasize the educational aspects of the audit process, before adopting criteria for a new topic, the director of medical education mails to each member of the committee one or two articles from the medical literature. At the first audit meetings a specialist speaks briefly on the topic and answers questions. He or she also acts as the screening physician and is an important resource when

variations are discussed. The director of medical education uses not only the data generated, but also the substance of the discussions in developing educational programs for departmental or staff meetings.

PROBLEM SOLUTION

The QACE program establishes a clear demarcation between the responsibility for *identifying* problems in suboptimal patient care and the responsibility for *correcting* those problems. The corrective action role is the prerogative of the clinical chief of service and his or her committee. The ability to meet the responsibility as a chief of service depends greatly on the chief receiving valid data from the various hospital sources that describe patient care.

After deciding on an action plan, the chief of service may delegate its implementation to others. For example, deciding that a departmental educational program is needed, the chief of service could ask the QACE committee and the director of medical education for assistance. If the chief of service decides that a discussion with the involved physician is in order, the chief may personally talk with the physician and not involve anyone else. Sanctions against any physician must be referred to the executive committee for final approval.

Figure 20-1 shows the delineation between the two roles of problem identification and problem solution. The dotted line from the clinical department to the UR, QACE, and pharmacy committees indicates the capabilities of these groups to implement actions.

HOSPITAL DATA MANAGEMENT PLAN

Most hospitals do not have a plan to integrate and utilize the multiple sources of data regarding pa-

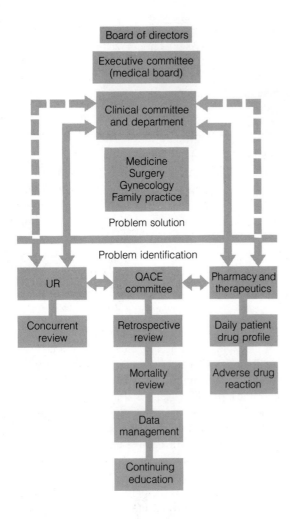

FIGURE 20-1. Hospital data management plan.

1. Bacteriology laboratory
2. Hospital epidemiologist
3. Infectious disease committee
4. Medical audit
5. Utilization review

In a recent study at one community hospital, a retrospective review of the complications of emergency colon surgery indicated an unusually high postoperative wound infection rate. In spite of this unacceptably high rate of infection, none of the sources that usually generate data regarding infections had reported the problem to the chief of surgery or the executive committee. Postoperative wound infections increase the length of hospital stay and thus escalate costs. A fragmented data system failed to identify the problem in a timely fashion and correct it. The QACE program represents our attempt to remedy the problem of uncoordinated patient care information.

The key elements of the QACE program are:

1. A central QACE committee is headed by a physician (at The Doctors' Hospital it is the director of medical education) and supported by a record technician and a secretary.

2. All data from a variety of hospital sources are channeled through the QACE committee for assessment and coordination.

3. A master display of all data and their status is kept.

4. Chairmen of committees, chiefs of service and staff, and members of the board receive data regularly on quality of care and utilization of facilities. Their monthly meetings focus on problems identified by data.

Finally, the QACE committee is responsible for following up on decisions for action made by

tient care. As a result, fragmentation usually results. Data may be inadequate, sometimes invalid, usually uncoordinated, and frequently poorly utilized. Prevention and control of hospital infections are examples. Data may come from the following possible sources:

chiefs of service and committee chairmen, to determine if they were implemented and effective. One of the major stumbling blocks to improving patient care through the review process is the failure to act when a problem is identified. For example, as a result of an audit on ulcerative colitis, the medical committee decided an education program for patients at time of discharge was needed. This decision went into the minutes of the medical committee. The chief of service assumed the nursing department would develop a protocol. There was no follow-up to implement the decision. One year later it was still a decision recorded in the minutes, but no action had been taken. From our experience, many decisions and recommendations often fall through cracks in the system.

The QACE committee meets twice monthly and reviews data from the various hospital sources. When problems are forwarded from the QACE committee to the appropriate chief of service, the chief responds by exercising one of the following options:

1. The department committee decides it is not a problem.
2. The committee decides it is a problem.
   a. The chief or the chief's delegate informally speaks to the attending physician regarding the care. Where two or three physicians are affected, the chief and director of medical education plan action.
   b. The topic is referred to the QACE committee as a possible subject for staff or departmental educational program.
   c. The decision is delayed to allow the chief to discuss the problem at the medical board or to obtain more information.
   d. Sanctions are recommended to the medical board.

LINKING QUALITY ASSURANCE AND CONTINUING EDUCATION

The idea of linking education to quality assurance is not new. This linkage has been fundamental to the philosophy of audit; however, the task of accomplishing it is sizable. In QACE we have begun to evolve a program that emphasizes learning by active participation in problem solving. The problem with most audit programs has not been in identifying problems in patient care but in assuring a change in behavior when needed. The aim of QACE is to identify performance problems and develop new approaches to the complex problem of improving performance.

CURRENT STATUS

The QACE program recently has been approved by the Washington State Medical Association Committee on Continuing Education for credit toward the AMA's Category I. The QACE program has contributed to an improved attitude of the staff toward the review of care. The comprehensive nature of the program in coordinating data from multiple sources has relieved the conflict physicians have felt about retrospective audits being the major, or only way, of assessing quality of care. Furthermore, the concurrent review of care in the UR committee is now affecting the care of patients presently in the hospital or those recently discharged. The committee has found that care seldom is ideal and that lessons learned from the review of care can benefit all the staff. The emphasis on the review of care as an important learning experience is gaining acceptance.

The QACE program provides a feedback loop to the various committees generating data that describe suboptimal care. For example, the UR and QACE committees receive a regular monthly report on the actions taken by the clinical committees on the problems referred to them (see boxed material below).

The new approach to mortality review reveals questions about the care of the dying patient that previously were not asked. For example, it usually was justified for a terminally ill patient to be admitted to the hospital from a nursing home. Now, the QACE committees receive a regular monthly re-priate. Medical deaths in the surgical department are reviewed by both internists and surgeons serving on the QACE committee. Previously they were reviewed only by the surgical department. The chiefs of service and their committees were angry at first and overwhelmed by the data sent to them requiring action. Recently, they have asked for help in interpreting data and planning departmental meetings to deal with problems. They frequently seek further information and are anxious to follow up on the effectiveness of their action.

The development of the hospital data management plan continues to evolve. Keeping track of problems identified by multiple groups, and subsequently the action taken, will continue to pose a major challenge to the QACE program.

We continue to gain new insights in linking quality assurance to continuing education. The staff is accustomed to weekly formal educational programs rather than active participation in problem solving. We continue to develop traditional continuing education programs but also seek new ways to emphasize the learning process of small groups solving patient care problems. We are developing an evaluation plan for the QACE program. This plan will help pinpoint problems in quality assessment and quality assurance based on

Quality Assurance Monthly Report   Date _____

Data Source	Medicine Department	Surgery Department	Gynecology Department
Mortality			
Pharmacy			
Utilization Review			
Tumor Board			
QACE Committee			

better understanding of the specific roles and responsibilities. The hospital data management system enables us to link problem identification and problem solution activities at The Doctors' Hospital.

SUMMARY

A comprehensive, coordinated quality assurance–continuing education program in a community hospital has been presented. We emphasized the importance of using a variety of hospital data sources in assessing the quality of patient care. A clear distinction was made between the responsibility of those who identify problems through the review process and those who solve problems. The need for a hospital data management system was underscored as well as the need to equate problem identification and problem solving with continuing education. Finally, we stated that the QACE concept gives us an opportunity to evaluate the effect of the program on patient care.

BIBLIOGRAPHY

Barnes, R.H. 1976. The evaluation of hospital medical staff performance: does health care review help? *AHME*.

Jacobs, C.M., Christoffel, T.H. and Dixon, N. 1977. *Measuring the quality of patient care: the rationale for outcome audit.* Cambridge, Mass.: Ballinger Publishing Co.

Miller, G.E. 1975. Why continuing medical education? *Bull. N.Y. Acad. Med.* 51:701–788.

Sanazaro, P.J. Sept. 1976. Medical audit: continuing medical education and quality assurance. *West. J. Med.* 125:241–252.

21

Quality Assurance–Continuing Education Model for Rural Hospitals in the Northwest

Robert H. Barnes

Medical care is no longer a privilege but a right, and no longer is it just a right, but care received must be of high quality and reasonable cost. Federal and state governments have initiated sizable efforts to monitor both the quality and cost of care. Blanket regulations have been imposed on all hospitals, regardless of their size, resources, or location. Furthermore, many state governments now require mandatory continuing education for physician relicensure. These regulations raise new problems for the medical staff, administrators, and boards of directors of all hospitals and have created some unique problems for small, isolated, rural hospitals.

In the Pacific Northwest small rural hospitals represent up to 50% of the total number of acute-care facilities. Of the 113 hospitals in the state of Washington, 40 have less than 50 beds, the great majority of which are located a considerable distance from a major metropolitan area. Oregon, Idaho, Montana, and Alaska present a similar picture, with nearly one half of all hospitals conforming to the general description of small, isolated facilities, many of which are struggling to survive financially. It has long been recognized that certain characteristics of rural hospitals make them different from urban ones. Two obvious differences are

the smaller number of beds and the staff size. Economic reasons may permit only one or a few physicians to locate in a rural setting and may make the small hospital a tenuous financial enterprise. In addition to the problem of geographic remoteness, there is professional isolation as well. Local continuing education programs linked to patient care problems are practically nonexistent. It is often difficult to obtain consultation, particularly for emergencies, and demand on the physician's time may be crushing. There is not the constant stimulus of ideas found in teaching centers or the sharing of knowledge between colleagues that is so typical of the doctor's lounge in the large urban hospital. If a key nurse gets sick or goes on vacation, there may be no replacement. The hospital often lacks trained staff to abstract and display data from charts. The medical staff may not have the time, skills, or motivation to develop and implement a quality assurance–continuing education program.

Specifically, the MCEs required by the PSRO and the JCAH have limited value in the rural hospital because of the small sample size of patients and limited number of procedures. Because this method of reviewing care has required a great deal of effort with minimal payoff in terms of education and improved patient care, many physicians have a negative attitude toward reviewing care. Alternatives to this procedure are needed. The roles and responsibilities of the administrator, the organized medical staff, and the governing board have not been well defined with respect to quality assurance. Trustees in particular are not familiar with the kind of information they should receive regularly from the medical staff to enable them to make informed policy decisions concerning the quality of care their hospital is providing.

My experience in rural hospitals further underscores the need for training physicians to develop, manage, and interpret multiple sources of data about individual patients as well as patterns of patient care. Even when deficiencies in care are identified, often there is no plan to implement corrective measures. Peer review in rural areas is clearly more difficult than in larger urban areas because of the closeness of the small number of physicians to each other.

Not surprisingly, many small, isolated hospitals feel that they are unable to handle the requirements for reviewing care, let alone the immense problem of providing adequate and appropriate continuing education for their physicians. Among the additional problems they see confronting them are the following:

1. The medical staff may not be comfortable in setting its own criteria for care or modifying sets of national or regional standards.
2. Even when the medical staff is dealing with common diagnoses or frequent routine procedures, the number of cases is small, making evaluation, detecting trends, and noting changes in behavior difficult.
3. Because of low occupancy and a limited budget, the small hospital may find it difficult to budget support for quality assurance activities.

4. A small staff may feel social and psychologic pressures that prevent them from sanctioning a peer who is also a friend and neighbor.
5. Geographic isolation may make it difficult to acquire the assistance needed to develop and implement new programs.
6. Limited health manpower may make it difficult to plan time away from the hospital for educational purposes.
7. The staff may not solve patient care problems identified by audit because of:
   a. Difficulty in one physician communicating with another where criticism is involved.
   b. Inability of a staff to improve the skills or change the attitudes of a peer.
   c. Lack of skills in changing patterns of care versus an individual case.

During the past 3 years, the Health Care Review Center has worked with nine rural hospitals to help them develop a meaningful medical audit process through the Tele-Audit Program (see Appendix C). These nine hospitals in central Washington vary in size from an institution with 16 beds and two staff physicians to facilities with 50 beds and 12 physicians. My experience with these hospitals has taught me the following:

1. The classic medical care evaluation study is of limited value in the small rural hospital. Alternative approaches to quality assurance need to be developed.
2. Peer review is difficult in a small group of rural physicians. Discussions about suboptimal care can create a threatening environment, disruptive to the normal support physicians provide each other.
3. It is difficult to obtain patient care data from sources other than MCEs, that is, phar-

macy, pathology, mortality review, or utilization review.

4. Once problems in patient care are identified, the skills and motivation to correct them may be lacking.

PROBLEM STATEMENT

The federal and state governments and insurance intermediaries require all hospitals to review the justifications for admissions to the hospital and prolonged stays in the hospitals as well as the quality of patient care rendered. The regulations do not take into account the unique characteristics of small rural hospitals previously described. A rural hospital quality assurance–continuing education (QACE) model needs to be developed. The lessons learned from such a model could be used to modify appropriately the regulations affecting these hospitals. At present there is a negative attitude by the practicing physician toward the mandated review of care because the amount of effort expended seems out of proportion to the small patient benefit. This is at least in part due to inappropriate methods of quality assurance being applied. Alternatives to present methods need to be developed. My experience teaches me that present patient care information is not only fragmented and incomplete but is often invalid. To improve patient care and control costs, the hospital staff needs appropriate and valid data and an information management plan to make better decisions. An effective model will include training of administration, medical staff, and governing body.

Many state governments require mandatory continuing medical education for relicensing of physicians. This regulation is especially threatening to the isolated rural physician. The proposed model for quality assurance would be closely linked to continuing education to meet this need of rural physicians. The physician would receive hour-for-hour credit toward relicensure by participation in the program.

PROGRAM GOALS AND OBJECTIVES

I. To construct a rural hospital model for quality assurance–continuing education
   A. Develop alternative methods of review more suitable to rural hospital settings: drug and mortality review and the use of nonspecific indicators.
   B. Integrate the patient care information obtained by review procedures into a management plan that will assure identification of suboptimal patient care and corrective action.
   C. Strengthen the communication link among administration, governing body, and the medical staff so that quality assessment will lead to quality assurance.
II. To train key staff in rural hospitals to review care
   A. Specify roles and responsibilities of: chief of health care review, coordinator of health care review, administrator, and trustees regarding the review of patient care.
   B. Conduct initial on-site training sessions for key staff just specified.
III. To develop a support system that assists in reviewing care and planning corrective actions
   A. Collaborative link with the School of Pharmacy and Drug Information Service.
   B. Role of Health Care Review Center as coordinator/manager of review activities and continuing medical education activities for the Central Washington Consortium of Hospitals.

IV. To evaluate the impact of this quality assurance–continuing education model.

    A. Assess the capability of the QACE model to identify and correct important problems in patient care, both in terms of patterns and individual practice.

    B. Assess the attitudes of participating physicians, nurses, administrators, and trustees toward this QACE model.

    C. Identify the unique constraints and capabilities of rural hospitals to review care, including critical mass of people, methods, and data to meet present regulations.

    D. Disseminate results of demonstration project to the Washington State PSRO, the Washington State Medical Association, the JCAH, and the HSQB.

CONSTRUCTING RURAL HOSPITAL MODEL FOR QUALITY ASSURANCE – CONTINUING EDUCATION

The ideal of a workable rural hospital QACE model is based first on the premise that valid data that describe patient care are available from a variety of sources within the hospital. Second, these data are displayed in a unified way for a review group. Third, this review group interprets the data to identify problems in patient care and makes recommendations to the staff for correction. Fourth, the group develops an implementation plan for the corrective action. Fifth, it determines a plan to evaluate the outcome of the action.

Development of Valid Data

The review processes, which have produced descriptive data in the past, have come from MCEs, admissions, continued-stay review, and mortality review. In this proposed model the use of "nonspecific indicators" to screen charts for possible patient care problems and the regular review of prescribed drugs are the main methods being developed as alternatives to past ones. Admissions review would be continued but on a selective basis, where problems with an individual physician are discovered by screening charts with "nonspecific indicators" or where a particular diagnosis or procedure is a known problem. As stated before, MCEs have limited value in the rural hospital; therefore, such a study would be done only when a problem has been identified by one of the other review procedures. It might be that in any given year, none, one, or two MCEs would be done. This would further help to avoid all the work involved when medical care evaluation study shows no problems. Even though there is value in documenting good care, this can seem purposeless to a staff after a few "no problem" MCEs.

Non-Specific Indicators

The use of "nonspecific indicators" is a part of the review process in which a list of key questions is applied to each chart concurrently to seek out potential or possible patient care problems that might not be detected otherwise. Some of these key questions might be:

    1. Did the patient die?

    2. Did the patient stay in the hospital 1 day?

    3. Did the patient stay in the hospital longer than the ninetieth percentile?

    4. Was only 1 unit of blood given?

    5. Did the patient receive an antibiotic without a diagnosis of an infection, or with no fever or culture?

    6. Did the patient return to surgery during the same admission?

    7. Did the patient return to the hospital within 2 weeks after discharge?

8. Did tissue review justify the surgery?

9. Did tissue review show a postoperative diagnosis consistent with the preoperative diagnosis?

There are other nonspecific indicators, but these are offered as examples. At the time of discharge these charts would be tagged by the record room. Occasionally the review of such charts would identify a topic for an in-depth review by medical care evaluation study, or it would identify a drug needing review. Mortality is included as a nonspecific indicator but would be reviewed in a more meaningful way than in the past. (See Appendix D for a modified way of improving the review of deaths.)

Because 1-day stays constitute approximately 25% of all rural hospital admissions among the central Washington consortium, the PSRO must negotiate the options in reviewing this large group of patients with the hospitals. Screening criteria must be adopted. The utilization review nurse would screen these admissions using the criteria. Any exceptions to the criteria would be reviewed by a physician advisor. The review committee then could review two randomly selected 1-day charts each month.

Patients staying beyond the ninetieth percentile are automatically reviewed by the utilization review nurse. Where there is a problem, a physician advisor is called. Each month the review committee could review two charts in this category, asking not only if the stay was justified but if a complication occurred, could it have been prevented, and was it properly managed? In the past most hospital committees have only asked if the stay was justified.

Management Plan

An example of what might be worked out with the hospitals is as follows: Each month the utilization review nurse and the record room would refer the following charts for review: (1) the deaths (usually one or two), (2) two 1-day stays, (3) two ninetieth-percentile stays, and (4) any charts identified by other nonspecific indicators. In any particular month, if a medical care evaluation study or an in-depth drug review is completed, this might be substituted for the activities just mentioned.

Forms to report these activities to both the executive committee and the board of trustees would be developed. These would document the charts reviewed, problems identified, decisions made to correct problems, and how and by whom the decisions would be implemented. Finally, a time to reevaluate the results of the action would be stated. The record room would be responsible for these. The hospital administration would receive a copy and would take an active part, along with the chief of staff, in seeing that once problems are identified, they are indeed corrected.

In the smaller hospitals the review committee would be the entire staff; in others a standing committee appointed for 1 year would do the work and make recommendations to the executive committee or the staff. (See Figure 21-1.)

Continuing Education

Continuing education is closely linked to the whole process. By definition, criteria setting, chart reviews, problem identification, and problem solving are parts of continuing education.

Drug Review in Rural Hospitals

Drug interaction and inappropriate use constitute a major hazard to the patients. There has been no plan in rural hospitals to monitor and evaluate the use of drugs. To do this locally would require personnel and skills not ordinarily available. I believe that a plan to review drugs has a high probability of

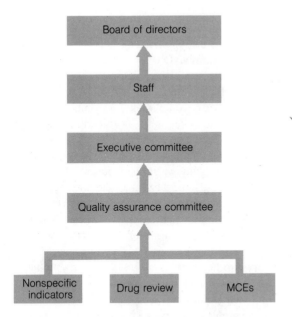

FIGURE 21-1.   Flow of patient care information.

improving the quality of care and reducing costs in the rural hospital. Because of the lack of a clinical pharmacist and local expertise to correct problems identified, this project seeks ways to overcome these barriers through linkage of the rural hospitals to an outside support system, for example, the School of Pharmacy, the University of Washington, and the Health Care Review Center.

A two-part program is planned for evaluating drugs in seven to ten rural hospitals.

Part One

STEP ONE A 3-month prospective display of drugs commonly prescribed in the hospitals would be made. The approach would be selective, focusing on drugs according to the following headings:

1. Expensive drugs
   a. High unit cost
   b. High rate of use
2. Drugs with high potential for inappropriate use
3. Drugs with high potential for adverse clinical consequences

STEP TWO Four drugs would be selected from lists obtained under step one to be reviewed during the first year.

STEP THREE In conjunction with the School of Pharmacy, resource physician specialists (both of which are at the University of Washington School of Medicine), and private practitioners, criteria would be developed for the appropriate use of the first 4 drugs.

STEP FOUR The criteria would be mailed with representative samples of the medical literature to the chief of staff of each hospital. The chief of staff would distribute copies of these to staff members for study before the first Tele-Audit conference.

STEP FIVE The initial Tele-Audit program would be planned and scheduled: (1) to discuss the use of the drug by the resource specialist and clinical pharmacist, and (2) to obtain agreement on the criteria.

STEP SIX Data on the use of the drug would be collected both retrospectively and concurrently. The data would most likely be collected on concurrent usage because of the difficulty in identifying patients who have received the drug in the past. A data display sheet would be developed in cooperation with the School of Pharmacy and the Health Services Research Center. An appropriate person would be trained at each rural hospital to accurately document the data on a daily basis.

STEP SEVEN Each hospital would mail the data display sheets to the Health Care Review Center. Review of the data display sheets would be done by the staff of the School of Pharmacy, the Health Care Review Center, and the resource specialist.

Variations from optimal care would be identified.

STEP EIGHT A second Tele-Audit conference would be held to discuss problems in the use of the drugs. This would include both cost and quality. Agreement on problems and corrective action would be obtained.

STEP NINE Concurrent monitoring of the drug would take place, and the hospital staff would receive feedback whether or not the problems had been corrected. This would be done by mail, telephone calls, Tele-Audit conferences, or by a combination of these.

The cycle of data collection, agreement on criteria and problems, and how the data are to be collected for three or four commonly used drugs would be completed during the first year. During the second and third years, this process would be stepped up to evaluate the use of five or six drugs each year, so that at the end of 3 years, between 13 and 15 drugs would be evaluated with a final analysis of the change in prescription habits and costs.

Part Two

Daily patient care profile sheets would be monitored concurrently. Once a week the daily drug profile sheets would be mailed to the School of Pharmacy for evaluation by a clinical pharmacist. The pharmacist would look for combinations of drugs that are potentially incompatible and that might cause adverse drug reactions. An example might be the simultaneous use of phenylbutazone (Butazolidin) with warfarin (Coumadin) sodium, which increases the hazard of hemorrhage. The School of Pharmacy would develop a select list of drug combinations that are known to be a national problems. Habit patterns of prescription writing that adversely affect patients could be spotted and reported to the staff. A discussion of any problem could be included in the Tele-Audit conference. Continued monitoring would determine whether or not the problem had been corrected.

IV

POTENTIAL

22

Nursing Care Evaluation

Sharon V. Davidson

EVOLUTION OF NURSING CARE EVALUATION

The evaluation of nursing care is thought of as a current concept. However, one of the original evaluations of medical and nursing care and its impact on recipients can be found in *Notes on Matters Effecting the Health, Efficiency, and Hospital Administration of the British Army,* published by Florence Nightingale in 1858. This work included comparing mortality experienced in the British Armed Forces during the Crimean War with experience in the civilian population. This work possibly brought to the attention of the government and the public the atrocious standards of care for military personnel, although by today's standards the data are crude. The report was nevertheless instrumental in bringing about basic reforms in living standards and health services in the British Armed Forces.

The evaluation of nursing care is an evolutionary process. The beginning of modern evaluation of nursing care focused on hospital environment. If the appropriate amount of equipment was present at the right time in the correct place, it was believed that high-quality nursing care was being rendered. Following the evaluation of the environment, organizational standards were examined within a hospital. For example, were medications given at the same time on each unit? Were the ratios of registered nurses to licensed practical nurses to nursing assistants to patients appropriate for adequate patient care? From these considerations, the educational requirements for the nurse were examined. If the nurse had the appropriate licensure credentials, it was assumed that the nurse would be administering adequate quality patient care.

JCAH

As the evolutionary process continued, the JCAH began to survey and encourage the nurses to evaluate the impact of nursing on the patient. They worked in probabilities or outcomes. It was no longer a "yes, they did" or "no, they didn't" situation. For example, some might say "yes, medication was passed on time," or "no, medications were not passed on time." "Outcome" was now the key word. Did the medication have a positive or negative effect on the total outcome of the patient? The JCAH brought with it retrospective reviews of nursing care through the use of process, structure, or outcome criteria for the evaluation of nursing care. They hoped to find through the audits patterns of nursing care based on validated criteria. No longer was there to be a subjective evaluation by one nurse of another nurse's nursing care. Instead, criteria were to be established that would be objective, that could be applied to the medical record following discharge of the patient, and a judgment could be rendered about the quality of care that was being provided patients within a given institution. The JCAH retrospective audits were originally developed for the physician who has primary responsibility for the care of the patient on a 24-hour basis. After the development of the retrospective audit for the physician, it was modified and applied to the evaluation of nursing care. It was appropriate in some places; however, the registered nurses work as members of a team. They do not have responsibility on a 24-hour basis for the patient. They share that responsibility with numerous other nurses on three shifts. The nursing service assumes responsibility on a 24-hour basis, and because of this, retrospective review of nursing care is not necessarily the best way to evaluate the provision of nursing care. A concurrent review of nursing care would lead to the improvement of care while the patient was still hospitalized. This concept is not to be confused with the JCAH process audit, and it can be completed on a concurrent basis. The JCAH had an emphasis and a responsibility in helping the professional nurse to begin to look at the impact of nursing care on the patient and to begin to question how nursing makes a difference. How can one measure nursing care, and how can one prove to administration, physicians, and other health care members that nursing is an important aspect in assisting the patient to achieve his desired outcomes?

PSRO

With the passage of PL 92-603, an emphasis was placed not only on the cost containment of medical care but on the quality of medical care being rendered. Even though the PSRO, primarily made up of physicians, M.D.s and osteopaths, considered involvement of nonphysician health care practitioners in the PSRO review, nursing was slow to respond. Section 730 of the *PSRO Program Man-*

ual speaks to the involvement of nonphysician health care practitioners and PSRO review:

Health care is provided by practitioners of a wide variety of health care disciplines. Review of care provided by non-physician health care practitioners should be performed by their peers. Thus the PSRO retains ultimate responsibility for the decisions made under its aegis. It should seek the participation of all health care practitioners in the development of criteria, standards, and the selection of norms for their professions in the establishment of mechanisms to review the care provided by each type of practitioner and in the actual review of that care. The PSRO's formal plan shall contain a plan for the involvement of nonphysician health care practitioners in the PSRO review system.

Perhaps unknowingly in the evolutionary process of the evaluation of nursing care, the PSRO in its guidelines provided a blueprint to the nurse for the development of a nursing care evaluation system. Components of this system included a review mechanism based on criteria, norms and standards, continuing education tied to the result of the auditing, a review process that would parallel and complement the one already set up for the physicians, and profile analysis that would allow for a comparative study from several institutions of the quality of nursing care within local areas. [PSRO influence came after the JCAH, which was already strongly imbedded, decreed that there would be retrospective review of nursing care.] Many institutions nationwide had begun to develop through their nursing service personnel criteria for the retrospective review of nursing care. The JCAH had provided numerous conferences for teaching nurses how to develop retrospective review criteria, audit their work, and utilize the forms that were available from the JCAH for nursing audit. When PSROs began, their impact required that the profession of nursing take another look at the auditing of nursing care and see what the key concepts were that should be included and how they could be included in the review of the quality of nursing care.

PURPOSE OF NURSING CARE EVALUATION

As the evolutionary process continued, the purpose of nursing care evaluation was examined. The result was a systematic approach to the evaluation of nursing care that not only would be compatible with the goals of the PSRO but would be a benefit to patients based on the concept of peer review and would encompass the principles of nursing quality assurance.

Nursing quality assurance can therefore be defined as a commitment to excellence in the delivery of health care. It is a program designed to determine the extent to which a specific nursing practice achieves selected objectives (criteria based on specified values). These specified values are then measured in terms of predetermined standards. Analysis of data collected exposes deficiencies or variations in nursing care. Continuing education programs can then be implemented to correct these variations and upgrade professional performance. Reevaluation will reveal the changes in professional behavior achieved through nonpunitive, educational measures. The overall effectiveness of the nursing quality assurance program and the identification of review priorities will be realized through profile analysis.

BENEFITS OF QUALITY ASSURANCE PROGRAM

With the great deal of work that goes into the development of nursing quality assurance, it is necessary to identify whether there are any benefits of a quality assurance program. Benefits realized could include: improvement of patient care; demonstration of deficiencies in hospitalwide policies or procedures; encouragement of coordination of physician-nurse planning for patient care; improvement of communication with other hospital departments or services; provision of better documentation of patient care; provision of direction for educational programs, pointing out where additional facilities, equipment or personnel are needed; research into particular aspects of patient care; and provision of methods of accountability to the governing body and to the public. Nurses themselves can realize benefits from quality assurance in the following manner: (1) a change in the amount and type of charting by using flow sheets or checklists for routine patient care; (2) identification of those observations that should be included in the nurse's notes (such as those that relate to the clinical criteria established for audit); (3) definition of the elements that should be included in patient care plans (such as meet audit criteria); (4) establishment of elements that should be included in nursing policies and procedures; (5) setting of priorities for in-service education, continuing education for nurses, or both; (6) justification of changes in staffing patterns; and (7) clarification of the status of the nursing department.

PLANNING AND IMPLEMENTATION OF QUALITY ASSURANCE PROGRAM

Understanding all of the positive benefits that could be realized from a quality assurance program in nursing would not make the program materialize. Continued work is needed to develop a comprehensive system of nursing quality assurance. The components of a comprehensive system of nursing quality assurance are identified as incorporating the following: (1) nursing care evaluation—(the combined analysis of concurrent and retrospective nursing review); (2) concurrent nursing care review or concurrent nursing audit—(the evaluation of nursing care of a patient while that care is being rendered); (3) retrospective nursing care review or retrospective nursing audit—(the evaluation after the discharge of the patient of the quality of nursing care that was rendered); (4) continuing education—(an educational program for members of the nursing staff presented to improve the quality of patient care based on the problems or deficiencies identified during the review process); (5) profile analysis—(the evaluation of the effectiveness of nursing review components, the identification of review priorities, and comparison with other local nursing groups). Planning and implementing the components of the nursing quality assurance system is a big task, especially since funding was not made available through the PSRO to help, and it is usually not a high budgetary priority within a hospital or health care facility plan.

I have mentioned before that the evaluation of nursing care is an evolutionary process. Because the profession of nursing is only one of the many professions involved in the health care setting, the most logical progression in the evolution of the evaluation of health care is toward an interdisciplinary health care evaluation system. One step toward the interdisciplinary process is the inclusion of nurses on medical audit or utilization review committees. Before nurses can actively participate they must understand the elements and data required for the assessment of quality of nursing care both concurrently and retrospectively.

Nursing Care Evaluation

Since the process for the review of nursing care should parallel the mechanism set up by the PSRO for the physicians, nursing care evaluation studies cannot be instituted until the nursing staff has developed and ratified criteria to be used in the evaluation of nursing care on a concurrent and ret-

rospective basis. Criteria can be developed along the lines of medical diagnosis or nursing problems. It is usually recommended to utilize the medical diagnosis in the majority of studies since retrieval of data is from the medical records department files, where charts are coded under a hospital adaptation of international classification of diseases (an H-ICDA number). If a nursing audit is done by H-ICDA numbers, it would also be possible to retrieve the nursing data at the same time that the medical audit information was being retrieved. It is also important to local nursing groups that they be able to know exactly which criteria sets apply to each diagnostic entity. For example, if a nursing problem were used as the basis of a nursing audit and one wished to look at the skin integrity of paralyzed patients, one would have to evaluate charts that had medical diagnoses of cerebrovascular accidents, spinal cord injuries, and neurologic disorders with paralysis, and one may find it necessary to go to many different diagnostic entities to evaluate one nursing problem. If one can clarify all of the diagnostic entities involved in evaluating any given nursing diagnoses or problems, then it is possible to compare groups of local nurses. However, this may become very difficult in that some groups may add to the criteria set diagnoses that had not been considered in the beginning without going back and assuring that there be similar data for comparison between groups.

Concurrent Review of Nursing Care

The process for the review of nursing care on a concurrent basis parallels that of doing an admission certification or continued-stay review of medical care. Concurrent review of nursing care should be conducted at 48 hours after admission and at the twenty-fifth and fiftieth percentile of the expected length of stay. The reason for this is that if nursing has not implemented the appropriate procedures by the fiftieth percentile, the possibility of having an extended stay in a facility or having less than desirable outcomes for the patient is greatly increased. The review of concurrent nursing care can be conducted by the PSRO utilization review coordinator or a PSRO-trained nurse on the unit. Experience shows that many of the PSRO coordinators are already reviewing the nursing care to make a determination on continued-stay review. Adverse determinations from the concurrent review should be referred to a nursing advisor for evaluation. As with medical review, the PSRO utilization coordinator, even though he or she may be a professional nurse, would not render negative decisions about the quality of nursing care. Only positive decisions would be made. Adverse determinations would be handled by the nursing advisor who would have at his or her disposal either supervisors or direct contact with the floor nurses to immediately correct any areas identified by the concurrent review as not being met.

Retrospective Review of Nursing Care

The retrospective review of nursing care should be consistent with the yearly determination of numbers of MCEs required by the HSQB. Retrospective studies can be spaced throughout a calendar year and can be used to evaluate care provided before the current year. One study should be in process at all times. It is helpful if the plan for the MCEs for the year is provided to the nursing audit committee, and they can map the nursing audit studies to be compatible with the studies being done by the medical care evaluation committee. It is much easier for the medical records department to retrieve data simultaneously for a medical audit and a nursing audit on the same charts than it is repeatedly to retrieve data separately from two different sets of medical records.

The medical records data analyst should retrieve the actual data for both the concurrent and the retrospective review of nursing care. The results of the nursing care evaluation studies are evaluated by the nursing audit committee, and the analysis is reported to the nursing administrator, the hospital administrator, the hospital board of trustees, and the PSRO.

Continuing Education Programs

Continuing education programs sponsored by the hospital in-service department or professional organizations or the continuing education departments of local universities should reflect the variations in nursing practice that were identified through the concurrent or retrospective reviews of nursing care. Reauditing at predetermined future dates would help to assess changes in professional behavior. At all times it should be emphasized and remembered that the thrust of review activities is not intended to be punitive but rather is to improve the quality of nursing care through the education of the nurse practitioner.

NURSING CARE EVALUATION CRITERIA

Criteria Development

Originally criteria were developed for the acute-care facility. As the criteria were applied and utilized, interest was aroused in a home health setting, in a long-term care setting, and in an ambulatory care setting for the utilization of criteria for the evaluation of the nursing care being rendered in various levels of facilities. Attempts have been made to develop criteria specific for a given level of care. The long-term care projects under the PSRO have developed criteria that they utilize on a shared basis for evaluation of nursing care. A group of nurses was brought together representing acute care, long-term care, home health agencies, and ambulatory care or the physician's office in the greater Colorado Springs area to look at appropriate types of care and to see if an understanding could be developed between the nurses at various levels as to what to expect from criteria from other levels of care. The result of this study was the recommendation for the development of criteria for three levels of nursing care, to be written simultaneously, that could be applied to any level of care. They planned for acute criteria, subacute criteria, and maintenance criteria, the belief being that if three levels of criteria were written at once, nurses (regardless of the facility that they work with) would be able to assess the patient and determine which of the three criteria sets was appropriate, realizing that the patient moves from acute to subacute to maintenance. It was discovered that in the maintenance category, which would normally refer to ambulatory care or to home health care, it was not uncommon to find a patient who was actually receiving acute nursing care but was not hospitalized. An example of this would be the diabetic patient who, according to the acute level of care criteria, should have administered insulin three times under supervision in the acute-care setting before being discharged. However, the patient was hospitalized only overnight, and the nurse in the physician's office then had to pick up the monitoring of the patient's ability to administer his own insulin. It could have been that the home health nurse or the visiting nurse might have been notified to make a home visit and to see that the acute-care level of nursing had been completed before the patient moved on to the subacute or maintenance level.

Formats for Criteria Development

Availability of criteria sets in the three formats just discussed will allow nurses to utilize their assess-ment skills, place patients according to the criteria most appropriate to their needs, and then assist them in movement along the health continuum. The basic format for criteria development for nursing care evaluation is illustrated on p. 211. The major categories used in the nursing care format are applicable to acute, subacute, and maintenance. The concurrent review criteria are applied when the patient is in the hospital or has an open chart. The first broad category is the identification of the patient's physical and psychosocial need or concerns. This is normally limited to five, but there may be variations in the number. If the patient's concerns are not dealt with or if the patient has an agenda different than that of the health team, it will be more difficult to accomplish the desired outcomes; therefore, in the nursing criteria, the patient's physical and psychologic needs or concerns that he has brought with him either to the acute facility, subacute facility, or maintenance setting are identified. The second broad category is the recommended nursing action consistent with the diagnosis. "A" under that lists the nursing services. What are the minimum nursing services that should be provided to this given patient? The second category, "B" under roman numeral II, is health education. What must this patient be taught for him to resume living at the highest point of his capabilities? The third broad category is indication for discharge. "A" is the adaptation of health status. Now the patient can be discharged from acute, subacute, or maintenance, and the criteria should reflect what has to be achieved for the patient to be discharged to another level of care or from nursing services altogether. "B" is an example of the community resources that are normally utilized with this particular type of patient. This is a reminder to the nursing staff that communication with other professionals is essential to provide continuity of care for the patient as he moves along the health care continuum. The three broad categories constitute the concurrent review of nursing care.

NURSING CARE CRITERIA

Topic _____ Code _____

Concurrent review criteria

I. Identification of patient's physical and psychologic needs or concerns (limited to five or fewer entries)*
II. Recommended nursing action consistent with diagnosis
  A. Nursing services (limited to five or fewer entries)
  B. Health education (limited to five or fewer entries)

III. Indicators for discharge
  A. Adaptation of health status (limited to five or fewer entries)
  B. Examples of community resources (limited to three or fewer entries)

Retrospective review criteria

I. Health
II. Activity
III. Knowledge

Complications

*These are suggested numbers of entries. There may be variations.

They are applied while the patient is receiving care. The second broad grouping is the retrospective review criteria. This parallels the requirements of the JCAH. They ask for, under the first category of health, those activities of health that the patient should have achieved as an outcome on discharge from acute care, subacute care, or maintenance. The second level is activity. In what activity can the patient be involved? Is he ambulatory? Can he perform activities of daily living alone? Does he need assistance with walking? The third broad category is knowledge. What health teaching has been completed, and what information should the patient or his significant other possess for him to continue making progress? The last category, which applies both to concurrent and retrospective review, lists complications. This section should also include the critical nursing management of complications. What must the nurse do before the physician is even notified? Nursing care evaluation criteria emphasize psychologic needs and concerns of the patient as well as health education, two areas that frequently are not assessed in the completion

of MCEs. Therefore, nursing care evaluation brings another component to the evaluation of health care that may provide data and information to improve the overall provision of care.

The general format for performing a nursing care evaluation study is similar to or consistent with that for completion of a medical care evaluation study. The major steps included are: (1) identify the study topic; (2) design the study, including setting objectives and developing draft criteria; (3) ratify the criteria; (4) perform data retrieval and display; (5) analyze the results; (6) analyze identified problem(s); (7) develop corrective action; (8) implement corrective action; (9) evaluate corrective action and (10) establish profile for analysis.

Other Necessary Forms

In addition to the nursing care evaluation criteria format, the audit committee will require the following types of forms: (1) a study format, (2) an abstract sheet, (3) a cost report, (4) a procedural checklist for audit studies, and (5) a nursing care evaluation study summary sheet. Data display sheets and analysis sheets will also be used by an audit committee. Many types of forms that can be utilized in nursing audits are available from different groups. Each health care facility should evaluate the available forms and adopt the forms that are easiest for them to use and that meet their needs. When a nursing group experiences difficulty in applying forms, they should modify them or design a form appropriate for their needs. The JCAH has forms available for retrospective audit.

Model Criteria Sets

Physicians have developed model criteria sets that are available through the PSRO to be ratified on the local level. Before 1977, nursing did not have available model criteria sets. There are, however, model criteria sets available for nursing for 85% of the admissions to an acute-care facility on the con-

current and retrospective review of nursing care. [1] Examples of nursing care evaluation criteria sets are shown on pp. 212–215.

A word of caution is necessary. Model sets are just what the name implies. They are an example or a guide that local nursing groups can use to develop or ratify criteria appropriate to the quality and quantity of nursing care being provided within their institution. Ideally the model sets will assist in the development, modification, and ratification of criteria for concurrent and retrospective review of nursing care. If the model sets as a basis for acute criteria are utilized, it should be easier to develop the subacute and maintenance criteria.

REFERENCES

1. Davidson, S., Burleson, B.C., Crawford, J.E.S., et al. 1977. *Nursing care evaluation: concurrent and retrospective review criteria*. St. Louis: The C.V. Mosky Co.

NURSING CARE EVALUATION: ACUTE

Topic ___Hypertension___ Code _____

Concurrent review criteria

I. Identification of patient's physical and psychologic needs or concerns (limited to five or fewer entries)
Relief from headache
Prevention of complications
Evaluation of elevated blood pressure
Fear of hospital environment, death, incapacity
Explanation of nature of disease, cause, prognosis, management, and plan for care
Monitor heart rate, rhythm, and vital signs
Observe for changes in behavioral characteristics, symptoms of strokes, decreased urine output, and chest pain

II. Recommended nursing action consistent with diagnosis
A. Nursing services (limited to five or fewer entries)
Maintain restful and serene environment
Initiate medical directions
Restrict sodium intake and monitor output in accordance with drug therapy
Teach risk factors
B. Health education (limited to five or fewer entries)
Explain diet
Explain disease process

NURSING CARE EVALUATION: ACUTE *(continued)*

Explain relationship of normal cardiac function to hypertension

Help patient develop plan of care to be self administered

III. Indicators for discharge
  A. Adaptation of health status (limited to five or fewer entries)
     Diastolic blood pressure decreased below 100 mm Hg
     1. Physician notified
  Urine output approaching 2000 ml/24 hours
     1. Secondary renal diagnosis, physician notified
  Diet restrictions as tolerated; exception: if not restricted
  Mentally alert; exception: preexisting condition, physician notified
  Ambulatory; exception: preexisting condition, physician notified
  Able to care for himself for activities of daily living; exception: preexisting condition
  Patient and/or significant other verbalizes understanding of diagnosis, diet, drugs, activity limitations, and importance of medical follow-up

Retrospective review criteria

I. Health
  Diastolic blood pressure below 100 mm Hg
  Urine output approaching 2000 ml/24 hours
  Diet restrictions tolerated
  Mentally alert
II. Activity
  Ambulatory
  Able to care for himself for activities of daily living
III. Knowledge
  Patient and/or significant other verbalizes understanding of diagnosis, diet, drugs, activity limitations, and importance of medical follow-up

Complications

Cardiac arrhythmia
Cerebral thrombosis
Myocardial infarction

NURSING CARE EVALUATION: SUBACUTE

Topic ____ Hypertension _____ Code _____

Concurrent review criteria

I. Identification of patient's physical and psychologic needs or concerns (limited to five or fewer entries)
  Fear of incapacity
  Understanding of disease process, especially drug and diet regime

Evaluation of blood pressure once a week
Fear of loss of sexual performance
Provision of emotional support through the grieving process
II. Recommended nursing action consistent with diagnosis

NURSING CARE EVALUATION: SUBACUTE *(continued)*

Topic _____ Hypertension _____ Code _____

A. Nursing services (limited to five or fewer entries)

Provide psychologic and emotional support for patient expressions of feelings and fears through the grieving process

Check blood pressure once a week

Monitor patient's medication and diet; observe for impending danger signs

Discussion of adaptation to sex

Design a plan for self-care

B. Health education (limited to five or fewer entries)

Explain or teach disease process, with danger signs to be alerted by proper diet, medications, and risk factors

Explain grieving process

Teach technique to implement plan of self-care

Teach alternative modes of coping, including sexual adaptation

III. Indicators for discharge

A. Adaptation of health status (limited to five or fewer entries)

Diastolic blood pressure below 100 mm Hg for 6 months

Follow plan for self-care

Identifies appropriate diet restrictions and medication action and dosages

Identifies and enumerates the elements of grieving process

Has reduced or quiet smoking—or has attended a smoking clinic to learn how

Retrospective review criteria

I. Health

Diastolic blood pressure below 100 mm Hg for 6 months

Complications not evident

Drug regimen and diet restrictions tolerated

II. Activity

Taking medications and diet as prescribed in medical and nursing regime

Actively adapting his life style appropriately

Following self-care program

Has quit or reduced smoking—or has attended a smoking clinic to learn how

III. Knowledge

Knows names of his drugs, dosages, actions, side effects

Demonstrates knowledge of disease process by correctly implementing self-care program

Knows ways or techniques to appropriately adapt life style

Complications

Hypertensive crisis

Angina

Edema in lower extremities

Pulmonary edema

Myocardial infarction

Cerebrovascular accident (cerebral hemorrhage)

Depression

Denial

Drug side effects

Congestive heart failure

NURSING CARE EVALUATION: MAINTENANCE

Topic ____Hypertension_____   Code _____

Concurrent review criteria

I. Identification of patient's physical and psychologic needs or concerns (limited to five or fewer entries)

Relief from headache, dizziness, edema, and impaired vision

Understanding nature of disease, cause, prognosis, and management with plan for care

Understanding of diet and drug instructions

Fear of incapacity

Prevention of complications

Concern for costs

II. Recommended nursing action consistent with diagnosis

A. Nursing services (limited to five or fewer entries)

Blood pressure, heart rate, and rhythm; weight each visit

Check for signs of fluid retention, headaches, dizziness, chest pains, and behavioral changes

Provide psychologic and emotional support, allowing client to verbalize fears

B. Health education (limited to five or fewer entries)

Teach risk factors and significance

Explain diet

Explain disease process and effects on body

Explain drug regimen

Discuss symptoms requiring professional medical intervention

Provide general health teaching

Determine that patient understands and implements correct choices in diet selection

III. Indicators for discharge

A. Adaptation of health status (limited to five or fewer entries)

Identifies need for drug therapy and identifies drug side effects

States an understanding of no smoking and decreasing stressful situations

Identifies symptoms that require further medical supervision

Diastolic blood pressure under 100 mm Hg for 6 months

Is referred to local unit of American Heart Association

Retrospective review criteria

I. Health

Blood pressure diastolic under 100 mm Hg for 6 months

Complications not evident

II. Activity

Returned to activity

Implements no smoking program

III. Knowledge

Verbalizes knowledge of drugs and diet, complications, and stressful situations

Verbalizes importance of follow-up care

23

Private Review

George Himler

Peer review of health services has two major components—utilization review and the evaluation of the quality of care. The quality audit serves a special and important purpose in assuring that efforts to control costs do not do violence to the standards of excellence that the health care professions have developed through years of self-evaluation and discipline.

The bulk of the utilization review currently being conducted is the function of the conditional PSROs and is applied only to patients whose care is funded under the Maternal and Child Health and Crippled Children's Services (Title V), Medicare (Title XVIII), and Medicaid (Title XIX) programs. By contrast, the MCEs being performed by the same PSROs either directly or by delegation embrace the care of all patients, regardless of the source of payment. Since medical care evaluation is universally applied, the discussion of quality assessment under a separate ''private'' heading is unnecessary. The balance of this chapter is therefore devoted to private utilization review, with the reminder that it is only one of the two major review activities and that the continuous evaluation of the quality of care is an indispensable complement to the utilization review function in a complete program.

PRESENT SCOPE OF REVIEW

Utilization review is now being performed principally by the PSROs, Foundations for Medical Care (FMCs), HMOs, or HMOs and Independent Practice Associations (HMO/IPAs). In March 1977, there were 106 conditional PSROs with negotiations in progress for the designation of 51 new planning PSROs, which will probably not begin review until February 1978. When this program is fully implemented and PSRO coverage becomes nationwide, there is an ultimate potential of 195 such agencies. The number of FMCs involved in review is more difficult to determine accurately, but a recent survey indicates that there are at least 100. Not all HMOs and HMO/IPAs can be counted as review agencies, because many have preferred to contract with existing FMCs or PSROs in their respective areas rather than create parallel review programs. Whatever the precise counts may be, it is clear that the PSROs, FMCs, HMOs, and HMO/IPAs that conduct virtually all of the private review now being done account for only a small fraction of private or nongovernment funded patients. In the average community, therefore, only about one third of hospitalized patients are subject to utilization review, and the great majority of these are Title XVIII and Title XIX beneficiaries.

In addition to the public-private fractionation, there is another stratification with regard to the practice setting to which review is applied. The PSROs and other review organizations have concentrated their early efforts on the acute-care hospitals, because that is where the major health service expenditures are made and the greatest cost reductions might be anticipated. Pilot projects for the study of the utilization of ancillary services, such as rehabilitation, x-ray, clinical laboratory, and respiratory therapy, will soon be added to the in-hospital review programs of some PSROs. A limited number of PSROs have ventured into the monitoring of long-term care in skilled nursing facilities (SNFs) and intermediate care facilities (ICFs) while even fewer will be adding systems for ambulatory care review. The techniques available for assessing the utilization of noninstitutional, or private, ambulatory services are rudimentary at best, and their application is quite limited. Home care has received virtually no attention, probably because there is relatively little organization among the agencies that render home services.

Although the FMCs, PSROs, and HMOs are the best known and, in the aggregate, by far the most numerous of the agencies engaged in review, they do not have a complete monopoly on technical skill or the actual operation of such programs. There are other entries in the utilization review derby.

In industry, a number of large employers have been active for years in devising and implementing review and cost control programs for their own employee health benefit plans. Some of these were developed and are operated in conjunction with local medical care foundations. Although they may be quite satisfactory for the management of the program for which they were designed, these systems are not exportable because they involve atypical populations and unique situations.

The Blue Cross and Blue Shield programs, individually and collectively, have made periodic efforts to analyze utilization in search of methods to control premiums. Their loss ratios and continual requests for rate increases in recent years bear witness to the difficulty of the problem and their inability to cope with it.

The insurance industry, too, has engaged in some review activity often through an FMC or HMO in the implementation of a medical care foundation type of delivery system. Their involvement has been individual and sporadic, however, and has not brought forth a broadly applicable review system or an agency capable of implementing it.

OBJECTIVES AND POTENTIAL OF PRIVATE REVIEW

Before discussing how utilization review can be extended to the private sector, I wish to examine what is expected of utilization review and determine whether it is likely to be worth the effort.

The primary expectation is that utilization review will result in immediate cost reductions by eliminating unnecessary or inappropriate care concurrently, that is, before it occurs, or by terminating it promptly once it has begun. The concurrent review is designed to limit medical services to those that are medically necessary and prevent unwarranted prolongation of hospital stay. In addition to the overall cost control element, the review system should detect program abuse or actual fraud and provide for the withholding of payment or the imposition of sanctions. Over a longer term, the data captured are used to modify patients' behavior and physicians' practice patterns to prevent misuse of facilities and services, as contrasted to outright abuse.

There are other outcomes of a review program, however, that if properly used will have a more important effect on the nation's health care delivery system and how it is financed. One of the major defects of health insurance as it is known today is that it encourages the hospitalization of patients who could be cared for equally well in a less costly setting. By failing to provide collateral coverage, current benefit structures tend to motivate both physicians and patients to choose hospitalization, purely on the ground that it is the only setting in which the patient will be reimbursed for the cost of his care. The data acquired by an efficient review system will suggest modifications of insurance coverage or program benefits to ensure the delivery of care in the least costly, most appropriate facility.

Finally, PL 93-641 has entrusted health care planning to a nationwide network of Health Systems Agencies (HSAs) and associated local and state planning groups. As these agencies work toward their 5-year health systems plans (HSPs) and their annual implementation plans (AIPs), they will have an absolute need for the type of data that utilization review and medical audit should and do provide. Because the HSAs are specifically prohibited from developing their own data systems (a prohibition that is hardly necessary in view of the parsimony with which they are funded), they will be forced to rely on existing review organizations to meet their data requirements.

As official planning bodies, administrators, and legislators grope for a way out of the morass of current health care problems and fumble toward better systems of delivery and financing, possibly national in scope, it is of the utmost importance that they have accurate, complete data and that they know how to interpret them. Even a nation as wealthy as the United States could ill afford another such planning fiasco and operational disaster as the Medicaid program. The data base required can be produced only by systems designed specifically for the study and evaluation of health care.

It was pointed out previously, however, that the majority of patients now being reviewed are either Title XVIII or Title XIX beneficiaries, and even at that, reviewed only for in-hospital care. That review is adequate for the purposes of program administration and control. Each group, however, represents a unique population, with a makeup that bears no resemblance to that of the public at large. Medicare provides benefits only for those over 65 years of age, those who are permanently disabled, and sufferers of end-stage renal disease. Medicaid, on the other hand, covers the indigent and medically underserved, many of whom have little or no health education and belong preponderantly to groups that are disadvantaged in terms of housing, nutrition, sanitation, and a number of other factors. The fact that Medicare and Medicaid patients are so atypical of the general public makes the data on their care useless for overall planning. This is a pursuasive argument for the extending of review to all patients, regardless of whether the payment for their care comes from public or private sources.

Along somewhat similar lines, it is evident that whatever planning is done cannot be for one care setting alone. The various elements of the health care delivery system and their use are interdependent and inseparable, and the data required for local and national planning must, therefore, of necessity be gleaned from the entire spectrum. Hence, aside from the benefits they hold for program management and cost control, there are sound theoretic and practical reasons for extending utilization review and medical audit to the entire private sector and all practice sites and modalities.

COST-EFFECTIVENESS OF REVIEW

The proponents of peer review are constantly being challenged to prove that the cost reductions resulting from utilization review are proportionate to the time, effort, and money expended in conducting the programs. A number of legislators still question the entire PSRO concept on the basis of lack of cost-effectiveness. The value of utilization review is difficult to prove immediately and conclusively. The major difficulty lies in the almost universal dearth of baseline data that can be used as a frame of reference. The data that are available in any one locale are spotty, incomplete, and often ill kept and are not adequate for objective, before and after, comparison and evaluation. Comparing review outcomes among the various review organizations is even less reliable because of the great number of variables in their patient mixes, which profoundly affect utilization rates. It does not follow that a plan having 800 days of hospitalization per 1000 subscribers or beneficiaries per year necessarily has a less appropriate experience or less efficient review system than one that has only 500 days per 1000 per year.

Nevertheless, there is a substantial body of evidence accumulated by long-standing FMCs and a few PSROs, to indicate that the benefit-to-cost ratio in the first year or two following the initiation of a good utilization review program is in excess of 8:1. Some of this evidence is anecdotal, but although it might not convince the purist who demands strict statistical proof, it is impressive in the aggregate.

There are other problems in evaluating review and deciding how much to do and where to do it. Review outcomes must now be judged in the face of a recent trend toward declining admissions. The cause for this decline is poorly understood, and there is no indication whether it will level off or increase. This adds to the difficulty of evaluating the efficacy of a newly inaugurated utilization review program.

In addition, it is an oversimplification to arrive at a cost benefit merely by multiplying reductions in hospital days in a given period by the per diem rate. First, the entire cost of a hospital day is not saved because there is a fixed cost to the hospital in maintaining an empty bed. Second, if the unhospitalized patient receives care outside the hospital, that expense will not be recognized unless the review system in effect covers that other category of care. Thus, it is clear that accurate cost information can be achieved only by systems that address all levels of care.

As a corollary, it is also evident that sought-for reductions in the cost of health care will not be realized fully until complete review data are used to modify institutional capacities, the types and ratios of services that are available, and the settings in which they are rendered. The entire health care structure must be brought into congruence with the demonstrated needs of the communities and the nation and with new concepts of delivery and financing.

A final factor must be considered in judging the cost-effectiveness of a review program. As it approaches its goal of "normalizing" utilization, further reductions are hard to achieve, but as the savings level off, the expense of review remains fixed. There is no evidence that if review were discontinued at this point, costs would rise to their previous levels. It must be remembered, however, that neither health care delivery nor review requirements are static, so that cost-benefit ratios cannot be judged on the incomplete review systems that are now prevalent. Review methodologies must be adapted to changing needs as the programs are expanded into new areas and as their original objectives are attained. If it is agreed that review will be truly effective only if it is applied across the board, it follows almost inevitably that the entire range of services cannot, and should not, be reviewed with the same intensity that is now being lavished on acute hospital care.

The current state of the review art does not permit the implementation of complete, integrated programs that simultaneously cover all segments of the health care system. As a practical matter, this has dictated a step-by-step approach, which may be fortunate. In the course of extending review progressively to ancillary services, long-term care, ambulatory care, and home care, the methods in use for each type of service already under review can be refined and focused to reduce requirements for personnel, funds, and facilities, thereby freeing resources for the new addition. The methodologies and data processing for each review area added in this fashion are compatible with those already in operation, thereby allowing the system to develop in an orderly, modular, and economic fashion. Thus, although it is true that ratios of cost-effectiveness can be roughly assessed with some validity for an agency reviewing an individual limited benefit program, the value determination for the review of health care as a whole will have to be deferred until the systems are generalized and perfected.

INCENTIVES AND PRESSURES FOR IMPLEMENTATION OF PRIVATE REVIEW

The mere demonstration of the theoretic and practical advantages of extending review into the private sector will not bring it about without other motivating forces and specific initiatives. Historically, the single most powerful stimulus for establishing review programs has been the rising cost of health care, as reflected in benefit payments and insurance premiums. The federal government was the first to move to protect its programs. Drawing on the prototype review systems of the FMCs, the DHEW instituted a study of review potential in the EMCRO program. Subsequently, PL 92-603 established PSROs as the review organizations for federally funded programs.

Industry, which pays massive sums to support employee health benefit plans, workmen's compensation, and disability, was slower to react as a group. Through the years, a number of individual large employers experimented with new delivery systems and cost control mechanisms based on utilization review. Usually these experiments were conducted in conjunction with FMCs, large multi-specialty clinics, and hospitals in one combination or another. Some were successful, some were abandoned, but all were limited, and no generally applicable methodology or wide distribution of capable review organizations emerged. With their needs in terms of cost and quality control still unmet, employers are now exhibiting an intense interest in utilization review and the agencies that can provide it.

With some exceptions, industry does not administer employee benefit programs directly. Most employers either insure with a Blue plan or a commercial carrier or self-insure under an "administrative services only" contract with a carrier. No matter what carrier they use, they have been vociferous in demanding that the carriers develop or adopt review systems that are effective in containing or reducing their expenditures for health care.

Again, some of the commercial carriers and Blue plans have been involved with experimental review systems for a number of years, but all have failed to develop effective programs or the organizational structure to implement them. Under ordinary circumstances, the carriers had been able to meet rising costs by passing them through in the form of increased premiums. Stiffening resistance from employers and much unkind treatment at the hands of insurance commissioners at rate setting time has finally convinced the insurance industry of its need for utilization review in the business it underwrites and the programs it administers. The incentives for applying effective review and cost containment programs to the private sector are now intense and unremitting. Reluctance to take risks and innovate is diminishing as the pain of continually rising costs becomes more acute.

SOURCES OF PRIVATE REVIEW

Since neither employers nor the insurance industry have been successful in devising review and cost control systems of wide applicability, it is apparent that they must look elsewhere for the services they need. The logic of utilizing existing review agencies has not escaped them, but their choice is limited. The only competent organizations of wide distribution are the FMCs, which have developed and improved their methodologies over many years, and the PSROs, which have had the benefit of many millions of dollars of federal development funding. Indeed, both employers and carriers have approached review agencies of both types and have initiated a few review programs on an area-by-area basis. This can be a satisfactory expedient for local employers but is not suitable for insurance carriers and employers who have offices and plants in many locations, distributed through multiple regions or nationwide. Carriers and employers of this size and distribution find it difficult or impossible to negotiate the many contracts that would be necessary to cover their widely dispersed operations. Furthermore, they do not have the capability of evaluating the local review organizations or of monitoring the review once it is in effect. They have begun to recognize the advantages that could accrue from dealing with a single entity that represents a substantial network of review organizations and that can evaluate and certify their competence, monitor their performance, and give them expert technical assistance where improvement is needed.

ORGANIZATIONAL INTERESTS IN PRIVATE REVIEW

At this point the organizational entities that represent to one extent or another the various interests involved in private health care delivery and review should be identified. It has already been observed that the FMCs and the PSROs together are the most numerous and widely distributed review organizations performing review at this time. Both the FMCs and PSROs have national organizations that with their concurrence could represent them in negotiations involving many localities in multiple regions or states. The voluntary and commercial insurance carriers have analogous associations, and there is now an association that speaks for industry, though it does not represent it in actual negotiations. At least an acquaintanceship with these organizations is necessary to the understanding of the forces at work in establishing private review. The following are merely brief sketches and do not purport to describe all the activities of each organization.

The Washington Business Group on Health has become a very articulate spokesman for commerce and industry in matters pertaining to health care and its financing. The group was formed in 1974 and involves over 200 large corporations. It does not officially speak for industry or even all of its own member corporations, but it does maintain a presence in Washington, D.C., is well sponsored, and can enunciate industry's concerns, attitudes, and objectives on all matters pertaining to health care.

The Blue Cross Association and the National Association of Blue Shield Plans (NABSP) are essentially federations of free standing, independent, local or state plans. They have been given authority to set standards, advise their member organizations, and represent them nationally in matters of broad policy, but neither has negotiating power for its members unless that power is specifically granted. Nevertheless, both associations will be influential in shaping the response of their member plans to proposals for private review.

The Health Insurance Association of America (HIAA) numbers virtually all the large commercial health insurance carriers among its members. Like the organizations discussed previously, it is concerned with all matters pertaining to and affecting health care insurance. The organization's activities are primarily directed toward the development of policy for the industry and representing it before legislative and administrative bodies. It does have one committee devoted specifically to utilization review programs that has been particularly active. The recommendations of this committee, although not binding on any of the member carriers, will certainly influence their individual responses to the demands their clients in industry are making for utilization review and premium containment.

The American Hospital Association is a federation of state and local hospital associations, each of which speaks for its own member hospitals. On a national scale it is active in participating in the setting and maintenance of standards, in establishing policy, and influencing legislation on health and hospital care and financing. It will never be involved in direct negotiations for private review, but its policy statements will certainly affect the reception the local hospitals give the review organizations.

The activities of the American Medical Association are too well known and numerous to set forth here. Structurally, it is a federation of state medical associations, each of which is autonomous. The AMA, aside from its myriad educational activities, is the accepted national political representative for the majority of its state associations and member physicians. Although it is not authorized to enter into specific negotiations, it is a powerful influence in shaping health care legislation. The AMA has accepted the principles of utilization review and quality assurance, although it has taken successful issue with a number of the provisions of the PSRO statute and the DHEW regulations.

In recent years, the various medical specialty associations have assumed varying degrees of activity and influence in the politics and socio-economics of health care. They constitute another axis or dimension along which physicians are organized, but their concepts and attitudes on peer review parallel those of the AMA in most instances.

The nonmedical health professions, such as dentistry and nursing, also have national organizations whose opinions on health care legislation should be sought. Their individual members have been active in review at the local level, and their continued participation and cooperation will be essential to the success of private review.

The American Association of Foundations for Medical Care (AAFMC) now has a membership of approximately 100 FMCs and HMOs. The first FMC was founded in the San Joaquin Valley in 1954 for the purpose of rendering health care on a capitation prepayment basis and performing utilization review to insure the financial integrity of its program. Thus, the FMCs had a 21-year start on the PSROs in review, but because they were engaged in the delivery of health care as well as review and did not have the stimulus of federal funding, they proliferated rather slowly. When they finally achieved a critical mass, they perceived the need for a national organization to serve as a medium for the interchange of information and techniques, to render them technical assistance services, to coordinate their activities, and to represent their interests nationally. The AAFMC was incorporated in 1967. The AAFMC will play its role in the development of private review through another organization, which is presented shortly.

Early in 1972, the leadership of the AAFMC anticipated the enactment of the Bennett Amendments, which ultimately were embodied in PL 92-603. It was recognized that the PSROs, when designated, would be performing peer review, a traditional, long-standing, and well-developed medical care foundation function. It therefore seemed indicated that AAFMC make the cumulative expertise of its member foundations available to the PSROs and provide the latter with an organizational structure to assist them in implementing the national program.

In November 1972, the AAFMC reserved the name American Association of Professional Standards Review Organizations (AAPSRO). The new association was incorporated on May 4, 1973. AAPSRO was initially controlled entirely by AAFMC because that was its parent organization. This arrangement was temporary, and by mutual agreement the bylaws were amended in May 1976, giving control of the AAPSRO to its own house of delegates and board of directors elected by the institutional and individual members. Again, AAPSRO, like AAFMC, will play a somewhat indirect part in private review. It is worth pointing out at this time that there is no legal deterrent to prevent PSROs from conducting private review. Although they are federally funded for the review of government programs, they are locally sponsored private corporations functioning under the authority of their own boards of directors. When they do engage in private review, the only requirement will be that they distinguish between public and nonpublic costs for purposes of accounting to the DHEW.

PEER REVIEW NETWORK

Since AAFMC and AAPSRO together represent the only functioning, effective health care review organizations that can claim anything approaching national distribution, the two boards of directors decided to incorporate those FMCs and PSROs that wished to participate into a nationwide review network for the purpose of extending review into the private sector. The response of the review organizations to an initial inquiry was enthusiastic, so that adequate participation by the local review agencies was assured. For various legal and operational reasons, AAFMC and AAPSRO could not operate the network directly, and it became necessary to create a new corporate entity that was called the Peer Review Network, or the PRN.

The concept is that PRN will negotiate directly with national and multistate accounts for review that it will subcontract to its participating local FMCs and PSROs. The local organizations will retain the sole right to negotiate local and intrastate contracts. Each review organization may participate or decline to participate in any PRN sponsored program. Blanket participation is not required, neither will PRN initiate competing review organizations in those areas in which existing ones decide not to service PRN programs. On the other hand, in those areas in which there are no review organizations, and there is a demand for review, PRN will lend assistance to groups of physicians who wish to found an organization for that purpose. As the national coordinating agency, PRN will assume certain unique functions. It will assess the capabilities of each review organization in the light of criteria that have already been developed before its acceptance into the network. It will monitor local network review on a regular, periodic basis and certify its continuing efficacy. It will provide developing and existing review organizations with technical assistance for the dual purpose of upgrading the quality of review and expanding the network's coverage.

Those corporations that contract with PRN for in-hospital review will receive the following:

1. Case-by-case certifications of the appropriateness of the admission, the medical necessity for the length of stay, and the suggested date for the termination of benefits, all for purposes of claims administration

2. Length of stay statistical data

3. Other aggregate data to document the effectiveness of the utilization and cost control program

4. Statistics to be used for overall planning

and the devising of more rational and cost-effective benefit packages; the specific contents and formats of the reports to be individually negotiated

5. The benefits, for their employees or subscribers, of the review organization's supervision of the quality assurance activities that are an integral part of the peer review process

6. Guarantees of complete confidentiality of their data

PRN's review services will be made available to all health insurance carriers, employer funded and sponsored health care benefits programs, union welfare programs, and any other large purchasers of health services.

PROBLEMS AND OBSTACLES

The expansion of review programs to include much or all of the private sector is not without its problems, which should be identified, because they must be addressed and solved.

First, the review network is still incomplete, which means that in some areas where review might be particularly needed, there are no functioning review organizations to undertake it. Although PRN has adopted the policy of not attempting to create review organizations in areas that lack them, it does have the capability of approaching physician communities and stimulating their interest in establishing and operating review agencies.

It is also apparent that not all the review organizations are equally developed and competent. As indicated earlier, AAFMC and AAPSRO each has a massive body of experience and a cadre of administrators, reviewers, data analysts, and physicians, active and skilled in the review field, to draw on for advice and assistance. This faculty is already organized and is rendering technical assistance to newly developing review organizations and those that require improvement and further development. The technical assistance capability is fundamental to the network concept.

Another problem in private review lies in the fact that review cannot be done at an acceptable cost for only a few patients in a given area. Initially, it will therefore be necessary to institute programs where the employer or carrier has a large penetration of beneficiaries or subscribers. Localities with small populations and few facilities may ultimately be annexed to adjacent, functioning review organizations for review purposes.

In communities with large populations but no predominant employers or carriers, negotiation will be needed to bring together enough of the funding organizations to form a beneficiary or subscriber pool sufficiently large for economical review. Once that minimum number is attained, other groups, large or small, can be added at will. Obviously, this is a long-term solution, because it will take much longer to accomplish than the installation of review programs in areas of high beneficiary concentration covered by single employers or carriers. Program development in areas of this type may have to be relegated to a subsequent mop-up period.

Program evaluation and reporting also can give rise to some thorny issues. Understandably, employers and carriers seek some assurance that they will benefit from the review process to a degree at least commensurate with its cost. That type of assurance can now be given only by quoting the successes of review programs elsewhere, which may or may not be applicable to their own unique situations. Because of the acuteness of their malaise, they are inclined to accept such assurances in contracting initially for review services. At the same time, they must be given some mechanism for the evaluation of review efficacy at appropriate intervals. This would pose no problems if they had adequate baseline data on their own plans, which oddly enough, most do not. In addition, they tend not to know precisely what type of statistical reporting would be most useful to them. It thus becomes necessary for PRN to suggest the types of data that are to be acquired and the services that are to accompany review.

The functions of certification of medical necessity and advice as to termination of benefits are reasonably straightforward and easy to identify. Some types of statistical reporting that are fairly universal in their application also come readily to mind. These could include such reports as:

1. Gross utilization figures on the number of hospital patient days per 1000 subscribers, with comparison data from baseline statistics or comparable subscriber/beneficiary groups

2. Analysis of the case mix for the reporting period

3. Breakdown of utilization data by line of business, age, sex, diagnosis, surgical procedure, and other variables

4. Average length of stay data, again with validly comparable statistics

5. Reports on ancillary service utilization by hospital and for the entire group

Beyond these and similar outputs, it will be necessary to customize reporting content and format to meet the unique requirements of the individual subscriber to the review service.

The PRN has approached the problem of poor or absent baseline statistics by instructing its actuaries to examine the types of data that most carriers and employers customarily collect and to devise a method of abstracting from them at least provisional statistics that could be used for initial comparisons. As far as reporting is concerned, the network will offer the standard reports of its participating review organizations and work with client organizations to identify and meet their special reporting needs.

The final area in which private review poses some questions, if not problems, lies in the attitude of the local hospitals in the review organization areas. Utilization review is not now mandatory except for Title V, XVIII, and XIX patients. Will the hospitals permit nondelegated review of "private" patients by the review organization or accept delegation and perform it themselves? There is no ready answer to this question, and it will vary from hospital to hospital and locality to locality. The hospitals are beleaguered by regulations and beset by hordes of reviewers and monitors from voluntary agencies and all kinds of government licensing and regulatory bodies. Their instinctive initial reaction will probably be that they will not voluntarily take on or permit another review program.

On the other hand, in some states obligatory utilization review is already being performed across the board, and the PSRO statute calls for medical care evaluations on all patients. The delegated hospitals' compensation for such review ranges from inadequate to nonexistent. They may be willing to recoup some of their review outlays by cooperating with a private review program that pays its way.

Another consideration may also persuade hospitals to cooperate. They are now subject to rate controls in several states. The proposed federal legislation on reimbursement ceilings may well box them in completely. They are constantly required to justify construction, daily rates, expenditures, and services. They may see a physician-sponsored, local review organization's appraisals as an assist in these efforts, especially as they realize the ultimate inevitability of across-the-board review.

INITIATIVES

It has been noted that the FMCs, PSROs, and HMO/IPAs may all legally perform private review and are willing and anxious to do so. Without binding commitment in responding to inquiries from PRN, they have accepted the principle of dealing with multistate or national organizations through the network, accepting its monitoring and certification.

Based on these indications, PRN has engaged in an active program to convince the major nongovernmental funders of health services, namely industry and the insurance carriers, of the advantages they would derive from the services of a competent, integrated network of review organizations. PRN has also responded to numerous inquiries from individual multistate employers and some insurance carriers.

Meetings have been held with the BCA and the HIAA, both of which were receptive to the PRN concept. Discussions are now in progress with both organizations to choose appropriate locations to set up test programs under the network. It therefore seems that the initiatives are originating, as they should, from industry, the insurance carriers, and the review organizations through AAFMC/ AAPSRO/PRN. These three components of the private sector recognize, albeit for somewhat different reasons, the urgency of implementing an effective and widespread, if not universal, review program.

These initiatives are taking place none too soon. It is evident that this nation will restructure its entire health care delivery and financing system within the next several years. The present administration has already announced its intent of introduc-

ing a national health insurance program next year. Presumably the federal planners are already actively designing the proposed program without the benefit of advice from an organized private sector, which could be as disastrous now as it was before.

However, even now, before the long-heralded national health insurance program, the federal government through the DHEW is in the process of drastically reshaping the health care system. The Hospital Cost Containment Act of 1977 (HR 6575, Section 1391) and the Medicare/Medicaid Administrative Reform Act of 1977 (HR 7079, Section 1470), if eventually enacted, would have a tremendous effect on the private sector, yet contributions from that sector in their planning phases has been ineffectual because they were fragmented and uncoordinated.

The private sector must break its long-established behavior pattern of merely responding to and testifying on government proposals and then living with the sorry results. One of the many lessons of Medicare and Medicaid is how difficult, costly, and protracted it is to undo the results of ill-conceived and poorly administered programs.

If the nongovernmental funders and providers of health services can find common ground in private review, they can go on to form a coalition of a size and status that can demand the legitimate role in planning that was denied them in the HSAs and go on to set standards of cost, performance, and administration for health care as it is today and as it will be in the future.

24

Ambulatory Review—
Overview of Current Methodology

Robert Hare

Until recently, review of ambulatory care has been limited primarily to the area of utilization and appropriateness of charges, with little attention given to quality assessment. This has been due to the many inherent difficulties associated with non-institutional quality evaluation, the relatively rudimentary state-of-the-art,[2] and the focusing of attention on the hospital setting by PSRO and JCAH requirements.

Two developments have created a sense of urgency of the need for the development of effective methods for quality assurance and utilization review of outpatient care: the rapidly escalating costs of health care with the possible advent of national health insurance, and the desire of professional organizations and groups to enlarge the scope of peer review to the office setting as a necessary requisite of a comprehensive quality assurance program and as a condition of recertification and possible relicensure.[1]

CHARACTERISTICS OF AMBULATORY CARE DELIVERY SYSTEM

If ambulatory care is defined as all the care provided the nonhospitalized patient, it is enormous in volume and is presented in a large and diverse group of settings. According to the National Ambulatory Medical Care Survey (NAMCS), it encompasses approximately one billion visits per year.[28] Of these, two thirds are made to physicians in solo or small group practices and the remainder in a wide variety of settings: the home; large group practices (including HMOs); federal, state, county, and municipal clinics; hospital outpatient clinics; surgicenters; union health centers; free-standing clinics; and many others.

Other relevant characteristics are defined by the survey. Ninety-five percent of all visits resulted in some form of therapy, and in 50% this consisted of prescribed drugs. In 2.9% of visits no follow-up was planned, and in 21.4% return was to be on a patient-initiated basis. About two thirds of the visits were the result of a specific symptom, and the remaining visits were for a wide variety of services, including routine examinations, immunizations, or administrative purposes.

The survey thus graphically describes a massive, heterogenous system delivering a broad spectrum of services in a wide diversity of settings. Visits are stimulated by a variety of problems, many of which are ill defined, defy diagnostic labeling, and frequently involve a single encounter with no definite plans for follow-up or evaluation of outcomes. Each of these tends to impose difficulties in the development of any system of ambulatory care review.

APPROACHES TO AMBULATORY CARE REVIEW

Review strategies may be broadly classified into: (1) those based on information obtained from the claim form or a modification thereof and (2) those that utilize data derived from the medical record and are frequently termed the "medical audit." It is the purpose of this chapter to consider the strengths and limitations of these approaches and to point out some of the requisites for a review system that can address the inseparable concerns of efficiency and effectiveness in the delivery of health care.

Claims-based Review

Review of claims generated by individual patient-physician encounters has been carried out by third-party carriers for many years. It has usually focused on patient eligibility, program coverage (administrative criteria), and the quantitative appropriateness of charges made by the provider.

In the early 1960s, with the advent of the Foundations for Medical Care and later the increasing application of computer technology, claims review became more sophisticated and began to deal to a limited extent with the issues of quality. The history of the foundations, with their important role as conceptual precursors of the PSRO program, has been well documented by Harrington and Egdahl.[10,14]

The earliest detailed analysis of the impacts of claims-based review on the practice patterns in ambulatory care came from the San Joaquin Foundation for Medical Care.[14,17] The basic approach consisted of clerical screening of each claim against utilization criteria, with second-level

physician review for final determinations, and the use of aggregated data for the development of profiles to reflect the care provided by the physician to a number of patients (physician profile) or care provided one patient over a period of time (patient profile) as a supplement to individual review. These techniques have subsequently served as a model for much of the utilization review carried out by third-party carriers.

In reviewing the experience of the San Joaquin Foundation for Medical Care, Buck and White reported small but significant decreases in the utilization of a number of services, including injections, office and hospital visits, and laboratory procedures, and found a statistically significant relationship between the percentage of billing claims adjusted by the peer review process and subsequent changes in practice patterns.[8] In addition to this "individual" effect, they recognized a "group" educational component stemming from provider awareness that the review process is occurring.

The experiences of two statewide professional review organizations—New Mexico and Utah—supporting the feasibility of quality assessment of ambulatory services based on computerized screening of Medicaid claims have been reported. Each operational system employs initial screening of all claims against process criteria developed by physicians in the area. This is followed by second-level professional peer review of all claims that fail to pass the screen. Each has reported significant provider behavior modification in the areas under scrutiny as a result of focused educational activity and denials of reimbursement.

Brook and Williams have reported an in-depth analysis of the impact and possible implications of the 2-year New Mexico Experimental Medical Care Organization (EMCRO) study.[5] This review activity focused on the appropriateness of the use of injections in the office setting. A dramatic decline in the number of injections from 46 to 16 per 100 visits was recorded by the end of the study. As measured by predetermined criteria, 40% to 45% of all injections given by New Mexico physicians (almost half of which were for antibiotics) were felt to be inappropriate throughout the period of observation. Particularly striking were the changes in practice patterns of the 6% of physicians who were responsible for 40% of the inappropriate injections. (The primary effect on quality of care was felt to lie in the greatly decreased incidence of iatrogenic complications.)

Utah's Physician Ambulatory Care Evaluation (PACE) program employs a similar sophisticated data collection technique, but review has been expanded to address patterns of practice involving a large number of problems or diagnoses.[20] Consensus screening criteria have been developed aimed at defining combinations of care that are either "critical to ideal care" or "inconsistent with ideal care." These may address indications or contraindications for given services or therapy, potential drug interactions, utilization limits, and other components. Second-level screen is also carried out by physician reviewers.

Individual variations from the criteria are evaluated in the context of patterns of practice as determined by physician and patient profiles. Deficiencies are reported to the physician directly, and claims are denied when there is no alteration in the practice pattern. When data indicate widespread failure to comply with criteria, formal educational programs are implemented.

Although the full quality of care and utilization impacts of the program have yet to be evaluated, Nelson is encouraged by the substantial decrease in the frequency of exceptions experienced by physicians subjected to direct educational feedback.

Limitations and Potentials of Claims-based Review

The New Mexico and Utah projects represent the most advanced current state-of-the-art, yet a number of review components, all or some of which are considered by many to be essential to a valid quality evaluation system, are missing. Among these are linkage between presenting problems, procedures performed and diagnosis, data validating diagnosis, compliance with short-term outcome criteria, and adequacy of follow-up. Because of the limitations imposed by the lack of availability of these and other quality indicators, there is much pessimism regarding the possible usefulness of claims-based review as a tool to measure quality.

On the other hand, with the majority of medical care provided in free-standing physicians' offices, the claim form represents the only readily available source of information regarding the ambulatory physician-patient encounter. This, coupled with the great expenditure of money and manpower required for audit based on review of office records, has led many to conclude that any national system of ambulatory quality assurance will have to rely, at least in part, on the claims approach.

Sanazaro suggests that reliance on such a system will serve only to identify and eliminate clearly substandard performance but feels this is a worthwhile goal in the absence of such mechanism at the present time for the great majority of patients receiving ambulatory care.[24] However, even to achieve the goal of assuring compliance with basic standards of care through this mechanism, he sees the need for broadening the scope of claims-based review through a concerted developmental effort.

Others have stressed the need for such developmental activity, giving particular consideration to possible modification of the basic claim form to include components needed for quality assessment, providing this can be done without adding prohibitive professional and clerical time demands.[9] One such study is now underway and will be able to benefit from the experience of the Multnomah Experimental Medical Care Review Organization and Multi-Use Data Projects. These efforts utilized an "encounter form," an expanded claim form including elements of the history, physical examination, laboratory tests linked to the presenting problem, and follow-up. Completed by the physician or an assistant, the format was found to be too time consuming for routine day-to-day use. It is possible that a solution may lie between the extremes of this type of encounter approach and the traditional claim form.

It would seem a reasonable goal at this time to focus developmental efforts on expanding the capabilities of claims-based review to meet the challenge of assuring compliance with basic standards of care proposed by Sanazaro, as well as serve as a much needed mechanism for identification of problems to be subjected to the intensive and costly approaches of office medical audit.

In-depth Evaluation of Ambulatory Care

The past decade has seen much evolution and refinement in the art of quality assessment and assurance. The ultimate goals of the latter have been defined by Sanazaro as "a near guarantee to every patient of appropriate treatment and fewest possible complications," and its appropriate boundaries were delineated by Brook, who stated, "Quality assurance activities that do not improve health status should be eliminated."[6,25]

Even in the organized structure of the hospital setting and with a vast amount of time and money devoted to mandated audit, the development of an ideal quality assurance system capable of achieving the above goal is still far from attainment. This awaits the solution to such fundamental problems as a better definition of the causal relationship between what is done to the patient (process) and its effect on the illness or condition (outcome), the development of effective methods to modify practice behavior to correct deficiencies, improved record keeping in all settings, and the development

of approaches to measure the art as well as the technical content of care.[6]

The question of the best method for quality evaluation is far from resolved, but basic models for all settings predicated on the present state-of-the-art have evolved. These call for (1) comparison of services provided against preestablished criteria for appropriate care (process evaluation), (2) comparison of results obtained against preestablished criteria for results expected when efficacious therapy is provided (outcome evaluation), or (3) a combination of both. The advantages and disadvantages of these approaches have been reviewed extensively in the literature.[4,29]

Some of the major problems posed by the ambulatory care setting can be considered in terms of the methodological requirements of these models.

Identification of Problem Areas

A wide variety of techniques are in use or under consideration for the identification of possible problem areas subject to in-depth audit. Each presents limitations, and development of a generally applicable approach awaits further research and development efforts.

As previously considered, use of review based on the claim form or a practicable modification thereof as a driver to more intensive study seems promising, based on the experience of a number of foundations. This approach is undergoing study at the present time.

Group-process identification of perceived problem areas is also undergoing trial in a number of settings and has been most widely publicized by Rubin.[23] His approach, used in a large group practice, calls for review of the medical record to trigger group discussion and selection of possible problem areas. Whether this methodology can be used in the unstructured setting of the PSRO area remains to be seen.

The promising "staging" concept proposed by

Gonnella is based on the premise that the seriousness or stage in the severity of a patient's condition at a given time is a good indicator of the outcome of previous treatment.[12] This approach is now under study at the hospital-office interface.

Selection of Subjects for Review

At least two characteristics of the ambulatory care encounter tend to limit the number of problems amenable to objective quality assessment today: lack of relationship of process to outcome and the frequency of undiagnosed problems.

The principle that subjects for review should be limited to those in which it has been shown by scientific study that the course of the condition can be predictably affected favorably or unfavorably by specific action of the physician has been stressed by Williamson and Sanazaro.[25,29] The latter has pointed out that only a small proportion of ambulatory care can be objectively documented as efficacious today in view of the frequency of self-limited and single-encounter problems.

These authors also suggest that the quality of care can best be measured in those conditions in which it is possible to make a precise diagnosis that can be validated by objective data and that measurement requires use of the medical record audit for in-depth evaluation. This limitation of the scope of ambulatory audit becomes particularly important when assessment of the overall quality of a physician's practice is attempted and requires selection of an appropriate constellation of problems to obtain an adequate valid sample.

Data Acquisition

In-depth medical audit at this time requires availability of detailed information from the medical record. Except in group practices and in settings with computer-based record systems, acquisition of this data is difficult and expensive.[25]

The shortcomings of the medical record—incompleteness, inaccuracy, nonstandardization, and inadequate coding and filing—particularly in the offices of solo or small group practitioners, has been described by Thompson and Osborne and many others.[26] Awareness of these deficiencies has lead to intensive efforts on the part of individuals and organizations to upgrade the record and improve its format, thus increasing its potential as a tool for quality evaluation.[15,21,27]

Despite these deficiencies, several studies have shown that a large percentage of charts from the office practices of volunteer physicians can be abstracted by trained, nonphysician personnel.[13,16]

This approach to data acquisition is widely used in ambulatory care audits. Considerable technical refinement in abstracting methodology leading to increased accuracy and validity has been reported.[13] Costs of this system are extremely high, necessitating limitation of its use to evaluation of important specific medical problems identified by other peer review methods or for the in-depth evaluation of the overall quality of a physician's practice.

A few highly sophisticated computer-based information systems for monitoring health care are in use and probably represent the most advanced state-of-the-art at the present time. Notable is that reported by Barnett in which concurrent review utilizing explicit criteria provides immediate feedback to physicians to change their management of patients.[3]

Use of Criteria

One of the most significant advances in quality evaluation has been the growing acceptance of the basic concept that care must be measured against objective (explicit) predetermined criteria in contrast to the individual subjective (implicit) judgments of the past. Also of great importance has been the evolution of the concept of appropriate criteria. The early optimal care ("laundry list") criteria containing all of the procedures that might be used in a given diagnosis have been largely discarded in favor of essential (critical) criteria, which include elements that apply to almost every patient with a specified condition.

Sanazaro points out that the ongoing arguments over "process versus outcome" become irrelevant if essential criteria are by definition process criteria predictive of objectively definable outcomes.[25] This underscores the desirability of developing, when possible, both essential process and outcome criteria for the medical audit and serves as the basis for the outcome-oriented JCAH Performance Evaluation Procedure (PEP) program and the American Society of Internal Medicine's assessment of performance research. The latter links consensus-derived outcomes to each of the process stages in which medical care is usually provided: history, physical, and laboratory (process) to diagnosis (outcome); short-term therapy (process) to short-term management goals (outcome); and long-term management (process) to long-term management goals (outcome). When the desired outcome is not achieved, the study utilizes logic branching technique to enter a new process cycle.

Modification of Behavior

For a quality review process to result in actual improvement in patient care, corrective action in the form of modification of behavior is usually required. How this can best be done is under study at this time and constitutes one of the more important agenda items for quality assurance research and development.

Although emphasis has been, and no doubt will continue to be, on continuing medical education (CME), there is little objective evidence of its ability to modify physician behavior.[18,19,22] In an effort to improve this performance, Brown has proposed the well-known bi-cycle model, which would structure the content of CME programs for the correction of specific deficiencies identified by peer review. This approach has been widely accepted (although less widely implemented), but firm evidence that it significantly improves physician behavior has not been reported.

Sanazaro suggests two possible explanations: that some physicians look on CME as an educational exercise divorced from their actions in treating patients and that a physician's knowledge is not necessarily related to the physician's actual performance.[7,11,25] As pointed out by Barnett, many studies of ambulatory care quality indicate that the most significant problem is the failure to perform systematically routine diagnostic and treatment activities and to follow up on identified abnormalities.[3]

These deficiencies point to the necessity of utilizing other approaches in addition to CME for assuring quality of care. Among those under study are direct physician feedback (primarily through use of the educational letter), peer pressure (through physician's awareness of being reviewed), denial of payment or fee reduction, and administrative changes. The traditional foundation approach and the advanced New Mexico and Utah models have incorporated the first three approaches with significant results.[5,20]

The potential role of each of these approaches in the PSRO system has not as yet been determined, but it is anticipated that group and individual educational efforts will be emphasized. Availability of statistically derived physician and patient profiles based on high-quality PSRO data holds the potential for identifying practices clearly and should provide a valid basis for such educational activities.[24]

Innovative approaches to shorten the feedback loop as that described by Barnett are clearly needed if maximal impact on practice behavior at the time one is seeing the patient is to be achieved, but concurrent review of this type awaits drastic modification of data systems in the solo or small group practice setting and is unlikely in the near future.[3]

SUMMARY

The basic concepts and tools of quality evaluation have been refined to a level consistent with the review of a small but important segment of care delivered in the ambulatory setting. This segment is limited to those problems in which the course of the illness under review is clearly affected favorably or adversely by the actions of the physician and focuses the immediate goal on detection and correction of basic deficiencies in care. Broadening of the scope of review awaits identification of additional problems with this causal relationship between process and outcome or development of new measurements of quality of care, such as determination of patient satisfaction.

Application of the audit and medical care evaluation techniques of the hospital has been shown to work well in organized group ambulatory care practices, but it remains to be seen whether they are either technically or economically possible in the solo or small group office where most care is provided. Pending this determination, it seems likely that any national ambulatory care evaluation system will rely at least for problem identification on claims-based computer screening.

Methodology for the assessment of the quality of a significant segment of a physician's practice at a level necessary for certification or relicensure is now in the process of development. Its ultimate feasibility has not as yet been established.

REFERENCES

1. *Assessing physician performance in ambulatory care.* 1976. Proceedings of a conference sponsored by the American Society of Internal Medicine. San Francisco.

2. *Assessing quality in health care: an evaluation.* 1976. Washington, D.C.: Institute of Medicine.

3. Barnett, G.O., Winickoff, R., Dorsey, J.L., et al. 1976. The role of feedback in quality assurance—an application of a computer-based ambulatory medical information system. In *Assessing physician performance in ambulatory care.* Proceedings of a conference sponsored by the American Society of Internal Medicine.

4. Brook, R.H., and Appel, F.A. 1973. Quality of care assessment; choosing a method for peer review. *N. Engl. J. Med.* 288:1323–1329.

5. Brook, R.H., and Williams, K.N.: Evaluation of the New Mexico peer system, 1971–1973. *Med. Care* 14 (suppl.):12.

6. Brook, R.H., Williams, K.N., and Avery, A.D. 1976. Quality assurance today and tomorrow: forecast for the future. *Ann. Intern. Med.* 85:809.

7. Brown, C.R., Jr., and Uhl, H.S.M. 1970. Mandatory continuing education: sense or nonsense? *J.A.M.A.* 213:1660–1668.

8. Buck, C.R., Jr., and White, K.L. 1974. Peer review: impact of a system based on billing claims. *N. Engl. J. Med.* 291:877.

9. Bussman, J.W. 1977. Personal communication.

10. Egdahl, R.H. 1973. Foundations for medical care. *N. Engl. J. Med.* 288:491.

11. Gonnella, J.S., Goran, M.J., and Williamson, J.W. 1970. Evaluation of patient care: an approach. *J.A.M.A.* 214:2040–2043.

12. Gonnella, J.S., Louis, D.Z., and McCord, J.J. 1976. The staging concept—an approach to the assessment of outcome of ambulatory care. *Med. Care* 14:13–21.

13. Hamaty, D. 1976. The American Society of Internal Medicine assessment of performance research. In *Assessing physician performance in ambulatory care.* Proceedings of a conference sponsored by the American Society of Internal Medicine.

14. Harrington, D.C. 1973. The San Joaquin foundation peer review system. *Med. Care* 11:185.

15. Hurst, J.W. 1971. How to implement the Weed System. *Arch. Intern. Med.* 128:456.

16. Kroeger, H.H., Altman, I., Clark, D.A., et al. 1965. The office practice of internists. I. The feasibility of evaluating quality of care. *J.A.M.A.,* vol. 193.

17. Krantz, G. 1961. The San Joaquin foundation for medical care. *Am. J. Public Health* 51:23.

18. Lewis, C.E., and Hassanein, R.S. 1970. Continuing medical education: epidemiologic evaluation. *N. Engl. J. Med.* 282:254–259.

19. Miller, G.E. 1975. Why continuing medical education? *Bull. N.Y. Acad. Med.* 51:701–706.

20. Nelson, A.R., and Cannon, J.Q. 1976. The PACE project: computer-assisted peer review of ambulatory services. In *Assessing physician performance in ambulatory care*. Proceedings of a conference sponsored by the American Society of Internal Medicine.

21. Page, O.C. 1976. Data acquisition and display in an ambulatory care setting: a systems approach in assessing physician performance in ambulatory care. Proceedings of a conference sponsored by the American Society of Internal Medicine.

22. Payne, B.C., and Lyons, T.F. 1972. Methods of evaluating and improving personal medical care quality: episode of illness study. Ann Arbor, Mich.: University of Michigan Press.

23. Rubin, L. 1973. Measuring the quality of care. *Group Practice* 22:7–14.

24. Sanazaro, P.J. 1977. *Issues, directions, and application*. San Francisco: Address before a conference of the Ambulatory Medical Care Quality Assurance.

25. Sanazaro, P.J. 1976. Medical audit: continuing medical education and quality assurance. *West. J. Med.* 125:241–252.

26. Thompson, H.C., and Osborne, C.E. 1976. Office records in the evaluation of quality of care. *Med. Care* 14:294.

27. Weed, L.L. 1971. Quality control and the medical record. *Arch. Intern. Med.* 127:101.

28. White, K.L. 1976. Results of the national ambulatory medical care survey in assessing physician performance in ambulatory care. Proceedings of a conference sponsored by the American Society of Internal Medicine.

29. Williamson, J.W. 1971. Evaluating quality of patient care—a strategy relating outcome and process assessment. *J.A.M.A.* 218:564–569.

25

Selecting Criteria for Review of Ambulatory Care

John S. Gilson

Application of the concept of public accountability to the ambulatory setting is extremely difficult, far more so than in the case of hospital care. There are, as I see it, two major differences. First is the absence of the hospital, with its aggregation of patients, physicians and records, which greatly simplifies the technical problem of quality assessment, and existing tradition of public accountability via the trustee, and varying degrees of experience with peer review.

Equally important, but less obvious, perhaps, is the fact that the goals of ambulatory care are more difficult to define. As a result so are the standards or criteria against which performance can be judged. Some physicians . . . insist that it is literally impossible to define the goals of ambulatory care. . . . In their view it is purely and simply an art . . . real art does not commit itself to external goals. . . . Despite the obvious difficulties the problem is not insuperable. . . .

Anne R. Somers
San Francisco, California
June 1976

No one has devised a widely accepted method for the review of ambulatory care. Consequently, it may seem premature to discuss the selection of criteria. On the other hand, initial consideration of what are or could be used as criteria could lead to a better appreciation of what kind of methods might likely prove useful and acceptable in reviewing ambulatory care.

Several different methods have been suggested for reviewing ambulatory care, and these have been discussed by Palmer.[2] Perhaps one of these, or some amalgam of two or more, may achieve professional consensus. However, until and unless this occurs, it would seem desirable to continue exploring a variety of methods for performing ambulatory care review and to continue exploring, in addition, the characteristic elements involved in providing the care itself. Ideally the methods used for review should either fit with these characteristic elements or derive from them; therefore this chapter first discusses some of the elements perceived as characteristic attributes of ambulatory care and then discusses some observations concerning those attributes and how they might affect the selection of criteria for use in reviewing ambulatory care. Third, the chapter discusses against this background some of the methods and criteria currently utilized for review, including commentary concerning features perceived as strengths or weaknesses. The chapter concludes with speculation concerning what directions might be taken and what methods and criteria the medical profession might consider for both short- and long-term approaches to the review of ambulatory care.

Although both Codman in 1916 and Lembcke in 1956 (after a 40-year gap) actively advocated review of medical care, their cause languished for lack of general acceptance.[3,4] Furthermore, they emphasized review of care in hospitals, not ambulatory care. The recent impetus for review of care came in the late 1960s as a consequence of two major factors: judicial decisions that questioned the adequacy of methods for assuring the quality of care provided in hospitals and a growing apprehension concerning the rapidly escalating costs of care (and of malpractice decisions), which in turn, raised questions concerning whether the quality of care was commensurate with cost. The judicial decisions and the interest in cost control both focused on hospital care where accreditation mechanisms were in place (JCAH) and legislative arrangements for subsidy were already functioning (laws covering Medicare and Medicaid). Therefore, the initial quality review mechanisms were naturally directed toward hospital care. However, putting the focus on the hospital and adding quality assurance as yet another objective for existing hospital functions also led to a premature assumption that hospitals understood what they were attempting to do and needed only to get on with doing it.

In retrospect, one might now perceive that the problems were actually much more complex. First, review of care was thrown into the company of compulsions imposed on the profession from outside, compulsions that many physicians believe should be rejected like any other foreign body. Furthermore, those compulsions related heavily to cost concerns, which many physicians believe should not be their direct concern. Finally, there was too little attention given to the fact that accomplishing reviews directed at quality is an entirely new function; any entirely new function requires new methods, and new methods need to be proved before they can gain general acceptance. For the latter to happen, it helps to base new methods on a broad understanding of the phenomena involved. Unfortunately, both for hospital and ambulatory care, deliberate studies of how care gets delivered—in contrast to what is

best to deliver—have begun only in recent years. Consequently, there is only a narrow base of understanding on which to build new review systems for quality assurance purposes. The medical profession has until recently invested its collective energies (and the public's resources) into discovering the best procedures to follow. The assumption was that knowing what to do would ensure that it got done, that being well-informed ensured high-quality performance. However, by now both the medical profession and the public have had enough contrary evidence to question that assumption. As a result there is strong social pressure on the profession as a whole to provide direct and explicit evidence bearing on the quality of its performance, a pressure that has been translated into an expectation that performance will be judged against agreed-upon criteria. The questioning, pressure, and expectation are all new, and the first attempts at satisfying them have yet to be evaluated.

For these reasons the central theme of this chapter goes beyond the four topics just discussed. The approach to reviewing the quality of hospital care may have been too superficial, too hasty, possibly misdirected, and too soon locked into a prescribed pattern. Before the confusion is compounded by taking a similar approach to ambulatory care, the medical profession might reconsider. Therefore, the theme of this chapter is that the review of ambulatory care will require a much better understanding of how big a task it is, that is, about the essential nature of ambulatory care itself, and the need for a cautious skepticism about easy answers.

SOME GENERAL ATTRIBUTES OF AMBULATORY CARE

In the same manner that the response of children to pharmaceuticals was long believed to be the same as the adult response except for requiring considerably less drug to produce it, the medical profession has behaved as though ambulatory care were a lesser derivative of hospital care, requiring primarily the same skills but much less of them. Not only were similar but lesser skill levels presumed but the ambulatory care endeavor was not subjected to scientific studies of how it was done; apparently it was not perceived as different enough from hospital care to be based on its own specific body of scientific knowledge. Perhaps physicians have thought of ambulatory care, as Somers said, as an art with indefinable goals. However, I suspect that seeing it mainly as an art, as a lesser derivative and an endeavor not worthy of its own scientific base, came less from a critical look at ambulatory care directly than from viewing it through lenses ground to fit hospital vision, through hospital-adapted pupils. As a result, the medical profession does not have as clear an understanding of the mechanisms by which ambulatory care gets accomplished or a widespread consensus about how physicians are expected to practice in their offices.

Ambulatory care, as Somers mentions, also lacks the "aggregations" long associated with the hospital: the standardized records, the policies and procedures that are virtually uniform across the country, identifiable roles (such as physician, nurse, and aides) and the mutually understood expectations associated with them, and so on. Even though some of this hospital pattern is changing, it still represents a common body of reasonably well agreed-upon practices. Ambulatory care in the usual office practice, on the other hand, lacks all of this. Records are in whatever style the practitioner chooses, as are policies and procedures, and the nonuniformity of roles is almost total, except, perhaps, for the physicians themselves. Ambulatory care is idiosyncratic.

These idiosyncratic realities pose serious problems, especially in selecting criteria for the review of ambulatory care. Hospital review has largely settled on a new variant of peer review that emphasizes the *evaluation of professional performance against explicit criteria.* Even though there have been difficulties both locally and nationally in designing explicit criteria for hospital practice, a body of reasonably well agreed-upon practice patterns in the hospital from which, in theory at least, criteria can be derived does exist. There is also a certain logic in preferring to evaluate performance against explicit criteria, and the reasonableness of that logic suggests that performance in ambulatory care ought to be similarly evaluated against explicit criteria. However, explicit criteria would seem easiest to derive in proportion to the presence of consensus and common practice patterns and difficult in proportion to the amount of idiosyncracy, and as described, ambulatory care is fundamentally idiosyncratic.

Perhaps in some of the situations common to ambulatory care, explicit criteria of the sort used in the hospital setting can be derived. Hypertension, urinary tract infection, and diabetes are a few examples that come to mind and are the conditions usually cited as prototype models for ambulatory reviews. But perhaps they come to mind because of a basic error: thinking in terms of doing ambulatory review as a derivative of hospital review, requiring only modification of the hospital model, not a basically different model. Or they may come to mind because they are conditions that have been shifted to the ambulatory setting only relatively recently and thereby still have an association with hospital-type care. However, the burden of this entire chapter suggests that *the hospital model may have only a limited utility in review of most ambulatory care* and that whatever its utilities may be, one should look directly at the characteristics of ambulatory care itself to see to what extent it may be generically different from hospital care. As a rule, hand-me-downs are well received only if they fit and are useful to the receiver. Some of the specific characteristics of ambulatory care of the sort alluded to by Somers are given in the following list. These characteristics are of two types, clinical and procedural, and both types are generally idiosyncratic.

Unique Attributes of Ambulatory Care

Clinical Attributes

1. Patient-defined end points
2. Vague, or unspecified, and unvalidated level of illness
3. Lack of diagnosis and "approximate diagnoses"*
4. "Paramorbi"†
5. Variable continuity
6. Considered as an art—negligible body of scientific knowledge
7. Wide mix of patients

Procedural Attributes

1. Patients not confined, not subservient
2. Lack of hospital disciplines and constraints
3. Lack of coding for access to records of comparable cases
4. Nonuniformity of procedural details: type of histories, sequence of workup, timing of intervention
5. A different function for the medical record
6. Self-taught using anecdotal data

*Approximate diagnoses: the patient's diagnosis is not fully identified but further diagnostic efforts are judged unnecessary.[5]

†Paramorbi: unwanted states other than disease—symptoms with an emotional cause misinterpreted as manifestation of a long-standing illness (such as aching attributed to osteoarthritis when the problem is ordinary aches and pains in an emotionally stressed individual). The opposite of paramorbi would be somatic illness caused or triggered by emotional components (such as peptic ulcer).[5]

Each point in the previous list is discussed for its probable effect on selecting review criteria.

Clinical Characteristics of Ambulatory Care

1. *Patient-defined end points.* Patient-defined end points are obvious but seldom recognized characteristics of ambulatory care, which may be its most significant hallmarks. Hospitalized patients become subservient to their illness (and often subservient to those caring for them) and become detached from direct contact with most of their daily concerns. Their illness and their caretakers largely determine what happens. For example, the caretakers decide when the hospital episode begins and ends and much of what comes between. However, in ambulatory care, the patient as a rule decides, albeit with varying amounts of advice, when the medical care episode begins and ends and may or may not comply with advice along the way. Although the physician in particular seldom acknowledges directly the dominant role of *patient-control of ambulatory care,* this feature should probably be explicitly recognized in designing or selecting criteria for the review of that care.

2. *Vague, or unspecified, and unvalidated level of illness.* In ambulatory care in contrast to hospital care, the level of illness present in any given patient is neither stated explicitly nor recorded as a rule; the impression itself is usually subjective and is often idiosyncratic. Even when the physician actually records a "diagnosis," that diagnosis is not as specific as it might seem and probably is a relatively poor indicator of what level of illness is actually present. This facet is further amplified later in the chapter. In addition, whether stated as an impression, recorded as a diagnosis, or not even mentioned, the actual level of illness perceived as present in an ambulatory patient is rarely validated by direct or indirect peer and institutional interactions to the degree that occurs regularly in the hospital. Thus the level of illness for patients remaining in ambulatory care is neither clearly nor precisely categorized except for being less than the hospital level, and its validity is uncertain.

In addition, the range of illness levels encompassed by ambulatory care is extremely wide. Hospitalization by itself carries the implication that the level of illness is somewhere in a very narrow range at the upper end of the scale. Therefore, the level of illness can usually be inferred with fair accuracy in hospitalized patients. On the other hand, the level in ambulatory care cannot be inferred with any such degree of accuracy.

The importance of stressing the wide range of illness levels relates to the use of diagnoses, especially the use of diagnosis-derived categories, as topics for review in ambulatory care. "Peptic ulcer" as a discharge diagnosis after hospitalization connotes a relatively serious level of illness that is likely to be reasonably comparable to the level of illness in another hospitalized patient similarly diagnosed. On the contrary, the conditions of two ambulatory patients diagnosed as peptic ulcer could have levels of illness so far apart that they would not be at all comparable. The illness in the more severe might be serious enough to approach hospitalization levels, whereas the other with mild illness might have ulcer symptoms hardly requiring medical attention at all. The points are that hospitalization itself is an approximate indicator of the illness level present, that the range of possible levels in ambulatory care is too broad for the setting itself to serve as a similar index, and that *similar diagnostic labels do not encompass similar levels of illness* with any reliability in the ambulatory setting.

3. *Either no diagnosis or approximate diagnoses.** The diagnostic label in ambulatory care not only poorly indicates the level of illness, the label itself is often absent. In contradistinction to the circumscribed hospital episode with its final diagnosis in the discharge summary, many ambulatory episodes are not given a diagnostic label at all. Instead they are recorded as problems, treated as such, and never given firm diagnostic labels whether the patient comes once or for a long series

*For definitions, see footnotes on p. 238.

of visits. Or they are carried on the record with what amounts to Krogh-Jensen's "approximate diagnosis," which under the circumstances, applies a diagnostic term without implying a final or established diagnosis. An example would be a physician who sees for the first time a patient with a history of moderately severe but brief widely intermittent attacks of epigastric burning without prior confirmation by x-ray examination, who then makes the working or "approximate" diagnosis of peptic or duodenal ulcer. Symptomatic treatment would probably be advised, but follow-up care might not be urged. In this case, peptic (or duodenal) ulcer would be an "approximate diagnosis." Usually that diagnosis would not be firm in the same way that the same term when used as a hospital discharge diagnosis would be firm. If patients seen in the office are given a diagnosis at all, it is quite likely that it will be an approximate diagnosis but not necessarily so specified. Therefore, *highly specific criteria,* as customarily used in reviewing hospitalized cases with firm diagnoses, are probably *inappropriate for reviewing groups of ambulatory patients selected by diagnostic categories.*

4. *Paramorbi.* Paramorbi, another Krogh-Jensen term (p. 238), represents another example of the difficulties in identifying sharply defined clinical categories in office practice.[5] As previously noted, paramorbi are illnesses traveling under an assumed name; the diagnosis is actually an alias. Even though the patient or the physician may interpret the symptom as organic disease, both the cause and the treatment of that symptom are found to depend quite often on influences affecting the patient other than physiology, bacteria, physical trauma, and so forth. In other words, they may depend on psychosocial influences that trigger emotional responses, which in turn, may be perceived as though they arose from somatic dysfunction. No matter whether the patient misperceives

the relationship, as in the example given on p. 238, or the physician misperceives it, as in the case of a postsurgical cardiac patient who reports easy fatigability on exertion instead of continuing apprehension, the ultimate problem with "paramorbi" lies in the *misperception* itself.

Neither paramorbi nor approximate diagnoses are unique to ambulatory care. The problem arises because they are ubiquitous in ambulatory care and much less common in hospitalized patients. By understanding how the specificity of diagnostic terms has been eroded when used in ambulatory settings or by clarifying the limitations of hospital terms when transposed into the ambulatory setting, one can see the emergence of another characteristic distinction that further distinguishes ambulatory from hospital care; *Not only are diagnoses frequently inadequate for estimating level of illness but they often do not even accurately characterize the illness itself.*

5. *Variable continuity. Variable continuity* is a feature that pervades ambulatory practice. Patients choose not to return, either because the problem resolves itself or because they seek other help. Physicians usually forego active follow-up and depend primarily on patient initiative to trigger continued care. For these and such reasons as difficulties related to gaining access to care and coping with the necessities of daily living, the *recording of an episode of ambulatory care is often tantalizingly incomplete,* especially for the recording of outcomes or what ultimately happened. Furthermore, ambulatory care often stretches out over long periods of time so that the medical care personnel as well as the prevailing patterns of good care may change significantly without being well reflected in the record. These variabilities in continuity will of necessity modify the selection of criteria for ambulatory care review; they will need to reflect the difference from the hospital model where short-time continuity is the rule.

6. *Considered as an art.* Until very recently, the lack of academic interest in the specifics of ambulatory care as a distinct discipline within medical practice has served to foster the impression that ambulatory care, that is, office practice, is an art. Furthermore, because it is a discipline that involves *all physicians regardless of specialty,* its uniqueness, whether art or science, is obscured. This seems to occur because ambulatory care *within each specialty* varies in its impact; it is virtually congruent with the full range of care encompassed by the specialty of family practice, and at the other extreme it may be considered as a completely subordinate activity for the consulting cardiovascular or neurologic surgeon. Therefore, ambulatory care, perceived as an art without much of an up-to-date artistic literature (a literature that lost its stature after Osler and Peabody), has tended to be self-taught, based on highly subjective impressions, and unanalyzed. For these reasons, it seems likely that *achieving consensus about criteria proposed for ambulatory review,* especially if ambulatory care is perceived as an art, *will be more difficult* than achieving consensus about criteria designed for the *science* of hospital care.

7. *Wide mix of patients.* Regardless of any specific triage arrangements that may exist, the mix of patients presenting to any type of ambulatory care setting seems quite naturally to be broader than the mix presenting to its hospital counterpart. For this reason, ambulatory care serves as a "sorting gate" for the undifferentiated population that seeks medical care or prevention. Besides serving such a triage function, ambulatory care also serves to complete some levels of care, continues others, and passes on the rest. Ambulatory care in every specialty tends to be more mixed than the corresponding type of hospital care. This attribute expresses in another way the diffuse and ill-defined nature of ambulatory care. It reemphasizes that *review criteria may be inappropriate*

if the hospital model is used outside the hospital setting.

Procedural Attributes of Ambulatory Care

The discussion of these distinctive clinical elements within ambulatory care can be extended by noting additional differences in procedural elements.

1. *Patients not confined, not subservient.* Patients not confined and not subservient obviously overlap with patient-defined end points but have procedural elements in their effect on appointment making, follow-up and compliance, arrangements for referrals, and so forth. It almost certainly would affect criteria selection both for the process type of criteria and for outcomes.

2. *Lack of hospital discipline and constraints.* Somers alludes broadly to the lack of hospital discipline and constraints. This lack covers the presence in the hospital of a body of rules, a chain of command, a set of well-recognized and largely unquestioned expectations of each other among those involved in care, and so forth. These are largely absent in ambulatory care settings, or if present, they are quite idiosyncratic. *Given these differences from the hospital, it would appear as though a different type, or at least a broader type, of review criteria will be needed.*

3. *Lack of coding.* If quality assurance is to explore the full range of ambulatory care (in contrast to looking primarily at already recognized or likely problem areas), there would seem to be a need ultimately for some ongoing system of categorizing clusters of similar entities so that all instances within the cluster can be identified. In other words, there is a need for some sort of coding system. Perhaps as Rubin claims, however, there are enough entities that can be readily identified as topics for review that do not require coding for

their discovery so that attempts to devise a coding system specifically for ambulatory care can be set aside, at least for the present.[6] Certainly from what has been stated already it would seem reasonably obvious that *hospital-type codes already in use may prove largely inappropriate and misleading if applied uncritically to ambulatory care.* Coding specifically for ambulatory care is not yet commonly available. This fact will for some time to come influence the process of reviewing ambulatory care, including the kind of criteria that can be selected.

4. *Lack of uniformity within the process of care.* In the hospital the roles of various personnel and the kinds of data kept, as well as the manner in which they are kept, are reasonably well standardized. In office practice, however, there is a lack of uniformity within the process of care. This seems to be true in both small group practices and many of the larger institutions, such as the Kaiser-Permanente Foundation, the Mayo Clinic, and Group Health Cooperative of Puget Sound, even though each one tends to create its own internal standardizations. But although the forms used in records or for requests may be standardized within an institution or any other type of ambulatory practice, the type and content of entries on the forms are not. Furthermore, the sequence of workup, timing of interventions and follow-up, and patterns of coverage tend to vary widely and idiosyncratically both within and between such institutions as well as in smaller practices. Again, *given the lack of procedural uniformity, it seems likely that criteria for ambulatory care review must be selected with these differences in mind.*

5. *A different function for the medical record.* In the hospital the medical record is compulsively complete, partly because of its primary function as a definitive archival document covering the care of advanced or serious, often critical, illness. *The hospital record is an official record.* Conversely,

the records kept of ambulatory care in a physician's office are working notes for the physician or group of physicians involved—a characteristic emphasized especially by Rubin in the course of serving as a consultant in quality assurance. As a result, the entries in the office record of ambulatory care are not stylized and complete as required by the hospital but are idiosyncratic. The entries tend to fit the need for recording as those needs are perceived by the recorder at the moment of entry. The entry characteristically satisfies the perceived needs of a limited audience of one physician or a small group, not the wide and unspecified audience of physicians and others who have come to expect and require entries in the hospital record according to a protocol that is quite uniform nationwide. *Without a major revision of record keeping, the office record will not be as useful a tool for review as the hospital record, and criteria must take this into account.*

6. *Self-taught process.* The self-taught process is another overlap from the clinical characteristics of ambulatory care. Among the providers of care, physicians tend to pick up largely on their own an individualistic understanding of how an office practice should function. Interchange of ideas among peers about office practice patterns is almost entirely casual and anecdotal, and there are relatively few objective reports in the medical literature of careful and deliberately designed scientific studies on the topic to use as any sort of guide except for an increasing number of articles in some of the controlled-circulation "throw aways." In a sense, this probably explains much of the lack of uniformity mentioned previously regarding the lack of uniformity and the different function of the medical record. Whatever benefits may come from this marked degree of diversity, the diversity itself also creates difficulty. As is evident from experience with hospital reviews, criteria selection is easier where consensus is strong; it will probably

be difficult, or at least different, where consensus is weak or obscure as it appears to be in the largely self-taught circumstances of office practice. *Ambulatory review criteria must be adapted to diversity in individual physician's practice patterns to a degree far greater than in the hospital.*

This discussion belabors the point that ambulatory care differs profoundly from hospital care. When the two phases of care are critically examined, they can be perceived as basically different even though sequentially linked. The importance of their basic differences lies in the need to avoid perpetuating the perception that ambulatory care is a lesser derivative of hospital care or that the understanding of ambulatory care and the ability to provide it can be presumed on the basis of hospital experience. The discussion also strongly suggests that the design and selection of review criteria for ambulatory care might well differ substantially from the way hospital review criteria are designed and selected.

Characteristic Attributes and Their Effect on Criteria Selection

The preceding characteristic attributes are not meant to be definitive but are meant to be at least indicative of the need to consider ambulatory care as an activity that is distinctively different from hospital care. Other differences could be mentioned, such as the wide variety of practice styles from one physician to another, the differences related to the type of practice whether solo or group, and the range of specialties or illnesses cared for. However, the differences discussed so far will serve to indicate how the many differences will probably influence the review process generally and especially influence criteria selection.

The main feature that crops up throughout the preceding discussion is the impression that ambulatory care generally is so different from care in the hospital that ambulatory care review probably needs its own model. Even though there are conditions such as those mentioned on p. 237 in which the hospital review model may still be the best available, and even though no one has a very clear idea yet of what will work in its place, it seems unwise to cling to the hospital model in the face of the diverse ambulatory care realities as perceived and described in the preceding section. The knowledge that the hospital model is clearly not appropriate for all settings of care may make people realize its faults even in the hospital setting. That realization may also temper the widespread notion that the biggest problems with review of care lie in enticing the professions to perform it or demanding that they do so. Perhaps the real problem is the presumption that people know how to review medical care at all.

Human flight seemed simply the problem of how to approximate the flapping wing, but very little progress was made until people realized that man and bird had evolved too far apart for that to work very well. But a different approach to flight, based on understanding the dynamics involved, dramatically succeeded and rapidly surpassed the bare hope of simply imitating birds. Perhaps a more reasoned approach to ambulatory care review may also open up a new developmental path that will ultimately facilitate review in other settings, including the hospital. If that were to happen, it might possibly help reveal the inherent worth of reviewing care generally. Regardless of these speculations, it seems clear enough that the thrust to extend review to the ambulatory setting merits a fresh look at what people are trying to do and how they are trying to do it.

The following is a list of subjective generalizations derived from the elements on p. 238, and the list speculates how each generalization might affect criteria selection.

1. Necessity to include patient perceptions as desired outcomes—"concordance"

2. Necessity to expand the dimensions of desired outcomes beyond those used in hospital review

3. Limited potential for diagnosis-based methods

4. Greater need for consensus within the review process

5. Need for less rigid or less precise screening criteria

6. Limited utility of the hospital model for reviewing care

7. Need for redefinition of criteria "dimensions"

Once again, the list is meant to be less definitive than provocative. The following discussion considers each generalization on the list.

1. *Patient perceptions as outcomes—concordance.* As previously noted, patient-defined end points are a hallmark of ambulatory care. This feature dominates ambulatory care and sharply distinguishes it from hospital care. In a sense, the act of accepting hospitalization amounts to an abdication of self-determination by the patient. When the patient enters the hospital, the physician takes over control. In part this may be due to the fact that hospitalization is accepted when the disease process is serious enough that a specially trained professional needs to take charge. It is similar to requiring a specially certified individual to take charge of certain modes of transportation, especially when they involve dangerous speed, highly intricate equipment, and so forth. In the ambulatory setting, on the other hand, physician control is nominal at most.

With physician control nominal and the patient playing a major role in deciding what as well as how much happens during the course of obtaining care, it seems logical to define *desirable outcomes* in ambulatory care in terms that also include *patient perceptions* (including expectations), not just the physician's perceptions and expectations.

Physicians' perceptions as a rule tend to focus primarily but not exclusively on how the mechanisms of disease are affecting the patient. At the more serious level of hospital illness, these perceptions related to the disease tend to have overriding priority for both patient and physician. Because the hospital physician concentrates on perceiving the disease and its effects, a desirable outcome tends to be synonymous with the physician's accuracy of those perceptions and the physician taking action appropriate to them. Stated another way, desirable outcomes and screening *criteria* that relate to them for *severe levels* of illness (hospital) are largely defined by how well the *physician perceives the disease*.

At the lower levels of illness that characterize ambulatory care, where physician control is nominal and patient decisions can play a major role in outcomes, the perceptions of the patient would seem to be an important element to be included in both outcome and process criteria. Lacking the physician's detailed professional background in pathology, physiology, and so forth, patients tend to focus primarily on *how they feel* in the face of moderate or mild illness and its treatment, *how their activities of daily living are altered* by those circumstances, and on the arrangements, whatever they may be, that must be made in their lives *to cope* with the effects of illness. Although patients have a deep interest in the disease process and often have great interest in having it explained to them, their own concerns especially at the lower levels of illness seen in ambulatory care relate very strongly to their *perception of how well their disease has been handled*.

This line of reasoning leads to the conclusion that both good outcome and good process in ambulatory care relate to how well the perceptions of patient and physician match—to the "concordance" between them. Hippocrates said it another way when he stated, "The physician must not only do what is right himself, but also to make the patient, the attendants, and the externals cooperate." If the physician's perceptions of the disease are "right" but fail to be concordant with the patient's perceptions of how well the disease has been handled, the patient's actions, which in ambulatory care are often definitive, are likely to negate the physician effort. The importance of this for criteria selection in ambulatory care comes from the conclusion that ambulatory care—the care of lesser levels of illness than those seen in the hospital—requires some estimate of the *concordance between physician and patient perceptions, including ways to estimate the perceptions of each individually*.

This generalization, if accepted, raises a number of other corollaries. Is satisfaction synonymous with concordance? It would seem that satisfaction could occur even without concordance, as with a poorly healed fracture that the patient accepts and seeks no further care, even though the physician expected a better result and might advise more therapy if the patient came back. Compliance is probably not synonymous with satisfaction for similar reasons. Compliance without a reasonable congruence of expectations and perceptions between physician and patient could easily be undesirable, such as taking medications even in the face of adverse reactions.

However, in a somewhat similar sense the quality of the triage function, or what could be called "placement," might be an additional facet of this same generalization. Even if the professional is satisfied with the arrangements for the technical aspects of the illness, the outcome, especially in terms of future *management of the patient by the patient,* may well be seriously adverse if the patient perceives that "placement" of the illness within the care system is faulty. Even though the patient may perceive that the outcome for the moment is satisfactory, future decisions by the patient may be seriously affected if the patient perceives that more should have been done or that what was done should have been done differently. This relates specifically to whether the patient perceives that proper consultations were requested, that all of the appropriate tests were done, or that adequate instructions were given for how to cope with future events. For these reasons concordance between the patient and the provider perceptions seems to encompass the desired outcomes better than the more limited term "satisfaction" or "compliance," although each is involved. *Patient perceptions and their concordance with those of the physician seem to be an important source of outcome criteria for ambulatory care.**

2. *Necessity to expand the dimensions of desirable outcomes.* Where the process of care is idiosyncratic, where diagnoses are approximate and paramorbi are common and where it is hard to set a point at which to identify the outcome, or even what outcome to identify, relating criteria directly to the disease process itself, as characteristically used in review of hospital care, seems inadequate. For these reasons, the dimensions of criteria as used in hospital review need to be redefined and expanded. Length of stay clearly does not apply; death is not usually a probability; com-

---

*Concordance is consistent with Parson's concept of the "sick role" described in his book *The Social System*, 1951, New York: Dodd, Mead & Co. It especially fits with ideas rated by Freidson in his book *Profession of Medicine*, 1970, New York: Dodd, Mead & Co. It especially fits with ideas such as those articulated by Freidson on pp. 226–228, in which the meaning of illness to the patient is discussed. However, the concept of concordance appeared to derive directly from efforts to characterize the unique features of ambulatory care as identified during several decades of practice and from observing patients' behavior. The concept was crystalized in discussions with Linda Howell, a psychologist and colleague in quality review at Group Health Cooperative.

plications are unusual, minor, or both; the disease usually gets resolved or achieves a steady state; and the attending physician may not be made aware of some or all of those outcomes, whatever they may be. From complaints made, suits filed, articles in the public press, and so forth, it seems obvious that there is some degree of error in the assumption that failure to return represents a reasonably favorable outcome. It is even unreasonable to make that assumption in closed-panel prepaid systems, in which most patients might be expected to return somewhere in the system if an adverse outcome occurred. Regardless of the system of care, patients may not perceive the adverse outcome as adverse, may misunderstand what to expect, may assume that whatever happens is supposed to happen, and so forth. In addition, it is clear that for a variety of reasons patients may be reluctant even to report adverse outcomes to those from whom they will need to turn in the future for care of possibly more serious conditions than the current episode.

These generalizations suggest that as a rule *criteria used in hospital review cannot be used for ambulatory review without major modification or expansion.* In addition, *identification of some sort of opinion sampling may be an essential feature in selecting criteria for ambulatory care review.*

3. *Limited potential for diagnosis-based methods.* Because of such factors as paramorbi and approximate diagnoses, as well as those patients for whom a diagnosis is not reached or recorded, methods of review that are dependent on either the diagnosis or on forcing a diagnosis if none is entered are both unrealistic. Because of the common absence of recorded diagnoses, combined with reasonable doubts about diagnoses that are recorded in hospital terminology, diagnosis-based review methods would likely have limited validity for ambulatory care. Furthermore, any grouping of cases collected because they were given the same diag-

nostic heading, even when all were cared for by the same physician, are likely to be a more diverse group and thereby less comparable to each other than a grouping included under the same diagnosis made in the hospital. Up to now, most of the review methodologies proposed specifically for ambulatory care require collections of cases grouped under diagnostic categories. This would seem appropriate for only a narrow spectrum of ambulatory care. Finally, *even if it were otherwise appropriate, general application of diagnosis-based review methods would seem to require a quantum leap in the amount and accuracy of record keeping in office practice, a change that would be enormously expensive and disruptive without any compensating evidence that doing so just to facilitate audits would actually improve quality of care.* See Brook and Davies-Avery for examples.[7]

The inadequacy of diagnoses as the foundation for ambulatory review creates a dilemma for most physicians. Physicians are so accustomed to thinking about the practice of medicine (particularly the review of care) only in the framework of diagnoses that they have difficulty in comprehending methods not based on diagnoses. However, there are useful numbering systems other than those to the base ten, at least one other dimension than Euclid's three, and other motors besides reciprocating. One alternative to diagnoses would be to *review by problems* regardless of how those problems might be specified or by whom. Another would be to *review by reasons for visit,* identified by either the physician or patient. (The National Ambulatory Medical Care Survey has developed a reason-for-visit code, which was recently revised and is under final review.[8]) There are undoubtedly other alternatives, but the point is that diagnoses have a sharply limited utility in the wide spectrum of ambulatory care, especially given current styles of practice and record keeping. Even if diagnosis-based methodologies are used, their limitations should not be

forgotten. Ultimately, if ambulatory care is to be studied as it really is, *review methods that are not based solely on diagnoses, and that differ substantially from the diagnosis-based familiar patterns used for hospital reviews must be created.*

4. *Greater need for consensus within the review process.* Virtually all of the characteristic attributes listed on p. 238 would suggest that the general level of consensus is much lower in ambulatory care. The idiosyncratic nature of ambulatory practice, the relative lack of physician control over the care process, the diverse and poorly defined level of illness, and the fact that ambulatory care is largely self-taught tend markedly to increase the amount of diversity in ambulatory care. Nevertheless, diversity is characteristic of medical care, and physicians almost instinctively resist consensus as antithetical to the nature of people and their diseases. Furthermore, with the application of science to the more serious levels of disease and illness (levels associated with hospital care), consensus such as it is tends to be concentrated in the hospital setting. Even so, review of hospital care has struggled to identify enough consensus to enable the review of the care provided to groups of patients instead of reviewing care case by case as the actual degree of diversity might otherwise require.

Review mechanisms for ambulatory care will need to cope with an even greater degree of diversity. Undoubtedly some of the existing diversity could and perhaps should be reduced; some of the diversity physicians perceive and accept as inevitable may actually be unnecessary. The diversity might even reflect poor care, but in the absence of an organized body of knowledge relating to ambulatory care, it will be difficult to decide just which elements, if any, are unnecessary. In the meantime, any review methodology will have to accommodate to diversity and seek whatever consensus can be identified. It would seem that *methods that ignore this diversity or that attempt to overcome it by imposing methods that presume consensus are doomed to serious difficulty.*

Because of these reasons, review of ambulatory care may appear to be even less precise and consequently less assuring than even the current hospital reviews. However, one should remember that a neat and precise system, even though full of measurable statistics, may not be measuring the entity under question. Physical dimensions neatly tabulated do not establish beauty either in people or artistic design; the measuring instrument must be designed to measure the entity being measured. Review of ambulatory care may need its own set of methodologies.

5. *Need for flexible or less precise screening criteria.* In the face of diversity, it is tempting to measure those things that are measurable rather than devising measuring tools appropriate to the characteristic being studied. In the case of ambulatory care, with the probable difficulty in achieving consensus about outcomes or even finding outcomes for which markers are readily available, there is likely to be an impulse to select *process criteria.* Process is usually easier to measure than outcomes, especially when outcomes are long delayed, as they are in ambulatory care. Although process can be seen as an intermediate outcome if viewed from another perspective, it is important to remember that it seems more generally valid to look on outcomes or intermediate outcomes as being more valid than process for use as screening criteria for review of care.

The distinction between process, intermediate outcomes, and ultimate outcomes is arbitrary. In fact, they are a continuum, and what appears as process from the outcome end of the continuum may appear as an outcome when viewed from the process end, but the distinction is still helpful. In the context of this discussion, the distinction is important to avoid the error of calling a process item an outcome without identifying clearly that the process item chosen is indeed by itself a desirable outcome. For example, if the desirability of demonstrating an adequate hemoglobin level was specified as an intermediate outcome, this would be appropriate if it were agreed that correction of the hemoglobin level was the desired outcome for the problem. However, if the assumption has been made incorrectly that anemia explains the weakness, and the weakness is not due to the borderline anemia but to depression, demonstrating an adequate hemoglobin level would not be an appropriate outcome criterion. The problem, therefore, is to avoid this type of tempting pitfall when the desired outcome is difficult to specify.

Given the nature of ambulatory care, one's expectations for precision must be moderated, especially any expectation that precision will be similar to that for hospital review. The scientific body of knowledge underpinning the patterns of ambulatory practice is less precise, the methods for achieving results are far more diverse, the complicating variables are much more numerous and less subject to control, and those variables can intrude at an unpredictable rate over a long period of time, and so forth. For all of these reasons *flexible criteria may be the best fit under ambulatory circumstances* even though they seem too flexible compared with the familiar criteria used in hospital reviews.

6. *Limited utility of the hospital model for reviewing care.* The hospital model concentrates on the details of medical management as recorded in the hospital medical record. It focuses primarily on the effects of physiologic malfunction within the body and less on the function of the patient as a person. It is associated in many minds with review of diagnoses. It assumes that a desirable outcome as perceived by the physician is desirable to the patient as well. The hospital model may work for some situations in ambulatory care, but it seems unlikely that it will prove widely useful for the

majority of ambulatory care. In light of the difficulties encountered with initiating hospital review, it would seem only to invite even greater difficulties if ambulatory review is approached as a close relative of hospital review. The point of this entire discussion is that ambulatory review compared with hospital review may be an entirely different breed.

REVIEW OF CURRENT CRITERIA

Although review of ambulatory care has not yet become even a *quasi-legal* requirement (which would carry the same pressures for compliance as those associated with hospital review), it seems clear that the same social pressures that initiated explicit review of hospital care will in time produce a similar requirement for the ambulatory field. Regardless of whether this takes a quasi-legal form (as exists with the JCAH) or the fully legal requirements under the PSRO amendments, or whether it remains for a considerable period of time as a moral obligation on the profession, it seems unlikely in this period of public accountability that a privileged profession can retain its credibility without some measure of accountability across the full range of services it provides.

The current emphasis on reviewing care for evidence of quality probably began with the report by Trussell and associates in 1962 on care received by Teamster families in New York.[9] Unlike Codman's efforts more than half a century earlier, others carried on the efforts of Trussell and associates, and this time the emphasis spread beyond the hospital to ambulatory care. Morehead and associates have developed the approach of Trussell and associates into a systematized method.[10]

The program begun in 1968 by the then titled American Association of Medical Clinics (now the American Group Practice Association) began as a voluntary activity by a physician-management association, which was apparently stimulated by a feeling of professional obligation and a wish to confirm the high quality they proclaimed for the services provided by their members. That viable program, using written criteria that depended heavily on subjective interpretation, has evolved into the Accreditation Council for Ambulatory Health Care of the Joint Commission for Accreditation of Hospitals. More explicit criteria were added about the time of the changeover, and other explicit criteria are under development, but the program continues with essentially the same foundation on which it began 12 years ago.

In the late 1960s, Payne and Lyons made a detailed study of the process of care in Hawaii.[11] In the early 1970s, the American Society of Internal Medicine funded studies of internists' office practices as preparation for assessing the quality of care.[12] Williamson and Millder studied the behavior of physicians in response to laboratory data, and went on to explore how quality itself might be assessed.[13] Individuals such as Hamaty demonstrated how office practice, separate from practice in the hospital, could be studied.[14] Eventually the EMCRO programs, especially those in Oregon and Hawaii, attempted to do the same in anticipation of or as implementation for the emerging PSRO organizations. These efforts have recently been reviewed by the Institute of Medicine of the National Academy of Sciences with the conclusions that efforts in the field of ambulatory care will be at least as difficult if not much more so than those in hospital care, that there is a dearth of knowledge about ambulatory care on which to base a program of review, and that moves that would tend to freeze current methodologies and inhibit experimentation are probably premature and deleterious.[5] The purpose of this chapter is to endorse that point of view and provide a variety of subjective observations based largely on experience in ambulatory care to support that opinion. Brook, with Davies-Avery, has once again sounded the same warning with well-documented evidence from a wide knowledge of the medical literature and his own experience to support his position.[7]

Even with (or perhaps because of) the legal and quasi-legal mandates, the profession generally has been reluctant to embrace review of care for quality assurance purposes. The effort is often viewed as an imposed "add on," not relevant to the main purposes of medical practice. Some hope and others expect that it will fade away because of ineffectiveness, be dropped because of high costs, or be recognized as unnecessary. From an historic perspective this seems unlikely. As with the oracles at Delphi, the church with the Reformation, royalty with the revolutions in the last 200 years, the aristocracy based on slave labor, and the economic privilege of great wealth in the depression, once the justification for a social privilege is questioned, the question persists to its resolution. The outcome is usually the withdrawal of privilege from the privileged group by the socially dominant force unless the privileged group can persuasively revalidate its privileged position. Therefore it would seem prudent for the profession diligently to seek the best possible professionally appropriate answer to the question of accountability (hence, the analysis in this chapter).

REVIEW MODELS

Several types of reviews, or major components in methods of review, as currently considered or in use are loosely categorized in the following discussion. Each of these approaches is valuable both for pioneering in this difficult field and for serving valuable but limited purposes. The comments are directed not at how well they serve their restricted purposes but at how well they fit some of the specific generic features of ambulatory care. In other words, the comments focus on the limitations of each approach, on the aspects not covered by the specific approach when viewed against the characteristics of ambulatory care generally.

Trussell-Morehead Approach

Trussell and associates used conventional wisdom to develop criteria against which care was compared.[9] Morehead and associates have extended the method to ensure a wider consensus—albeit a consensus from a wider representation among the same sort of academically oriented experts—to a method now applied widely for review of neighborhood health centers and ambulatory care facilities generally.[10] This system is characterized by a large number of criteria that represent the conventional wisdom of the academic physician; the recorded details of actual practice are compared with these criteria. To the extent that the conventional wisdom of the academic physician derives from a wide body of validated knowledge, this method and any other method dependent on a consensus view of conventional wisdom would be the best available. Conversely, however, any such method would be seriously flawed to the degree that the particular conventional wisdom has its roots in tradition, authority, or both. Despite the obvious flaws that arise from the limited knowledge of ambulatory care as a science, the characteristic feature of the Trussell-Morehead pioneering approach, namely consensus around conventional wisdom, has become a major component of most of the other types of review in the discussion that follows.

Accreditation Council for Ambulatory Health Care Model

The Accreditation Council for Ambulatory Health Care (ACAHC) (a new council of the JCAH) as a beginning is concentrating on accrediting group practices or other institutionalized arrangements, that is, arrangements with three or more sharing a practice, that provide ambulatory care.[16] It requires the group to have an active ongoing audit process, but wisely in my opinion, leaves the details of method completely optional.* This leaves at least one accreditation door open to permit experimentation and innovation outside the gambit of PEP-type, hospital-adapted, diagnosis-based reviews. The legal door, the PSRO, is still officially ambiguous about what it intends to require in ambulatory review and is sponsoring a group of demonstration projects that may result in regulations that will permit a variety of approaches. These trends are consistent with the points advanced in this chapter.

The approach used by the ACAHC appears quite similar to that of the Trussell-Morehead approach except for the group chosen to express the consensus. In contrast to Trussell-Morehead, the ACAHC, and the American Group Practice Association before it, developed its consensus using the conventional wisdom of physicians in full-time, service-oriented, nonacademic practice. The criteria for accreditation are significantly different in their thrust and in the amount of procedural detail specified. The ACAHC standards seem comparatively loose but also seem more consistent with the characteristics of ambulatory care as discussed in this chapter.

Commission on Professional and Hospital Activities Approach

The Commission on Professional and Hospital Activities (CPHA) has made only exploratory moves

*The term ''audit'' conveys too many meanings. It has come to imply any review similar to that of the PEP (JCAH) program as used for hospital reviews and is synonymous with any review activity at all, that is, it implies both a specific and generic review activity. Obviously the ACAHC uses the term in its generic sense. Otherwise the term is carefully avoided in this chapter.

toward involvement with review of ambulatory care. From its traditional core of data derived from medical records and its diagnosis-based data displays, its capabilities seem poorly adaptable to the characteristics of ambulatory care as previously described. In fact, the CPHA preoccupation with process data, that is, with procedures carried out in the course of care rather than trying to identify at least intermediate outcomes, makes its relevance even to hospital review seem limited.

American Society of Internal Medicine Method

The American Society of Internal Medicine (ASIM) effort and similar efforts of other specialty societies reflect the nature of their training and practice: diagnosis based, hospital oriented, and physician centered. However valuable the CPHA and ASIM approaches may be, their value for ambulatory care would seem to be severely limited to a small portion of the ambulatory care spectrum where diagnoses are reasonably definitive and the physician is in control of the care process. In other words, their value is primarily for that portion where the illness level is close to requiring hospitalization. For reasons already discussed in this chapter, *these approaches and most of the other currently proposed methods will probably not prove out as models for overall review of the full spectrum of ambulatory care.*

Similar conclusions seem applicable to the *methods based on the use of billing forms.* Other EMCRO efforts and those by foundations for medical care as well as most efforts by professional societies other than ASIM fall into this category. Unfortunately, billing for ambulatory care was not designed to fit the realities of ambulatory care but instead is heavily influenced by the many factors previously described associated with the hospital viewpoint. The most serious limitation is again the failure to deal adequately with clinical situations where no diagnosis is appropriate, where the diagnosis is approximate (in other words, an alias) but not so specified, and where paramorbi are recognized but ignored to fit billing purposes. However, despite its severe limitation as a broadly adequate generalizable model, this type of model can be valuable in more limited but still important ways, as shown by the studies of Payne and more recently Brook and Williams in New Mexico.[17]

Criteria Mapping Model

The method of criteria mapping as proposed by Greenfield and associates deserves particular mention in this relationship.[18] Criteria mapping identifies decision points in the care of specified illness with *alternate pathways* through them. This approach attempts to minimize the enforced and unrealistic rigidity of using uniform process criteria and overcomes the expedient of weighted process criteria used by Lyons and Payne. Its advantage would seem to be its direct linkage between actions taken and the resulting outcome, especially as it highlights that relationship. Thus it reduces substantially some of the main drawbacks to the reliance on process criteria.

Practice Profile Method

The practice profile approach, as proposed by many medical care foundations and the discharge abstract services, such as CPHA and California Health Data Corporation, seems to be a device to identify areas of potential problems or poor fits between training and actual practice experience. If the profiles for ambulatory care were to reflect an appreciation of the many difficulties associated with using hospital-type diagnoses, the method would appear to be helpful by showing the "practice load" faced by the practitioner. Regardless, *it is better as a way to define topics for review* than as an aid for selecting criteria. In other words, pro-

files are valuable as a first step in the review process but do not by themselves directly influence criteria selection.

Tracers Model

Tracers as advocated by Kessner, Kalk, and Singer are another method of identifying topics for review.[19] Tracers are conditions that can be viewed as characteristic examples of typical care, and therefore the care given for these conditions can be considered as reasonable approximations of the general level of care. Regardless of their value, tracers, like profiles, do not affect directly the selection of criteria for review either for ambulatory or hospital care.

Preventable Illness Model

Preventable illness, as proposed recently by Rutstein and associates, also serves as a method to identify what to review.[20] In addition, it probably indicates directly a level of care. By establishing conditions that should not occur under conditions of high-quality care, the method also *defines criteria* for the care provided for a specific illness. The method itself is an agreed-upon group of specific outcome criteria. Although most of the conditions so far listed by Rutstein and associates usually end up in the hospital, most usually have a significant period of ambulatory care before admission. To that degree, these conditions represent criteria for ambulatory care but for relatively rare conditions.

Health Accounting Approach

The health accounting concept proposed by Williamson and associates is a fundamental advance.[21] It attempts to establish for a given condition the responses that can be expected under high-quality care and to consider those responses to be, in effect, intermediate and ultimate outcome criteria for that condition. The degree to which those criteria are met would indicate the level of quality for the care provided. This is ideal in theory as well as in practice, but at present it can be applied only to those conditions that are well enough studied so that there is broad professional consensus, in other words, for specific diagnostic entities that usually represent a high level of illness and have been thoroughly researched. As indicated previously, such conditions are at present characteristic of only a small portion of ambulatory care.

Kessner, Kalk, and Singer link their tracer approach to a type of health accounting to form a more complete system. The staging concept advanced by Gonnella, Louis, and McCord is related to health accounting by identifying explicit stages that mark levels of illness; progression from one stage to another can thus be used as a criterion against which to compare care.[22] Schroeder and Donaldson have proposed another variant of health accounting by linking diagnostic accuracy (estimated from chart review) and outcomes (estimated by polling a general sample of the population that includes those having the condition whether treated or not).[23] The Albemarle EMCRO has taken another similar approach by attempting to use only those process criteria that have been validated by critical research.[24] Finally, Sidel and associates have proposed a review that is linked to a follow-up survey to determine outcomes.[25] Each of these is related generically to the Williamson and associates' health accounting concept and share similar potentials and drawbacks. At this time (and for a long time to come) they remain attractive theoretic models that may eventually lead to very effective and practical methods. However, all of them depend heavily on diagnosis and consensus, both of which are uncommon features in much of ambulatory care as presently practiced.

It is noteworthy that two of these approaches (Schroeder and Donaldson and Sidel and associ-

ates) incorporate a *specific follow-up beyond that initiated by the patient* (and recorded by the physician). Such a follow-up inquiry, done specifically to obtain quality-related data, seems logically consistent with the characteristics of ambulatory care just described and the generalizations drawn from them. *Criteria related to patient perceptions subsequent to care seem essential for adequate review of ambulatory care.*

Comprehensive Quality Assurance System

The Comprehensive Quality Assurance System (CQAS) initiated by Rubin in the late 1960s for use in the Kaiser-Permanente system in the San Francisco area differs significantly from all of the preceding.[6] It involves four very pragmatic steps: (1) identifying a problem in care (whether in the hospital or at the office) that everyone agrees is a problem calling for correction, (2) setting criteria for care that if met would correct that problem, (3) using available data or setting up special data collection mechanisms to assess performance bearing on those criteria, and (4) taking corrective action on the basis of the assessment.

Rubin has repeatedly demonstrated that agreed-upon problems are common wherever they are sought. Consequently, he believes that other more structured methods of review are needlessly complex given current realities in medical practice. He often states that the CQAS method does not measure quality but just solves problems.

CQAS differs from other proposed methods in not trying to survey a segment of care in a broad sweep to document a general level of care and to pick up any problems noted during that sweep. It does try to identify problems directly from readily available sources, either from people who know where problems exist or by a quick review of a sample of medical records (''micro sampling'').

Although not limited to ambulatory care, CQAS does fit relatively well with the characteristics of ambulatory care described earlier in this chapter.

Batalden and O'Connor in an elegant demonstration have used a variant of CQAS very effectively in a large ambulatory care private clinic.[26] Like Rubin, they have demonstrated the acceptability and productivity of the approach in a service-oriented group practice. Batalden and O'Connor's approach, like the CQAS, is quite pragmatic and fits well with the characteristics of care listed on p. 238. However, neither attempts to measure quality but to improve it.

A review of current criteria and related approaches used for reviewing ambulatory care might stop here, but there is another related concept that deserves mention and that applies equally to reviews of hospital and ambulatory care. Data developed in the review of care, both in scientific research and quality assurance, have traditionally come from a study of *cases seen.* Consequently, the criteria against which such data are compared tend to be selected against a conceptual viewpoint heavily focused on cases seen. However, another viewpoint rooted in public health is beginning to spread into the study of personal care and seems specifically valuable for quality assessment. That viewpoint emphasizes the study of outcomes against the *population at risk,* in other words, *population-based studies,* in contrast to studies based on cases seen.

Examples of such studies that provide data relating to quality (and consequently to the selection of criteria against which data can be compared) are few but increasing. The halothane studies were one beginning. Lewis' study of varying incidence of surgery and another of the same type by Vayda, are others.[27,30] Some aspects of the study of surgical services in the United States (SOSSUS) used a population-based approach.[28] Recent publications by Bunker and Brown on utilization of specific types of surgeries by a population group, by Vayda comparing Canadian surgery rates with British rates, and by Shorr and Nutting on the continuity of ambulatory care are still others.[29-31] Taking these as a group suggests that population-based studies could be important indicators of quality.

In studies on appendectomy, by Watkins and Howell done on a defined member population at Group Health Cooperative of Puget Sound (Seattle) the population-based method has been specifically adapted to include an audit component (to meet JCAH specifications). However, the major result from this approach has been a look at quality of care from an entirely different perspective. The studies have indicated that the conventional wisdom concerning the inverse relationship between number of normal appendices removed and perforation may be wrong, at least in this setting. But regardless of the specific findings, the study suggests that reviews of care to assure quality may well include studies of the entire population served to provide another type of data highly relevant to quality. Such studies might stimulate entirely different types of criteria for use in reviewing care, especially if they change present understandings of what really works. There is an obvious logic to population-based studies of health care, and the logic seems as compelling in the review of ambulatory care. At this point, however, this approach is still so new that further exploration and demonstrations are necessary before it can be actively considered as an available practical method.

HOW TO SELECT CRITERIA FOR REVIEW OF AMBULATORY CARE

The preceding discussion outlines difficulties and points out inadequacies. Each of the methods discussed has merit and should be used. The previous discussion serves primarily to identify the limitations in each method, especially their limited applicability across the broad spectrum of ambulatory care. The important point for now is to *avoid the temptation to anoint any one method as the best for ambulatory care generally.*

Selection of criteria is dependent on the particular method chosen for use. It seems advisable from the previous discussion to *avoid the controversy over whether process or outcome criteria are best* (except for death, either can be defined as the other). It would be preferable to concentrate on reexamining each suggested criterion for its actual relevance to the quality of care regardless of whether the criterion is considered as process or outcome. It is desirable to strive, as in the Williamson and associates model or the Albemarle EMCRO project, to *avoid unvalidated criteria wherever they can be identified and to be aware of the limitations when nonvalidated criteria are used.*

Wherever possible, *criteria should be selected or designed to reflect patient's perceptions and expectations as they compare with those of the physician.* This implies that some *deliberate postevent follow-up* will be necessary. Follow-up occurs unpredictably in most ambulatory care circumstances, and even when it does happen, it seldom addresses directly the perceptions and expectations of either party. Doing so would, therefore, require an essentially new activity specifically for quality assurance purposes, and this may not seem practical. On the other hand, reliance on current criteria, especially those inadequately validated (that is, those validated only by custom or authority), may ultimately prove even less practical and even more costly without being at all relevant to quality. Therefore, it seems appropriate at least to take advantage of what postevent follow-up may exist or may be readily contrived and relate criteria selection to such follow-up wherever possible.

It also seems worthwhile when any of the available methods are used to reconsider them in the light of the ambulatory care characteristics described at the beginning of the chapter. If review of the broad spectrum of ambulatory care is desired, it should be recognized that *methods based on diagnoses, and especially on billing diagnoses, may have serious limitations, that diagnosis-based coding systems are probably not as useful as they seem, and that office records as they now exist will only suffice for a part of the data necessary to evaluate quality in ambulatory care.*

What then is the best method? For those in a position to do research each of these methods merits further development. *Those methods related to health accounting appear to have the most potential* for becoming tools best adapted to evaluate the full spectrum of ambulatory care. Of the available methods this seems the most generic, despite the obvious difficulties presently holding it back. From a different perspective, *population-based studies could prove to be similarly effective* in providing data concerning quality of care. *Both health accounting and population-based studies come close to measuring quality directly.*

For those who perceive at this time the need to review ambulatory care for their own purposes or to anticipate legal or quasi-legal requirements that are already in sight, the CQAS seems the preferable method. It is entirely pragmatic. It requires only minimal and temporary alteration in existing patterns of care. Furthermore, it fits into customary patterns of medical and administrative thinking. In addition, it addresses problems, an approach that avoids many of the adverse connotations associated with other quality assurance methods. Finally, it does not presume to measure quality directly, but that may be a premature assumption for any method. For these reasons, the *CQAS and the selection of criteria that if met will solve agreed-upon problems seems about right for the present* and perhaps for a long time to come, especially for review of ambulatory care.

REFERENCES

1. Somers, A.R. 1976. *Public accountability and quality protection in ambulatory care*. Keynote address before the Conference on Assessing Physician Performance in Ambulatory Care sponsored by American Society of Internal Medicine, June 18–19, 1976, San Francisco.

2. Palmer, R.H. 1976. Choice of strategies. In Greene, R. *Assuring quality in medical care*. Cambridge, Mass.: Ballinger Publishing Co., Chapter 3.

3. Codman, E.A. 1916. *A study in hospital efficiency: the first five years*. Boston: Thomas Todd Co.

4. Lembcke, P.A. 1956. Medical auditing by scientific methods. *J.A.M.A.* 162:646–655.

5. Krogh-Jensen, P. 1977. Classifying disease in general practice. *J. R. Coll. Gen. Pract.* 27:232–234.

6. Rubin, L. *Comprehensive quality assurance system: the Kaiser-Permanente approach*. Alexandria, Va.: American Group Practice Association.

7. Brook, R.H. and Davies-Avery, A. *Quality assurance and cost control in ambulatory care*. Series P-5817. Santa Monica, Calif.: Rand Corp.

8. DeLosier, J. Personal communication.

9. Trussell, R.E. et al. 1962. *The quantity, quality, and costs of medical and hospital care secured by a sample of Teamster families in the New York area*. New York: Columbia University School of Public Health and Administrative Medicine.

10. Morehead, M.A., et al. 1971. Comparisons between OEO neighborhood health centers and other health care providers. *Am. J. Public Health* 61:1294–1306.

11. Lyons, T.F., and Payne, B.C. 1972. *Method of evaluating and improving personal medical care—episode of illness study*. Ann Arbor, Mich.: University of Michigan Press.

12. Hare, R.L., and Barnoon, S. 1973. Medical care appraisal and quality assurance in the practice of internal medicine. DHEW Pub No HSM 110-70-420. National Center for Health Services Research and Development.

13. Williamson, J.W., Alexander, M., and Millder, G.E. 1967. Continuing education and patient care research. *J.A.M.A.* 201:938–942.

14. Hamaty, D. 1970. West Virginia voluntary peer review service, *W. Va. Med. J.* 66:307–309.

15. Institute of Medicine. 1974. *Advancing the quality of health care—key issues and fundamental principles*. Washington, D.C.: National Academy of Sciences.

16. Accreditation Council for Ambulatory Health Care of the Joint Commission on Accreditation of Hospitals. 1976. *Interim standards*. Chicago: The Council.

17. Brook, R.H., and Williams, K.N. 1976. Evaluation of the New Mexico peer review system, 1971–1973. *Med. Care* (suppl.): 14

18. Greenfield, S., et al. 1975. Peer review by criterion-mapping: criteria for diabetes mellitus. *Ann. Intern. Med.* 83:761–770.

19. Kessner, D.M., Kalk, C.E., and Singer, J. 1973. Assessing health quality: the case for tracers. *N. Eng. J. Med.* 288:189–194.

20. Rutstein, D.D., et al. 1976. Measuring the quality of medical care. *N. Engl. J. Med.* 294:582–588.

21. Williamson, J.W., Aronovitch, S., Simonson, L., et al. 1975. Health accounting: an outcome-based system of quality assurance. *Bull. N.Y. Acad. Med.* 51:727–738.

22. Gonnella, J.S., Louis, D.Z., and McCord, J.J. 1976. The staging concept: an approach to the assessment of outcome of ambulatory care. *Med. Care* 14:13–21.

23. Schroeder, S.A., and Donaldson, M.S. 1976. Feasibility of an outpatient approach to quality assurance. *Med. Care* 14:49–56.

24. Decker, B., et al. 1974. *Comparison of explicit medical care criteria in EMCRO*. Boston: Arthur D. Little, Inc.

25. Sidel, V.W., et al. 1977. Quality-of-care assessment by process and outcome scoring: use of weighted algorithms. *Ann. Intern. Med.* 86:617–625.

26. Batalden, P.B., and O'Connor, J.P. *Interstudy annual report to the W. K. Kellogg Foundation*. Minneapolis: St. Louis Park Medical Center Quality Assurance Program.

27. Lewis, C.E. 1969. Variations in the incidence of surgery. *N. Engl. J. Med.* 281:880–884.

28. Nickerson, R.J., et al. 1976. Doctors who perform operations: a study in hospital surgery. *N. Engl. J. Med.* 295:921–926, 982–989.

29. Bunker, J.P., and Brown, B.W. 1970. The physician-patient as an informed consumer of surgical services. *N. Engl. J. Med.* 282: 135–144.

30. Vayda, E. 1973. A comparison of surgical rates in Canada and in England and Wales. *N. Engl. J. Med.* 289:1224–1229.

31. Shorr, G.I., and Nutting, P.A. 1977. A population-based assessment of the continuity of ambulatory care. *Med. Care* 15:455–464.

26

Ambulatory Care Quality Assurance:
An Operating Model

Paul B. Batalden
J. Paul O'Connor
Marion P. McClain

Regular review of medical care has been increasingly accepted by physicians and required by consumers through their representatives in both public and private sectors. Although the impetus for this has been mandatory peer review, physicians themselves are becoming more interested in and curious about assessing their own practices. As presently mandated and operated, most peer review occurs in the hospital via utilization review (UR) and medical audit. For effective peer review, however, all medical care delivered to all patients must be reviewed. Moreover, although effective at first in decreasing hospital stays, UR is expensive and can be circumvented.[7] The initiatives undertaken by the ACAHC of the JCAH and the PSRO demonstration projects supported by the BQA reflect growing awareness of the need to broaden the sphere of review. The increased interest in examining ambulatory care affirms the fact that most care is delivered to most patients most of the time in the outpatient setting and that effective adequate ambulatory care can decrease or eliminate the necessity for expensive hospitalizations.

Better medical services at less cost can occur through the review of ambulatory care along with traditional UR than through hospital UR alone.[7] For instance, available and high-quality outpatient care can reduce hospitalizations of chronically ill patients with such diseases as diabetes or congestive heart failure.

Ambulatory care quality assurance initiatives are of limited value unless they spark the interest of physicians and continue to encourage them in their efforts to examine their practices. Physicians, not the federal or state bureaucracies, must fashion a workable and valid program for assessing medical care delivered in the ambulatory setting. Although various approaches to ambulatory care quality assurance have been tried and several reviews of those efforts are available, this chapter is limited to the description of the current Quality Assurance Program at the St. Louis Park Medical Center in Minneapolis, Minnesota.

The St. Louis Park Medical Center (SLPMC) is a 25-year-old, multispecialty group practice currently comprised of 93 physicians in 16 clinical departments and four satellite facilities. In 1976, there were approximately 387,000 patient encounters with about 85,300 patients at the SLPMC. Of the approximately 180,000 active clinic patients (seen within 5 years), a closed-panel prepaid health plan accounts for about 15% of the total patient activity.

After several months of planning, the Quality Assurance Program (QAP) at the SLPMC was begun in late 1975. The planning stage served as a basis for the implementation of the review program. Monthly evaluation sessions by the entire QAP staff are conducted to review the status of the program implementation and operation. This internal assessment has proved invaluable in the daily management of a program that by its nature consists of many separate activities.

During the planning stages, assumptions about medical care and its delivery were promulgated, and goals were set for each phase of the program and for its overall intended effect on physicians at the SLPMC. Assumptions about the quality of medical care fundamental to the QAP are:

1. Providers of health care are concerned about the quality of their services.

2. A successful and useful QAP must encourage providers' curiosity about medical care and its delivery, building on their ideas and concerns.

3. All employees and systems, because they affect the medical care of patients, must be involved at some point in the program.

4. Because they are the focus of the delivery of care, patients must also be involved.

5. Cost is ultimately related to quality, and the trade-offs between cost and quality in medical care need to be assessed.

6. To promote behavior change, an operating system must allow for feedback to providers about the medical care delivered.

It is further assumed that less than optimum quality of care usually results from gaps in performance rather than in knowledge. It is, therefore, a key goal to change provider behavior (and in some cases, patient behavior) to provide more effectively for high-quality medical care. Although educational intervention for physicians traditionally has been used to correct deficiencies in performance, this approach has limited value in the daily practice of medicine.[4] Knowledge is not the sole determinant of effective medical care, and unless new knowledge is perceived as relevant and useful in daily practice, it is not translated into new behavior. Many beliefs and attitudes as well as knowledge are responsible for determining the performance of a particular behavior.[2] Thus, a method for changing behavior while acquiring new knowledge if necessary is crucial to genuinely change behavior. In addition, educational intervention often ignores the patient's role, implying that patient concordance with treatment is automatic and that compliance by the patient is optimal. Patients perceive physicians in terms of their performance, not their knowledge of medical care, thus equating performance with quality.

Clearly then, for lasting change and a higher quality of care to result from any quality assurance activity, behavior must change. It is the goal of the QAP at SLPMC to promote and provide for such behavior change.

The QAP at SLPMC is a three-phased effort, both to determine the present status of health care delivery and to improve such wherever it is appropriate, at a reasonable cost. The first phase of the program focuses on the design and implementation of a problem-finding and problem-solving mechanism. The second phase seeks to develop and install a systematic method for describing and analyzing what physicians actually do in practice at SLPMC. The third phase is directed at understanding patient expectations of medical care and modifying patient and physician behavior to correspond more closely to appropriate expectations. Information from the second and third phases is integrated into the phase I problem-solving mechanisms. The overall concern of the QAP is to improve the quality of care through effective behavioral change, whether it be provider, patient, or the system in which they interact that changes.

PHASE I

Phase I is essentially the core of the program and consists of methods to identify and remedy problems. Its focus is the quality assurance meeting that is held at noon with a different department each week. This meeting is led by the medical director of the group and consists of department physicians, physician associates, nurses, and administrative staff. The associate administrator of the clinic and the QAP staff also participate in each meeting. The meeting is carefully structured to ensure optimal use of the full hour that has been allocated. (See Figure 26-1.)

Before each meeting, the QAP staff gathers

material in the following ways to facilitate departmental review:

1. A random sample of medical records from patient encounters 6 to 8 weeks before the meeting is selected to allow adequate follow-up of most problems in the chart notes.

2. A telephone survey of 20 patients drawn from that same random sample is conducted.[1] This structured telephone interview includes questions about access to care, diagnoses, treatment, medications, and patient understanding. The results of this survey of patient perceptions of medical care delivery are summarized for use at the meeting.

3. The most frequent diagnoses in that department are identified from a master patient care index to assist in the selection of a common problem.

4. Interviews are also conducted with key

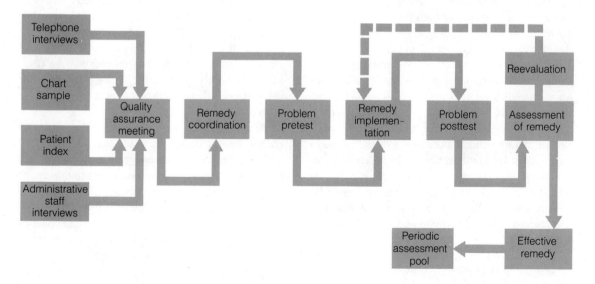

FIGURE 26-1.   Medical care problem solving.

clinic personnel who are in direct contact with patients and staff. Those interviewed are the pharmacists, patient educators, patient counselor, billing office personnel, HMO patient representatives, and inservice educators.

The material gathered from these four activities is summarized for the meeting participants to aid departmental self-examination.

Each meeting regularly begins with a brief orientation, including a review of new developments in quality assurance and the status of problems chosen previously by that department. Following this, participants can recall problems concerning the quality of medical care in their department. The medical records are then reviewed by the participants using implicit criteria. The records, as in daily practice, are reminders to participants of what they would like to do better. From the combination of chart review, departmental member recall, and the QAP staff–identified problems, a list of problems is generated. Problems include a wide range of topics and cover both the curing and caring aspects of medical care, that is, not only the content of medical care but the systems involved in delivering care are reviewed. By consensus, the group then selects one problem for remediation. An acceptable level of performance is agreed on by the participants, and a member of the department is chosen or volunteers to serve as the remedy coordinator and to facilitate acceptance of the remedy. Target dates for implementing the remedy and for assessing its efficacy are selected. Finally, a follow-up session is planned with the remedy coordinator and other relevant staff to define the remedy and further determine any special requirements.

At the follow-up meeting, the remedy coordinator and QAP staff explore the problem, design or refine the remedy, and determine the method of implementation and assessment of both problem and solution. If needed, the remedy coordinator obtains concurrence from other department physicians on the statement of problem and remedy, remedy methodology, and methods of assessment.

Quantitative parameters are uniquely identified for each problem to assess dimensions of the problem and effectiveness of the remedy. The problem is usually pretested using the parameters. This procedure provides baseline data to determine the extent or frequency (or both) of the problem. Only in this way can it be said with some measure of confidence that the quality assurance process has improved the care provided to patients.

A simple but efficient monitoring system has been developed to identify the status of each problem selected. The responsibility for remedy implementation belongs to the remedy coordinator. Through the monitoring process (which is people intensive, not paper intensive), the QAP staff assists and prompts the remedy coordinator in whatever manner is required.

After the effectiveness of the remedy has been assessed, the results are shared with the members of the department that identified that problem. To promote lasting change, effectively resolved problems are placed in a pool of problems to be reassessed randomly in the future. Inadequate remedies are reexamined and modified as necessary until the problems have been resolved.

Although 15 to 20 problems usually surface in each meeting, only one is selected for the QAP process. Problems generally fall into one of six categories: medical care content, continuity of care, medical records problem, resource use, communications, and system. Table 26-1 summarizes the problem areas and the percentages of problems falling into each group.

Problems chosen for remediation cover a wide range of subjects and reflect the diversity of specialities as well as the degree of organization of the SLPMC. Examples of problems chosen are: lack of a regular and consistent format for the ini-

TABLE 26-1.   Summary of Problems Identified and Selected for Remediation

PROBLEM	NUMBER IDENTIFIED (PERCENTAGE)	NUMBER SELECTED (PERCENTAGE)
Clinical care content (such as recognition/management of hypertension)	90 (18.1%)	15 (29.4%)
Continuity of care (such as lack of identified primary care physician)	87 (17.5%)	10 (19.6%)
Medical records (such as chart content/organization/ accessibility)	122 (24.6%)	7 (13.7%)
Resource use (such as nonproductive professional time)	54 (10.9%)	3 (5.9%)
Communications (as between mental health counselors and referring physician)	53 (10.7%)	4 (7.8%)
Systems (such as lack of flexible registration system to effectively and efficiently meet anticipated growth)	91 (18.3%)	12 (23.5%)
TOTAL	497	51

tial workup of new diabetic patients in all departments dealing with these patients, overuse of physician services by patients with the common cold, lack of a system for identifying a primary physician, lack of systematic feedback to referring physicians within the clinic, ineffective use of allied health providers, and the need for an instrument to systematically gather patient histories from patients with low back pain.

The problems cover both medical care content and systems and deal (at least indirectly) with the issues of cost and quality. If patients are taught when to use physician services and when not to (for instance, for upper respiratory infections), more appropriate use of services and lower costs to consumers can occur. When resources such as allied health personnel are properly utilized, the provider productivity can be directly increased without rapidly escalating costs. When medical care content is of a high standard and consistent within the system, patients benefit from increased quality without necessarily paying higher premiums.

Typical examples of problems that have been worked on through the phase I process and for

which an assessment of the remedy has been carried out are:

1. Administration and recording of immunizations of patients seen for routine physical examinations, well-child examinations, and injuries increased in one department from 36% to 69%.

2. A system to encourage patients to select a primary care physician was 100% effective in another department.

3. Patient participation in patient education programs from one satellite increased from one to 14 referrals a month.

4. Development of a comprehensive follow-up system for one satellite increased return visit compliance from 77% to 87%.

5. A patient-generated questionnaire for low back pain improved the method of history gathering for that problem.

Some problems that surface at the weekly quality assurance meetings cross departmental lines or are common to many departments. These are often dealt with on an administrative level rather than through the regular QAP channels. Problems regarding the content of care are dealt with through interdepartmental QAP meetings on a given topic, such as hypertension. In these cases, explicit criteria are used to review medical records before the noon QAP meetings to facilitate the finding and selection of problems. Some common problems deal with issues of concern to the Medical Staff Committee, such as organization and content of the medical record, for which the QAP serves as staff to the Medical Staff Committee. Other problems that cross departmental lines deal with administrative systems, such as evaluating new physicians. Again, the QAP staff serves as staff for administration. Although many of these problems do not bear directly on the delivery of medical care, they represent important areas in providing high-quality medical care; thus, their remediation can improve the quality of care.

In the phase I process, a conscious effort has been made to obtain information about the medical care process from many and varied sources. This has been done in an effort to understand from a variety of viewpoints the care provided. Not only the actual content of the care provided but also the systems for providing that care and patient-physician interaction can then be examined. The goal is to promote and provide for change, in whatever manner, to improve the quality of care provided at SLPMC.

PHASE II

The objective of phase II is to describe ambulatory care as it is actually provided and to index that care in a systematic way. To review ambulatory care, it is necessary to understand it. In contrast to the closed and well-controlled hospital situation, the office setting is open, loosely controlled, and made up of a wide variety of settings, including the solo practitioner, the single specialty group, the large, multispecialty group, and outpatient clinics in hospitals. Because of this diversity and because the patient has the option to enter or leave the system and to accept or reject treatment, it is difficult to understand, much less control, the outpatient setting in the same way that the hospital experience is understood and controlled.

A major barrier to the analysis of ambulatory care is the difficulty in identifying patients and certain elements of their care, such as diagnoses or procedures, and storing pertinent information in a systematic way so that it is easily accessible. The SLPMC had two major sources of computerized patient information: the patient file and the guarantor file. The patient file contained demographic data and was stored by a unique patient number (the chart number). The guarantor file contained data on diagnoses, procedures, dates of care, physician, department, location of care (hospital, main clinic, or satellite), and account type (prepaid, medicare, nursing home, fee-for-service, and so forth) and was stored by account number, with unique patient numbers stored within the accounts. A new computer file, the master patient activity file (MPAF), was created to merge information from both of these sources and to store it by chart number. Thus, it became possible easily to locate patients seen within a given period of time for a given diagnosis or procedure at a specific location or department or by a certain physician and to separate patients by account type. By simple manipulation of existing computer files, a powerful tool for indexing patient care was created. The expense of developing and updating the file periodically has been offset by savings in computer run time costs when dealing with the MPAF.

Among the other barriers to understanding ambulatory care is the documentation in the charts. Once the charts have been located by using the MPAF, they then need to be reviewed to abstract the care given. Ambulatory records are notorious for lack of organization and documentation. At SLPMC, the record is organized, however, and most progress notes are typed. One record serves for all encounters for each patient within the system and stores all relevant laboratory data, x-ray data, hospital abstracts, correspondence, and other data pertaining to medical care. Although the problem of lack of documentation is a real one and has to be dealt with, as providers become more aware of the problem, they tend to be more accurate and complete in their charting.

Problems for review in the ambulatory care setting are necessarily different from those in hospitals because of the differences in the settings and the review organizations. Thus, criteria for reviewing care have to be developed within a framework that accounts for these differences. As reviews of care at SLPMC have been conducted, a workable format for carrying them out has been developed.[6] Many other problems occur when ambulatory care is reviewed and must be dealt with as they appear.

It is the overall goal of phase II of the program to begin to understand something of the ambulatory care experience by carefully exploring care delivered in the setting—a moderate-to-large, multispecialty group practice. The first step in this process is describing what usually or rarely occurs to patients at SLPMC. To effectively change behavior in accordance with the goals of phase I, it is necessary to be able to understand and document regular practice in this setting. Without clear evidence of their usual practice behavior, physicians often lack incentive for changing the behaviors in their practices that are essential to assure high-quality medical care. Also, it is impossible to provide objective feedback regarding attempts at changing behavior without documentation.

Phase II of the program also provides the opportunity for clinic physicians as well as the QAP staff to carry out health services research, case studies,

system studies, and the like. Since approximately 15% of patient activity comes from a closed-panel prepaid health plan using the same providers as the fee-for-service activity, SLPMC offers a natural experimental setting for examining health services from the perspective of different modes of payment. Ample opportunity exists to study other aspects of health services, such as the cost of performing minor surgery in the office rather than in the hospital, the cost of finding abnormal laboratory or x-ray tests in a health screening package, the amount of primary care provided in a specialty department, and why patients choose to use a satellite facility.

Indeed, such projects have been undertaken. Presently, we are following a representative group of HMO patients and a matched fee-for-service cohort (matched by age, sex, and length of use of SLPMC for medical services) to understand the use of medical services by both groups more accurately. We have completed a study of the treatment of pilonidal cysts on an outpatient basis, contrasting that to in-hospital treatment for recurrence rates and cost to the patient. We have done several studies regarding the amount of primary care delivered in various specialty departments, all of which have a commitment to providing at least some primary care.

We are also in the midst of a study on the use of satellite facilities to try to understand why patients choose to use them. One other study examined the cost of finding a previously unknown abnormal laboratory or x-ray test in a health screening package. More work is underway on this topic to explore the subject further and to try to explain some of the findings in the study.

We have carried out studies of patients with hypertension, breast cancer, abdominal aortic aneurysms, and other diagnoses, examining treatments given and ongoing management as well as success rates. The content of the annual physical has been another topic for study. Through this phase of the program, we have also tried to aid clinic physicians who wish to carry out patient care evaluations; many of these studies were stimulated in this manner.

Another subject of interest and study is medication use. Since we do not have a formulary or own an in-house pharmacy, information regarding the prescription of drugs must be gathered at the time of the encounter. We are presently exploring ways of modifying our patient encounter form to provide a link between the medication and the diagnosis for which it is prescribed, thus facilitating future studies of medication.

Because most of our activity is fee-for-service, we need to generate diagnoses for claims documents. After systematically reviewing each of 11 available coding systems for ambulatory care, we test coded a sample of 1,400 reasons for visit and 1,700 diagnostic impressions and concluded that although imperfect, the ICDA-8 and the H-ICDA coded our ambulatory diagnoses as well as or better than other available codes.[3]

The goal of phase II is to describe and index care given in a multispecialty group practice and to examine that care from a different perspective than is done in phase I of the program. Physicians have shown considerable interest in these projects, because it is an easily available, systematic way to allow examination of the care they provide. Wherever problems are found through these studies, that information is fed back into the phase I problem-solving process to improve the care given in our setting.

PHASE III

Patient expectations of medical care provide critical information for any operating ambulatory care quality assurance program. These expectations, in part at least, determine patterns of use and satisfaction with care among patients. Understanding these expectations can lead to more effective interaction between patient and provider, and thus indirectly to higher-quality medical care. This phase of the program deals more directly with the *caring* rather than the *curing* aspects of medical care. By better understanding patient expectations, we can attempt to modify patient and provider behavior toward appropriate and achievable medical care and medical care delivery. Several efforts have been made to assess the expectations that patients have of both medical care encounters and the medical care system, but the quantifying of something as nebulous as *expectations* is difficult, because no simple method is available.[8]

Our first efforts to understand patient expectations were on the basis of a written questionnaire consisting of five open-ended questions regarding patients' experiences at SLPMC with both the medical center systems and the personnel. The questionnaire was distributed in various ways to achieve varied patient response and to attempt to discern which method solicited the greatest number of responses. We found the questionnaire method to be only partially useful because few patients responded, and for the most part they appeared to be satisfied with care. Their expectations of that care were tapped only indirectly.

A modification of a technique for determining "communication blocks" (information transfers that do not occur) of potentially harmful consequence was used at one of the satellite offices of SLPMC.[5] Episodes of care for patients seen there for a 4- to 6-week period were abstracted from information in the medical record. Patients were then interviewed by telephone by a registered nurse who followed a structured telephone interview format. The nurse then compared information about that episode of illness from the medical record and from the patient's recollection, using criteria developed for an earlier project to determine the existence of communication blocks. Two-hundred fifty patients were interviewed in the satellite study, and the information gathered in that study was fed back into the phase I QAP problem-solving process. A problem (return visit compliance) was chosen and did, in fact, improve from 77% to 87% for patients at that satellite.

Physicians at the satellite were eager for the kind of information provided by the telephone survey. After the structured interview was changed to query patient expectations more directly, and after a statistical study showed that 20 telephone calls were sufficient to raise valid problems, this technique was integrated into the routine of the QAP phase I process. Currently, before any QAP clinical department meeting, 20 patients are interviewed by telephone about the care received in that department. Patients are chosen at random from those seen within a 6-week period before the meeting so that their recollections of the encounter are still relatively fresh. This information is then fed into the phase I process at the departmental meeting as a method of raising problem areas. This has proved to be a powerful means of providing patient feedback.

We are currently exploring other techniques for assessing patient expectations. Among these is the use of marketing techniques for assessing consumer expectations of medical care. The differences between being a *patient* with expectations of medical care and a *consumer* with expectations of a product are great, with only a degree of overlap. Many techniques available to market researchers would be inappropriate in the medical care setting; however, we are exploring the adaptation and possible use of some of these insights into the assessment and quantification of patient and provider expectations of medical care.

This is a complex area because each patient is different and each has had a wide variety of experiences with medical care and its delivery. For instance, it is probable that the expectations of medical care for the parents of a 6-month-old child with severe diarrhea in the middle of the night differ from those of the parents of a 6-year-old with an upper respiratory infection; both differ from the expectations of medical care of a woman who is pregnant for the first time. Thus, there is still much work to be done to develop a usable instrument to understand and quantify these and other patient expectations. This deficiency should not, however, preclude inquiry into this area.

The second phase of the program deals more directly with the medical care content—predominantly the *curing* aspect of medical care. Phase III has begun to grapple with the patient's viewpoints and role in ambulatory care, often focusing on the *caring* elements of medical care. By the inclusion of both facets in a systematic problem-solving program, a comprehensive review of ambulatory medical care is being attempted.

PROGRAM MODIFICATION

Originally, the QAP included a plan for its modification with a separate phase for program changes and renewal. In reality, however, modification occurs continually in the refinement of the first three phases of the program. To gain the physicians' acceptance of the program and to pique their interest and curiosity, the insights gained from implementation of the program have been routinely integrated into the current operations. When all three phases of the program are fully implemented, the need for a concentrated effort at modification may again present itself.

The phase I process has changed somewhat from its initial form. Before the weekly meetings, 20 telephone calls to patients of that department are now carried out routinely; the frequency distributions of diagnoses have been dropped from the meetings; pharmacy and in-service education personnel are now interviewed as part of the administrative interviews; and a primer memo now goes out to all meeting participants before the meeting, summarizing some highlights of the premeeting information. The telephone calls were added to the process as a way of including patients' perceptions of medical care into the phase I process of finding and solving problems. Although lists of most frequent diagnoses in a department were intended to help identify a common problem, it became clear that they were not as useful as had been anticipated, and after a frequency distribution of diagnoses for each department had been obtained, they were discontinued. Pharmacy and in-service education were added to the administrative interviews because many problems raised in various departments dealt with issues relevant to either of them. The primer memo was added to stimulate thought before the meeting and, thus, the discussion about common problems at the meeting. It also reminds the participants that the quality assurance meeting is scheduled and that they are to attend. The overall effort at modifying phase I premeeting input has been to streamline it where possible and to add significant information.

The format of the meeting itself has been altered to some degree as well. The meeting now opens with a brief orientation regarding new concepts in quality assurance, such as Williamson's concept of "achievable benefits not being achieved" (ABNA). Also included is a brief status report on the problems that the department has chosen in previous meetings. Since new departments as well as affiliate provider groups have been added to the schedule, the number of meetings per year for each department has been decreased from two to one. The new schedule also allows for more intensive work on each problem and on an increasing number of research projects in phase II. Once a problem has been chosen, clearer definitions of acceptable performance standards are now required to reach a consensus about desired levels of performance.

The orientation for physicians and other participants serves two purposes: one is to acquaint staff members about quality assurance and new ideas in the literature, and the other is to focus the meeting on the theme of quality of care and those problems or issues in that department that relate to quality. The status report tells the department members how well they have been doing in implementing solutions to problems they had identified and allows them to decide whether they are satisfied with the current performance on that problem.

We have found that once a problem has been chosen and an acceptable level of performance has been agreed on, more emphasis on developing criteria to assess the problem and solution is necessary. Quantification of the problem and solution has provided concrete evidence of the existence of the problem and of the utility of the remedy.

Phase II has also been modified. The initial idea of developing routine utilization reports about ambulatory care has been dropped; it is unnecessary in view of the feedback from phase II studies into the phase I problem-solving process. A very positive reaction to the development of a systematic method for studying ambulatory care in our setting has been the unexpectedly strong interest in doing ambulatory care reviews. We have modified the methods for conducting ambulatory care reviews largely because of gaining more experience with our setting and the special problems ambulatory care presents for review. Conducting reviews of both inpatient and ambulatory care for patients with specific diagnoses (such as diabetes or asthma) has been considered as a way to review the special link that exists between hospital and outpatient care. The premise of this kind of review is that high-quality available ambulatory care can and will reduce the need to hospitalize these patients, and conversely, premature release from the hospital may create heavy demand for ambulatory care.

Phase III is still undergoing development, and some of the approaches to understanding and dealing with patient expectations have been altered in response to new ideas in the literature and after finding that first efforts did not necessarily elicit useful results. In particular, the written survey of patients was not nearly as useful as hoped, but telephone interviews have been more successful than anticipated. As a response to new ideas and to some of the psychometric literature, adapting market research techniques and insights is being considered as a tool to aid in understanding patients' perceptions of medical care.

The ability to index medical care and quantify information gathered through studies of ambulatory care has been applied in other aspects of the operations of the SLPMC. Studies such as long-range planning, future physician needs in the metropolitan area, staffing at SLPMC itself, and redesign of the medical record have been facilitated by the existence of a system that allows accurate indexing of care. These issues affect the quality of care at SLPMC, and thus much of this work has been done by the QAP staff.

MEDICAL RECORD

Problems with medical records were often mentioned at the weekly quality assurance meetings. Participants at seven of the first nine meetings raised this issue, and 122 of the 496 (24.6%) problems raised in the first 18 months of operation of phase I related to problems of the medical record. Among the more frequent complaints were: disorganized data, lack of readily available medications data, incomplete diagnosis lists, and loss of significant data. Because this problem came up so

often, the Medical Staff Committee of the SLPMC created a task force to study the present record and to consider possible redesign of the medical record. The QAP staff served as staff to that subcommittee.

The present record consists of progress notes that are usually typed on loose-leaf paper and filed in chronologic order. Laboratory and x-ray reports are filed behind the progress notes in reverse chronologic order. Correspondence, insurance claims, physical therapy forms, and all other reports and forms are filed behind the laboratory and x-ray reports. One record serves for all encounters with the SLPMC providers, including, in addition, information on hospitalizations by clinic physicians and emergency room visits. All hospital information is filed at the back of the chart behind a divider.

Data and suggestions from many sources were gathered for the use of the task force. Sample charts from 17 clinics and hospitals were received from the 28 organizations contacted. Departmental suggestions and reactions were sought regarding new and present forms. Organizations using top- and side-bound charts were surveyed for their experience with those records. Cost estimates from printers and suppliers along with a planned phasing in of the new chart formed the basis for an extensive cost analysis of the implementation of the new record. Operational problems and their possible solutions were studied to consider the actual implementation of a new chart.

Two surveys of all the physicians were conducted as part of the task force study to determine which, if any, of the hospital information would be eliminated and to determine what kind of binding (loose, top, or side binding) would be preferred. All physicians, therefore, had a voice in some of the redesign of the record, which was important to their acceptance of the final product.

The new record will consist of all the same relevant information, but some hospital forms will be eliminated. Many new forms in the record will facilitate transfer of information. The filing order will be somewhat different, and dividers will separate progress notes, laboratory and x-ray data, hospital data, and correspondence. The new record will be sidebound; progress notes will be color coded uniquely by department and shingled so that the diagnostic impressions at the bottom of the notes will form a current problem list. A medications list will be filed on the inside of the cover of the chart for easy availability. Progress notes, filed in reverse chronologic order, will make the more recent visits more accessible. The new forms and the binding will make information more readily available and reduce the chance of its loss.

We continue to explore and review the relation between hard-copy medical record and electronic data storage. An improved patient information and registration system has been developed for prepaid plan members. An assessment of the feasibility of developing a brief hospital discharge abstract from the hospital billing information for inclusion in the medical record is in the final stages. Other possible connections between the medical record and the computerized data base remain to be delineated.

PROBLEMS AND INSIGHTS

Operating a program such as the QAP, which is comprehensive and intended to change behavior on the part of providers, cannot be without problems. The unwillingness of providers to look very deeply for problems or to accept negative findings from a review of care has been faced. Also, some providers have not understood that quality assurance is ongoing and not a single, isolated event. Some of these problems resolve themselves as providers become more familiar and comfortable with the process. Some of the unwillingness to search for problems does abate, especially if the curiosity of the participants can be sparked in some manner, such as by broad input into the quality assurance meetings. Involving providers in reviews of care (from setting the criteria and actually reviewing some records to determining the desired change to be undertaken on the results), can diffuse some of the sensitivity to negative findings, and providers can become more aware of problems that exist. The natural resistance, some of which will probably never disappear, to finding negative aspects of medical care is understandable. In addition, behavioral change comes slowly, particularly with physicians who are traditionally quite independent. However, providers can come to accept problems found through review if they are actively involved in it. More than 90% of the group physicians have participated in the program through at least a noon meeting. This compares favorably with the hospital in which a quality assurance committee of a few physicians carries out the quality assurance activities for the entire hospital. The participation by providers in finding and solving problems is a key to motivating genuine behavioral change. The QAP has begun to involve providers more closely in these reviews in response to this problem.

Physician interest in the quality of ambulatory care has clearly been stimulated by the second phase of the program. Fourteen percent of the group's physicians have sought QAP help in conducting special projects and reviews of care. Several of these physicians have done more than one review. Also, the QAP biostatistician has served as a consultant to several others in the medical center regarding research or specific problems.

Beyond the success of phase II in sparking interest in studying ambulatory care, feedback from phase II studies and from phase III surveys into the phase I process has provided interesting and useful information for finding problems. Feedback to physicians about results of studies, both formally and through their participation in those studies, has given impetus to behavioral change that might otherwise have occurred more slowly. The most successful aspect of the QAP in changing provider behavior has been the provision of feedback from many sources—patients, reviews of care, administrative interview, and any other source—about the care provided, thereby creating a mechanism for solving problems once they have been found. Without the problem-solving/evaluation process, behavior cannot be systematically changed.

The planning stages of the QAP have been invaluable. Without clear and explicit statements of assumptions and goals of the program and without a guide to implementing the program (work plan), the QAP would not have developed and become operational as quickly or smoothly as it has. In the planning stages, a clear commitment from the medical center's board of trustees and physicians was obtained, and all have been kept informed through periodic reports about the progress made in implementing the QAP. Because the program was planned to be flexible enough to accommodate the various personalities of the physicians and differing needs of the medical center, it has stimulated many responses to the quality assurance concept and has promoted behavioral change on several levels.

The QAP has had experience in dealing with departments and facilities outside the immediate SLPMC by taking the phase I operations into other settings. The prepaid plan includes groups of affiliated providers, including small family practice groups, small multispecialty groups, and a mental health group practice. We have gained several insights into operating a QAP in these settings, among which is an appreciation that many prob-

lems (such as medical records; patient access to care; and consistent, continual, and comprehensive care for patients) are common to medical care, no matter what the setting. Also, improving simple systems rather than creating elaborate ones is more efficient and gains acceptance more readily. The more physicians become involved in the problem-finding and problem-solving review of care, the more likely they are to accept the results and to work for a reasonable, useful solution.

The support of the president of the board of trustees, the medical director, and the clinic administrative staff has been absolutely essential to the implementation and operation of the QAP. The support within the medical center has immeasurably aided the goals of the program: to find and solve problems, to understand and analyze ambulatory care in our setting, to involve patients in the process, and to provide feedback to providers about all of these, thereby promoting behavioral change. Ambulatory care quality assurance in our setting is based on lasting and genuine behavioral change promoted through feedback to providers from efforts in all phases of the program.

REFERENCES

1. Batalden, P. B., McClain, M. P., O'Connor, J. P., et al. *The telephone interview as a problem-surfacing technique in an operating ambulatory care quality assurance program.* (In preparation.)

2. Fishbein, M. 1976. Persuasive communication. In Bennett, A. E. *Communication between doctors and patients.* Oxford University Press, pp. 99–127.

3. Friedlob, A., Caro, D., Shimitz, R., et al. 1976. *A review of medical care classification systems for use in ambulatory care.* Minneapolis: St. Louis Park Medical Center Report to the National Center for Health Services Research.

4. Greene, 1976. *Assuring quality in medical care:*

the state of the art. Cambridge, Mass.: Ballinger Publishing Co.

5. *Innovative technology in a rural area: application to an urban setting.* Dec. 1976. Final report to the Department of Health, Education, and Welfare, Administration, National Center for Health Services Research.

6. McClain, M. P., and Batalden, P. B. Ambulatory care review for quality assurance. (In preparation.)

7. Morehead, 1976. Ambulatory care review: a neglected priority. *Bull. N.Y. Acad. Med.* 52:60–69.

8. Ware, J. E., Jr. 1975–1977. et al. Rand paper series publications No. P-5660, P-6576, P-5716, P-5599, P-5440, and P-5415. Santa Monica, Calif.: Rand Corp.

27

Comprehensive Quality Assurance System: Another Operating Approach

Len Rubin

Too often review of quality and cost in the ambulatory setting is approached as an impossible, formidable task with little likelihood of success. On the contrary, my experience with the Comprehensive Quality Assurance System (CQAS) has shown that it is an opportunity to be free from the traditional formal hospital approaches that are losing adherents because of increasing evidence that they do not work. The inability to apply these standard techniques to ambulatory care has enabled a deeper, more significant approach to quality assurance to emerge. Although there are many examples of this enrichment in quality assurance, just a few are sufficient to demonstrate its significance. One is the need to stop attempting to assess an "episode of illness" and to examine care provided to the total patient as an individual, not as the housing for a diseased organ or the locale for a surgical procedure. The multiplicity of circumstances that impact on patients, such as diagnoses other than the one being studied, should lead one to suspect that considering pure single disease states in quality assurance will not result in success. The pure disease approach resulted from "Sutton's law,"* which

*"Sutton's law" refers to the apocryphal story of the famed bank robber, Willie Sutton, who when asked by the police why he kept robbing banks all the time (and kept getting caught), stated, "That's where the money is."

means, "that's where [how] the data is." Another important example of enrichment was the obvious opportunity to demonstrate the proper place of the medical record as an active tool used in the care of patients, not as a document that may be completed after all care is provided.

HISTORY, SCOPE, AND MAJOR CONCEPTS

The CQAS, the single criterion approach to quality assurance, was begun in 1969 to identify educational needs in ambulatory care to assure improved quality in that setting. The author had the mistaken notion at that time that hospital quality assurance activities were effective and that attention needed to be directed to ambulatory care and to the interface between ambulatory and hospital care. It rapidly became apparent that techniques used in the hospital setting were neither applicable to ambulatory care nor very effective in hospital quality improvement.

Because of the apparent vagaries of ambulatory care regarding such aspects as well-defined episodes of care and coding of diseases, better systems had to be devised to accomplish the task. As these techniques evolved, it became apparent that they offered many advantages over the classical systems in use for quality assurance in the hospital.

New approaches for problem identification, topic selection, medical record retrieval, data retrieval other than medical record retrieval, and other aspects of quality assurance were developed and implemented. Additional weaknesses in the traditional hospital quality assurance mechanisms were discovered and rectified by the CQAS.

The term "comprehensive" is significant in the CQAS and refers to the fact that the CQAS addresses care in a truly comprehensive manner irrespective of practitioner or provider (physician, nurse, technologist, medical record personnel, and so forth), setting (ambulatory, hospital, long-term care, and so forth), type of inadequacy (process, outcome, overutilization, or underutilization), or timing of review (concurrent or retrospective). The CQAS thus addresses poor quality as well as waste in any setting regardless of the responsible agent. It is interesting to note in this regard that a single system has been used for several years in hospital and ambulatory care as well as at the interface between the two for the same three main objectives of the PSRO program. These are: necessity of care, quality of care, and performance with the least expense consistent with quality.

In the CQAS, quality is defined as "what we (and peers) believe is right *today* in regard to *an element* of care." "Good quality" unfortunately cannot be based on ultimate "good." It should not be considered poor quality to use a diuretic on a hypertensive even though this medication may be considered ill-advised next year. In the past, routine smallpox vaccination, sympathectomy for essential hypertension, routine radical mastectomy, low-residue diets for diverticulitis, and a host of other activities were considered good care, and rightfully so at that time. Before that, blood letting, leeches, and enemas were popular. It is likely that much of the present scientifically proved or generally advocated therapeutic activity will

similarly be discarded in the years to come. However, because of this likelihood, the accepted and "proved" activities obviously should not be considered poor quality at this time.

Quality assurance has to do with comparing "what we do" with "what we think today we should do" and attempting to minimize the difference. Quality assurance does *not* have to do with current uncertainties, controversies, and disagreements in medicine. Clarifying these disputed areas has to do with another important field of medicine, namely, research. Quality assurance must be clearly differentiated from research. Research tells of new ways of doing things or which of several ways is better. Quality assurance is directed at being sure that what individuals do today is what they believe they should do today.

It is difficult to leave this discussion without at least some reference to "process and outcome," although, as has been stated by many authors, it is wasteful to dwell on this subject.[1,2] The concept continues to be a nuisance, however, primarily because the word "outcome" is contained within statutory language and directives from "voluntary" accrediting agencies. Although the intent of such recommendations was laudatory, mainly to avoid inconsequential process criteria, the existence of such recommendations regarding "outcomes" has a serious and adverse effect on quality assurance activities because of motivational conflicts that exist. The above references give adequate reason why lengthy discussion of this concept is unwarranted. Suffice it to say that the CQAS addresses poor care regardless of how that care may be classified by the myriad of systems for defining "process and outcome." In no way does the CQAS look at process as an unfortunate necessity "because outcome cannot be addressed." As is shown by examples later on, process is equally important to assess and improve. Furthermore, if *improvement* is desired, *process* must be addressed because behavior, which is to be changed, always has to do with process.

Management Considerations

Many pitfalls in the operation of a quality assurance program must be recognized, or failure is sure to follow. Failure may be expressed in many ways, including failure for any activity to occur, or meaningless, wasteful, pro forma, expensive activity not resulting in improvement. Occasionally fear or hostility toward the review activity is so intense that discovery of poor care is hidden. The following items are worthy of special comment:

Quality assurance is part of medical care delivery and is not optional. The reason for performing the quality assurance activity must be explicated by management so that it is understood that since quality assurance is a professional responsibility it will be done, and secondarily that it should be done in a way to satisfy extramural agencies. If management allows the quality assurance activity to be optional, it will not have any force, and although it may satisfy regulatory agencies, it is not apt to result in any improvement. If management conveys the idea that quality assurance is being performed primarily to achieve regulatory requirements, the activity will be looked on as a necessary evil to be done in a perfunctory manner, and again no improvement will result. Management must make it clear that improvement is the primary objective. Recent activities in quality assurance that have had demonstration of good care as a primary objective have neither proved good care nor resulted in significant improvement.

It is extremely important for management to exert its authority in establishing the objectives (improvement and accreditation) for the quality assurance program. Care must be exercised not to exert its authority in regard to specific criteria for the practice of medicine. The latter must be on a peer basis. Demonstration of the need for improvement by revealing suboptimal performance is a management responsibility.

Responsiveness by management is essential. Because of the enormous amount of work that has been done nationally in regard to quality assurance activities without any substantive widespread demonstrable beneficial effect, quality assurance activities have a bad image at this time, and it is felt by many that they are wasteful and cannot be successful. It is, therefore, important for management to demonstrate to staff that quality assurance activities can be successful in improving care without resorting to punitive actions. Management must react to recommendations that are made as a result of quality assurance activity and, if feasible, institute necessary and desirable changes. If changes cannot be made, other appropriate response must follow. Failure to respond quickly will be proof to the staff that the entire activity is merely a token. Similar conclusions by the staff will be reached if the management attitude toward quality assurance is poor as manifested by assignment of inappropriate personnel and insufficient funding. Assignment of the management of the quality assurance activity to inexperienced neophytes from the medical care team rather than with the care exercised in selecting personnel to head major professional departments informs the staff of the low priority management has assigned to this operation. Quality assurance activities must be considered part of regular administration and not an optional appendage, such as research. Quality assurance activities are woven into the fabric of any professional organization and must be applied to all care by all providers. As with any other management activity, it is important to monitor the quality of the quality assurance performance as well as its costs.

The objective of improvement rather than demonstration of good care tends to demotivate and must be actively countered. The following discussion presents the view that demonstration of overall good care is neither feasible nor desirable as a primary objective in quality assurance. Such demonstration of good care would tend to maintain the status quo rather than be instrumental in improving care. The act of identifying "what's wrong" is at the very core of an improvement process, but the consequence of its constant repetition is a serious disincentive that will affect both management and staff and must be recognized and must itself be managed.

The word "element" in the definition of quality is important because it is necessary to consider quality one element at a time. Medical care consists of an infinite number of elements that have all degrees of correlation with each other, from perfect correlation to no correlation. Corrections and changes in one element may or may not impinge on another element. Each must be considered separately. In addition, high performance in one element gives one "no credit" in regard to another element. For example, getting a perfect drug history from a patient does not make up for doing a poor determination of the blood pressure. These elements may be looked at as an infinite series of numbers. The only way to show improvement is to compare performance in regard to *one element* that is being performed in a suboptimal manner before and after corrective measures have been instituted. When it is known that performance in one element is unsatisfactory, high-quality care cannot be claimed by demonstrating high performance in other elements.

Since care consists of an infinite number of elements, there are infinite degrees of freedom for making errors or performing suboptimally. This can be demonstrated by contemplating the many facets that have to be considered in the treatment of hypertension starting with determining the blood pressure, doing it correctly, recording it, recognizing an abnormal value, selecting the proper therapy, making sure the patient is not allergic to it or

is not already taking it for some other purpose, and so on. Because of the enormous number of elements of care, it is neither feasible nor possible to measure enough of them to establish that high-quality care is being performed. There is always a myriad of elements not examined. A lower than anticipated number of myocardial infarctions or cerebrovascular accidents in no way indicates that all of these elements are being performed correctly, because many circumstances may advantageously affect these conditions. Nor does it give any assurance that other "outcomes," such as preventable iatrogenic pharmaceutical reactions, are not present in excess. There is no reason to assume that labeling or tracer techniques in which elements of quality in one condition (in which the practitioner might be interested) are applicable to another condition even when consideration is limited to very specific areas. Recent experience with frequently used techniques demonstrating "good care" in a variety of diagnostic categories in the hospital setting attest to the futility of this approach. Sampling from the infinite pool of quality elements does not allow generalizations with high confidence. Nor is the converse true. Just because an institution has been shown to have suboptimal performance in regard to one element of care does not allow the inference that all care is poor.

Since demonstration of overall high-quality care is not feasible, quality assurance activities must be directed toward improvement. When this is done, the negative aspects of health care delivery are emphasized, because in an improvement process those are the only ones in which one should be interested. Constant attention to "what's wrong" turns out to be rather demoralizing to staff because practitioners tend to forget that most of the infinite number of elements of care are performed well. The demoralization results in a defensive attitude that leads to "justification" of serious transgressions. This undesirable reaction may be found in management as well as staff and has to be actively countered by reminders that an improvement process concerns itself only with what is wrong and properly pays no attention to the vast number of activities that may be performed in an exemplary fashion. Failure to address this problem will result in either cessation of quality assurance activities or relegating them to pro forma "busy work." There are historic precedents for this in the early work of the American College of Surgeons wherein the poor results of their first assessment resulted in the documents being burned. One must keep this aspect of quality assurance in mind, because it is extremely important to recognize and face it at the management level lest all the suboptimal performance discovered be swept under the rug.

It is not rare to find a professional staff so justifiably proud of its accomplishments that the thought of suboptimal performance is not acceptable. It must be pointed out to such groups that perfection is clearly not at hand and that professionalism is synonymous with continual self-appraisal and improvement. Even in the most prestigious and highly competent medical provider setting, abundant evidence of the need for improvement is always present and this evidence should be shown to the staff. However, one should be aware of both its motivating and demoralizing potential.

Quality assurance is not research. Additional common barriers and pitfalls include the tendency to equate quality assurance activity with clinical research. Although it is true that research may lead to improved quality, quality assurance is an activity akin to quality control and is quite different from the concept of medical advances. Quality assurance should be concerned only with those elements of care for which there is a currently accepted correct manner of performance or result. Whenever questions arise in regard to elements of care in which "the right way" is not known, one is

delving into research or surveys and not into quality assurance. For example, one is dealing with research if these questions arise: "How often does hematuria occur with anticoagulation?" "Is it better to do the A incision rather than the B?" Criteria for measurement must be statements, not questions.

There is significant precedent for confusing research with quality assurance as the latter process is considered in PSRO and related activities. Codman's work, often quoted as a forerunner of quality assurance, was actually clinical research. Codman questioned whether what was being done was good and devised a system to examine the results of care a year later. He did not know what was right. He did not have a criterion. He asked questions, and only after his research had been completed and conclusions drawn concerning "the right way" could a quality assurance program have begun. If his results had been inconclusive, and no way was clearly better for any particular procedure, a quality assurance program could not even have been initiated.

Although Codman's intention was most laudable (he had serious reservations about the conduct of medical practice), many diversions from quality assurance into research are examples of avoidance behavior. It is much safer for the staff of an institution to deal with aspects of medicine in which there is as yet no right or wrong. It is uncomfortable to deal with admittedly suboptimal performance, and it has often been observed that having identified a significant problem, efforts are diverted to an associated research activity rather than an improvement activity.

Management must be cognizant of these two incentives for entering research and must handle them appropriately. Management must also recognize that it too may succumb to the avoidance technique just described. It is not pleasant for professionals to concern themselves with an activity that is so occupied with error. Although research is a proper activity for health care practitioners, it is a totally separate activity from quality assurance. When these activities are confused, quality assurance is not done, and often poor research is the result.

Good medical records are an integral part of good medical care. Because so much of quality assurance has to do with the recorded facts of medical care as noted in the medical record, it is quite common for medical staffs to object to the entire procedure on the basis that this will improve medical recording but not medical care. It must be stressed and demonstrated to the staff that medical records are part of and not an appendage to provision of health care. It is not only in group practices that certain vital information must be recorded. Even in a solo practice good records are part of good care. There is no assured way for a pediatrician to remember the last head circumference of an infant to know whether the skull circumference is changing significantly. Similarly, changes in blood pressure or body weight during therapy must be recorded to be tracked. Neither is it feasible for a practitioner to remember all the medications prescribed or taken by a patient over time. These considerations are totally apart from the significant role medical records play in avoiding waste by duplication of tests and their role in malpractice protection.

Because medical records are part of medical care, they too are subject to audit, and as a result many improvements in medical records have occurred. There is little doubt that significant portions of medical records are without redeeming features and exist as anachronisms. Other portions serve only for medicolegal purposes and have little to do with care. However, a large part of the medical record is necessary for good care and is part of good care. Improved medical records frequently signify improved care.

Costs for quality assurance, as for any other activity, must be monitored. The financial management of a quality assurance program has hazards at several points. When the activity is planned, if outside funding (through grants, for example) is solicited, the entire project may be undermined from the very start. As mentioned previously, it will signify to the staff that the activity does not enjoy a high priority. Management must ''put its money where its mouth is'' as far as quality is concerned. Grant funds are the hallmark of an optional program and carry the implication that should the funds not be available, the program would cease. Another hazard of extramural funding is the thinking and planning invariably associated with such source of funds. It is characterized by relatively lavish expenditures for personnel, supplies, and so forth and not characterized by the more penurious approach used for normal line operations. The result of this is to denigrate the value of quality assurance, because it does not appear to be cost effective. The idea of transferring this expense to normal operations when the granted funds are exhausted becomes administratively prohibitive.

Once the operation is budgeted through normal channels as for any other integral part of medical care delivery, it is important to maintain the usual cost controls. Failure to do so will have an adverse effect on staff because of apparent cost ineffectiveness. In this regard, it is especially important to be alert that the process does not become the basis for generating an enormous data base of dubious value. Economy in the operation of the quality assurance program is as important as economy in any other area of operation.

REQUIREMENTS FOR CQAS

It is common to hear references to the inability of performing quality assurance in ambulatory care because the records fail to have a fixed format, clearly defined episodes of care, diagnostic coding, and all the other attributes of a hospital medical record. Besides being aware of these frequent misconceptions, one should realize that the CQAS does *not* depend on:

1. Coding of any sort (diagnosis, impression, or chief complaint).
2. Any abstract.
3. Any specific chart format (cryptic notes on 3 × 5 inch cards are as easily audited as typewritten problem-oriented records).
4. Electronic data processing or the use of computer in any form.
5. Any data base.
6. Style of practice (although developed in a prepaid group, it has worked successfully in fee-for-service group settings).
7. Encounter forms.
8. The presence of specific impressions or diagnoses listed for each counter.

The requirements for the CQAS are simply two or more physicians who agree to review each other's performance and to follow up with objective measures of performance in relation to agreed-upon criteria relating to suspected problems so that corrective actions can be instituted. Although this entire presentation clearly implies that the activity take place within a group practice setting, it is not in any way a requirement. It is entirely feasible for any two or three physicians to get together mutually to review their work for the purpose of identifying problems, and then for them to return to their own offices to set up criteria for themselves that they and their office staff can measure. Trained data retrievers are not necessary, though they are desirable.

CQAS CHARACTERISTICS

There are a number of additional characteristics of the CQAS. First, it has an extremely short lead time. Second, it is an economic operation. Third, it meets the requirements of governmental and voluntary agencies. Fourth, it addresses overutilization as well as more traditional aspects of quality. Fifth, it is based on the philosophy of improvement rather than just demonstration of good care. A discussion of each characteristic follows.

First, in most situations, the extremely short lead time can be as short as 1 day from the time a decision is made to start the CQAS. Peer review and problem identification can be instituted without any prior preparation of forms, protocols, and so forth.

Second, in a large prepaid health plan, the cost for CQAS operation is 25^{c} per health plan member per year, or about 6^{c} per patient-physician visit. Once a problem is detected and a criterion or standard is written in regard to the problem, the cost for accurately and objectively measuring performance is between $12 and $20. These figures indicate the low direct cost of the CQAS. Since only suspected problems are addressed, cost effectiveness is also quite good, because there is little waste on elements of care that are not being done poorly. No dollars are wasted attempting to demonstrate good care either in regard to specific elements or in regard to a specific diagnosis by measuring half a dozen aspects of the condition.

Third, a quality assurance program that improved quality but did not also satisfy regulatory agencies would be advocated with less than great enthusiasm by management. As shown in Figure 27-1, the standard audit cycle is the basis for the CQAS. If performed correctly, it meets the requirements of the PSRO and both the hospital accreditation program and the ambulatory accreditation program of the JCAH.

PSRO BASIC CHARACTERISTICS OF
MEDICAL CARE EVALUATION STUDIES

1. Focus on known or suspected problem
2. Focus on well-defined topic in accord with explicit objective
3. Written criteria

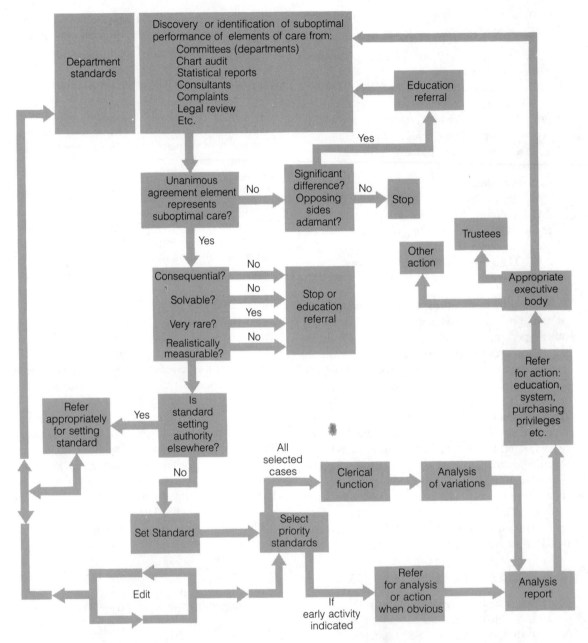

FIGURE 27-1. Medical center comprehensive quality assurance committee.

4. Data collection—size and composition of patients appropriate to objective
5. Peer analysis of discrepancies
6. Specific written recommendations where indicated (for education, organization/administrative changes, or other means for quality and utilization improvement)
7. Documentation of when, where, and by whom actions are to be implemented
8. Follow-up evaluation where indicated
9. Follow-up in reasonable time limited to key indicators of action
10. Periodic reporting to board

FOR JCAH HOSPITAL ACCREDITATION: ESSENTIAL CHARACTERISTICS OF MEDICAL CARE EVALUATION STUDIES

1. Criteria (standard) setting directed to problems
2. Measurement of practice against No. 1
3. Peer analysis
4. Corrective action
5. Remeasurement of No. 2
6. Reporting of results to responsible agent(s)

ACCREDITATION COUNCIL/ AMBULATORY HEALTH CARE ESSENTIAL CRITERIA FOR MEDICAL AUDIT

1. Repeated, ongoing activity
2. Actual review of performance
3. Peer based—all physicians can participate
4. Recommendations for improvement distributed appropriately

Fourth, because the CQAS addresses overutilization as well as more traditional aspects of quality, the same system may be used to assure proper expenditure of resources. This is discussed in greater detail in Chapter 28. For both quality and appropriate cost containment, the CQAS can be conducted in either a concurrent or retrospective manner depending on the nature of the problem being addressed.

Finally, the CQAS is based on a philosophy of improvement rather than just demonstration of good care.

PHILOSOPHY
CQAS

1. Find out what is wrong and fix it (objective).
2. Demonstrate good care.

Traditional

1. Demonstrate good care.
2. If bad care is discovered, address it.

Most traditional quality assurance activities have as their primary objective demonstration of good care. A secondary objective is improvement of whatever poor care may have been discovered. Although the CQAS has the same two objectives, they are reversed. The primary objective is to determine what in the medical care provision activities is suboptimal and to fix it. If a suspected problem is not confirmed objectively and proves to be an oddity with essentially a zero frequency of occurrence, the secondary objective of the CQAS (demonstration of good care in regard to an element) has been achieved.

Because quality assurance is basically an improvement process, it is important that local problems are addressed. One institution cannot improve an element of care that it is performing well but that is being performed poorly elsewhere. As a consequence, local criteria or standards are essential not only because practice patterns may vary but because criteria should be written only for elements for which there is some reason to believe improvement is desirable.

SPECIFIC TECHNIQUE FOR CQAS

The overall plan of the CQAS is similar to many other audit procedures in that a problem is identified with the objective of improving care in regard to that problem. A written criterion for that element or problem is then established with subsequent objective measurement of performance against the criterion. If suboptimal performance is shown before institution of corrective activity, validation of the measurement is done by peer analysis of discrepancies. After corrective action has been instituted, remeasurement of performance against the criterion is carried out, and the results are appropriately reported to the governing bodies.

The operation of the CQAS varies from more traditional quality assurance activities in a few major areas:

> 1. It uses a unique method for problem identification called microsampling.
>
> 2. It addresses each problem or element of care as an individual item.
>
> 3. It extensively employs different methods for retrieval of information.
>
> 4. It uses the concept of clinical rather than statistical significance.

These features are described in detail because other steps in the quality assurance program (peer analysis, improvement activities, reporting to governing bodies, and so forth) are in no way different from other systems of quality assurance.

Problem Identification

Discovery or identification of suboptimal performance of elements of care may come from any source (see figure 27-1). This may take the form of standing or special committee reports, statistical reports of any variety, complaints from members of the health care team or from patients, medicolegal review, serendipitous observations during patient care, chart audit, or any other source. One of the systematic and organized methods used exten-

sively in the CQAS for problem identification is a specific chart audit program called "microsampling." The name was selected because a very small number of charts (10–20) usually will reveal more significant problems than an institution can correct in many months.

Record Selection for Microsampling

The essence of microsampling is that records are selected not with regard to medical information, such as diagnosis, age, or type of complaint, but with regard to being sure that all health practitioners, various days and times of service, and various forms of encounters (appointment, drop in, telephone, and so on) are included. It is important not to confuse medical record selection for microsampling with the record selection process, which comes later for objectively measuring performance in relation to a specific standard or criterion. The intent here is to find problems that cover any aspect of provision of care from accessibility (Do patients telephone multiple times before they are seen regardless of the complaint or the diagnosis?) to diagnosis, to therapy and follow-up.

Records are usually picked by selecting a specific date and time about 6 weeks previously from the appointment log (being sure to select some appointment times and some drop-in times). Occasionally records may be similarly picked from telephone logs, being sure to give specific selection rules so that all personnel during the working day will be sampled. A very fruitful selection can also be made by selecting ambulatory records of patients who were discharged from the hospital 4 to 6 weeks previously regardless of diagnosis or reason for admission.

Regardless of which list or log is to be used for selection purposes, very specific instructions must be given. Examples might be: all 5:00 P.M. appointments on May 16 and May 19; every tenth telephone call logged on May 20; and first and last discharge from each hospital service starting May 20. If two discharges did not occur pick a second discharge from May 21. It is extremely important to give very specific instructions and not to use the word "random." Allowing medical record or other personnel to help set the selection rules during record retrieval invariably results in undesired bias. It is quite appropriate for medical record personnel to participate in setting the rules for chart selection in conjunction with the quality care committee but not independently or in a random fashion. If specific instructions are not given, it will be found that such records as incomplete records, "no shows," the record "not in file," and other such categories are rejected. It is in these types of records that the most flagrant problems are discovered. The record "not in file" is almost certain to have problems; the fact that the record is not readily available is the first. Selecting records that are several weeks old allows review of performance rather than just charting and also allows review of additional important aspects of care. For example, in a case in which the patient reported red urine 6 weeks previously, one would expect to find a urinalysis properly filed in the record whether or not the physician indicated a urine test was to be ordered. Properly instructing the patient in a way that the patient did comply, having the laboratory perform the test, and having medical records properly file the report are more important than whether or not the charting was properly done in the physician's note regarding ordering a urine test.

Reviewing ambulatory records of patients who have been hospitalized rather than "never hospitalized" seems to provide a greater yield of problems that are not necessarily related to the reason for hospitalization. For example, it is frequently found that hospitalized children have not had proper immunization, usually because they are sick so often that the injections keep getting postponed.

This is quite different from "staging," in which the condition requiring admission is assessed.

Additional reasons for selecting records in this manner previously have been described at length.[3]

Reviewing the Record

Having selected ten to 20 records in the systematic manner previously described, health care professionals (physicians, nurses, medical record personnel, administrators, and so forth) review the records to find problems within their knowledge that they are fairly certain their peers will endorse. These problems usually are either obvious major errors under any circumstance or errors as shown by internal inconsistencies within the record for that particular situation.

The essence of microsampling is that the good features of the old "one-on-one" review have been salvaged, and the process has been converted into a highly objective procedure. In microsampling professionals use all their clinical skills to ferret out internal inconsistencies within a record without any preconceived notions regarding what is being sought or based on theory. A discussion of the differences, however, follows.

It is important to point out that whenever health care practitioners are used for quality assurance medical record review, there are only two functions they should be performing. One is identifying problems, and the other is validating discrepancies found by medical record analysts after criteria have been set (peer justification). The latter function is described in detail later on.

Problem identification is described here in microsampling. It consists of perusing a chart for the purpose of finding evidence of suboptimal care in any area without having constructed criteria based on theory or deciding ahead of time what one will seek. Because of the infinite degrees of freedom practitioners have for making errors, no constraints should be applied at this time, so that any kind of problem may be identified. In regard to such problem identification activities, for the first few years the CQAS employed a format shown in Figure 27-2, but such a format is antithetic to the expenditure of professional time in quality assurance activities. The form shown in Figure 27-2 is specifically *not recommended*. It creates tunnel vision on the part of the professional, directs attention only to preconceived notions, repeatedly brings up the same types of problems, and is construed after a while as busy work. It results in inappropriate expenditure of practitioner time and a poor job in that significant problems are missed, and even the requested data are poorly retrieved. Once a problem has been identified or a criterion set (as manifest by the very existence of a list as in Figure 27-2), it is not necessary to have a health care practitioner determine frequency or compliance. That is a job for medical record personnel.

The reviewer of a record in microsampling makes no note of what is "right." Proper care and good record keeping are expected and occur most of the time. Attention to them cannot possibly lead to improvement. The reviewer seeks out only those items that indicate significant deviations from desirable practice and that he or she is fairly certain will be agreed on by peers.

It is important to point out that not only are errors in quality in the classical sense (that is, biomedic) being sought but also any evidence of wasteful practice that severely affects quality as a second-order phenomenon. It is not only in HMOs where the organization is at financial risk that this is important. On a national scale, overutilization is of such concern as to adversely affect quality because of necessary restrictive regulations and expensive bureaucratic procedures. In addition to these two aspects (quality and overutilization), microsampling is useful in problem identification for some types of medicolegal risk control that similarly have an adverse second-order effect on quality and costs.

The boxed material below shows the free form of the microsampling data sheet in use for several years. The lack of directives, routine, and protocol removes all tunnel vision and allows health care practitioners to use all their professional talents to identify any suboptimal performance.

COMPREHENSIVE QUALITY ASSURANCE SYSTEM
MICROSAMPLE DATA SHEET

Code _____ Index date _____ Hospital Clinic Facility _____
Reviewer No. 1 _____ Reviewer No. 2 _____ Today's date _____
Age _____ Sex _____ Reason for index contact _____
Refer for action _____
Note: Enter just "what's wrong"
       Not "who's wrong"
       Not "what's right"
       Look for problems in quality, waste, medicolegal area

OUT-PATIENT CARE REVIEW REPORT

CODE NUMBER	DATE INDEX VISIT	AUDITOR	RE-AUDITOR

SEX ☐ Male ☐ Female	AGE	NO SHOW	CANCELLED

I INDEX VISIT (ITEMS 1-8)

1. DIAGNOSIS/PROBLEMS	OLD			2. MEDICATIONS	CURRENT		
	New	Known	"Buried"		New	Known	"Buried"
a.							
b.							
c.							
d.							
e.							
f.							
g.							
h.							

Significant Buried Diagnosis   ☐ Yes ☐ No   Significant Buried Rx   ☐ Yes ☐ No

3. Is entry legible?   ☐ Yes ☐ No

4. Is entry adequate?   ☐ Yes ☐ No
   If no, explain_____

5. Is Diagnosis/Impression, etc., rational and relevant to problems of   Not Given   ☐ Yes ☐ No
   that visit? If no, explain_____

6. Is Treatment/Medication, etc., rational and adequate?   Not Given   ☐ Yes ☐ No
   If no, explain_____

7. Were Lab/X-ray procedures appropriately ordered and done?   Not Given   ☐ Yes ☐ No
   If no, explain_____

8. Was Disposition rational and appropriate?   Not Given   ☐ Yes ☐ No
   If no, explain_____

II GENERAL CHART REVIEW, ITEMS 9-13)

9. Has there been excess physician utilization?   ☐ Yes ☐ No
   If yes, explain_____

10. Has there been insufficient physician follow-up?   ☐ Yes ☐ No
    If yes, explain_____

11. Has there been excess utilization of Lab/X-ray, etc.?   ☐ Yes ☐ No
    If yes, explain_____

12. Has there been inadequate action regarding Lab/X-ray abnormalities?   ☐ Yes ☐ No
    If yes, explain_____

13. Miscellaneous deviations (Industrial, etc.)   ☐ Yes ☐ No

COMMITTEE DISPOSITION

☐ Refer to Dr._____   For Action_____

☐ Refer to Dr._____   For Information_____

☐ Refer to_____   For Action_____

☐ Refer to_____   For Information_____

☐ Referral not indicated

REASON

TABULATION

06991 (REV. 12-73)

[Watermark across form: NOT RECOMMENDED—SEE TEXT]

Figure 27-2. Sample form used by CQAS in the past.

One may rightfully conclude that this is no more than the old one-on-one review that medical professionals have been doing for many decades. Until now this is precisely what it has been with one significant exception. In no way is microsampling directed toward any individual. The entire review is done with the idea of "what's wrong" rather than "who's wrong." In this way errors involving systems and communication between providers and that are not any one person's fault are also discovered. It does not matter who was responsible for not following up in a timely manner on a patient with gross hematuria. There is no reason to point an accusing finger at a physician or at the laboratory for a delayed report or at medical records for delayed filing and so on. The entire attention is on what is wrong. Subsequent analysis (as is described later on) will determine *where* corrective action is necessary. The old "one on one" was directed more at the perpetrator of the wrong than at improving care to the patient. Microsampling has been found to be sound and with very little practice is conducted without defensiveness and hostility.

An interesting observation has been made in this regard over the past 10 years of doing microsampling. It has not been published because it lacks the "scientific validity" one expects to find in most journals. This observation is depicted in Figure 27-3. If a normal Gaussian distribution of physicians based on quality is assumed, from "bad" to "good" by whatever criteria used (board certification, few malpractice claims, few patient complaints, peer respect, high productivity, how many "physician patients" one has in one's practice, and so forth) the solid bell-shaped curve results. One would expect that the number of errors would be highest for the "low-quality" physician and lowest for the "high-quality" physicians as shown by the dash line. My experience over all these years is that the "best" physicians are responsible

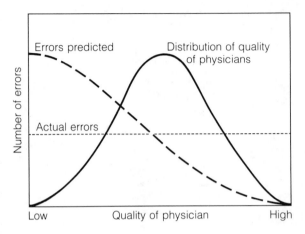

FIGURE 27-3. Relation of errors to other measures of physician quality.

for as many grievous errors as the "worst" physicians, as shown by the dotted line. This may seem strange, but it is a consistent finding. During microsampling sessions, one hardly ever hears the comment, "Oh, you would expect Dr. X to have done that." What is heard at essentially every session is, "How in the world could Dr. X have done that? He's our best surgeon [or internist, and so forth]." There does not seem to be any ready explanation for this confusing finding. It is not apparent whether it results from the fact that the "high-quality" physicians actually receive the more difficult cases, are usually more productive and therefore at greater risk, or do not bother themselves with repeatedly seeing patients who are essentially well and therefore not in need of any treatment. There may be other explanations, but there is little question about the observation. It is interesting to note that the dotted line of actual errors observed (and it must be remembered that this is merely an observation and not a scientifically valid precise measurement) mirrors very closely the malpractice curve.

The implications of this observation are note-worthy in several respects. First, it indicates that improvement is possible and necessary for all prac-titioners. Second, it indicates one reason why it is desirable to conduct microsampling in a way that divorces it completely from the concept of assign-ing "fault" or attribution at this stage of quality assurance.

This observation ties in with another considera-tion regarding improvement of health care deliv-ery. As shown in Figure 27-4, the solid vertical line in the normal Gaussian distribution of physi-cians providing various levels of quality of care (as shown by the solid bell-shaped curve) illustrates the mean level of care delivered. If one should en-tirely remove from practice the 1% tail of the poorest practitioners in a community (as shown by the dotted area, and which would happen if im-provement activities were directed only toward these physicians), the mean level of care provided

to the community would improve by a miniscule amount (as shown by the vertical dotted line). However, if all physicians in a community im-proved slightly (by improving only a few signifi-cant elements of care that each performed in a sub-optimal manner), the distribution curve of quality of care delivered would approximate the Gaussian dashed curve as shown, and the mean level of care would change significantly as shown by the verti-cal dashed line. This argument assumes that most physicians are doing a creditable job most of the time. The argument falls apart, of course, if one makes the assumption that the tail of the distribu-tion curve of bad physicians who should be com-pletely stopped from practicing approaches 20% to 30%.

The next step in microsampling is the second difference from the old "one-on-one" review. It is called "serial unanimity" and converts a highly subjective process into a fully objective one. Hav-ing recorded the problems discovered, the review-ing practitioner exchanges the medical record and his or her list of discovered problems with another practitioner of the same or different discipline who has a similar list of problems based on that prac-titioner's review of another record. Each practitioner reviews the second record in a manner identical to the first review, but in addition, the findings of the first reviewer are either validated or contested by the second reviewer. The second reviewer may add problems he or she detected to the list. After the second review, the two practitioners confer briefly to identify all items on which both agree. Each has power of veto. These agreed-upon findings are then presented to the remainder of the quality assurance committee for their approval or disap-proval. An example of such a list is shown in Figure 27-5.

The microsample data sheet shown contains all real examples taken from such reviews. The code B06 is a code for the patient's number (usually a

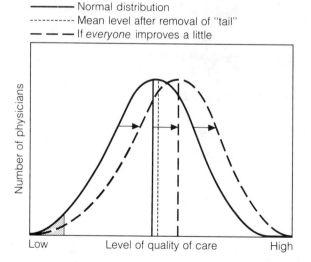

——————— Normal distribution
----------- Mean level after removal of "tail"
— — — If *everyone* improves a little

FIGURE 27-4.   Effect of removing poor physicians compared with minor improvement of all physi-cians' performance.

Code **B06** Index date **3/25/77** Hospital (Clinic) Facility *Anyplace Clinic*

Reviewer #1 *Dr. Smith*   Reviewer #2 *Dr. Jones*

Age **52**   Sex **♀**   Today's date **5/2/77**

Reason for index contact *Depression*

Refer for action *Gyn re pap smear*

1/17/77 Inderal given prn

3/25/77 Has paroxysmal tachycardia + is on thyroid for "history of low BMR"

11/2/76 - Entire entry: "Viral URI
Rx. Keflex"

10/7/76 History rectal polyps · recent rectal bleeding - referred for sigmoidoscopy but not done.   Sigms sheet filed in c̄ x-rays

6/10/76 Entry: "Probable viral syndrome
Urine neg
Poly cillin 250 qid"

Pap smear 1/15/77 - Gr III — no repeat, no referral, no follow up.

FIGURE 27-5. Microsample data sheet.

simple code, for example, James *Bond* No. 345*06* becomes B06). This is to be sure for medicolegal purposes that the data is not filed in the medical record. It does enable calling the patient back if he is still at risk. Index date is the date of the visit (or hospital discharge) that caused the chart to be pulled (from the appointment sheet, and so forth). This is necessary so that both reviewers know where the starting point is. Without it they may review adjacent discharges or visits in depth, and confusion results. The example shown is just a clinic chart review. Both hospital and clinic may be circled if the review is of both. The entire CQAS procedure, from microsampling to action following measurement, is the same for ambulatory or hospital review. Age, sex, and reason for index contact are the only summary features necessary for the quality care committee to set the scene. "Refer for action" is used when the patient is still at risk and ought to be called back, or some other action taken. Another example might be a misfiled significant laboratory report in the patient's chart that could lead to mismanagement. In the latter, the "refer for action" would mean medical records. As previously mentioned, these are taken from actual occurrences.

Note the two handwritings, one for Dr. Smith and one for Dr. Jones. Dr. Jones discovered the sigmoidoscopy report buried in the record. He also discovered the abnormal Pap smear that had no follow-up. No attempt is made to completely review the record. The efficiency of the system drops off sharply after 10 to 15 minutes on any record. It is not necessary to do a complete review. There are enough problems discovered in a short time to keep the group busy educationally and with system improvements without looking further. Moving on to a new record after 10 to 15 minutes is more interesting, and totally different types of problems will be found (perhaps of a child, older male, surgical case, and so forth). Physicians tend to get im-

mersed in a case and want to spend half an hour or so on each record. This has to be curtailed because efficiency falls off. After 15 minutes, the discussion is not apt to center on errors but on better ways, or alternative ways, the particular case could have been handled. Right and wrong is not clearly demarcated at this point, and quality assurance in the sense of the objective is no longer the target.

The question at this time is not, "How should this have been done?" but in this specific case under these specific circumstances, "Was this right?" This step must be done with the medical record at hand just in case a finding is challenged or additional information desired, but it does not involve a third review of the medical record. Not having the record at hand allows members of the committee to make unjustified suppositions, to become defensive, and to sweep the problem under the rug. Again, each member of the quality assurance committee has a veto. At the conclusion of the session, a list of problems has been created for which all members of the committee agree improvement should be sought. Assignment of fault is still not part of the system. Gaining serial unanimity or objectivity is then repeated with the appropriate department or medical center group. In essence, all the practitioners who may have responsibility for an element of care must agree that in the particular situation described in the particular record, the performance was not desirable. Thus a list of unanimously agreed-upon problems is created. Problem solving, or stating "what's right," is not yet part of the system.

It may seem as though getting large numbers of physicians to agree on anything is futile. A few real examples will demonstrate that this can be achieved. It is not likely that a physician will defend the following:

1. Entire entry: "viral infection—cefazolin sodium (Keflex)"

2. Twenty-one days of daily chemistry panels on a patient not on any dangerous drugs and about whom no determination was ever abnormal.

3. Administering long-acting insulin every 4 hours as necessary depending on urine, to a newly discovered postoperative diabetic patient

4. A 10-year-old boy who had three determinations of hemoglobin over a period of a few years, all of which were under 10 gm without note or procedure in regard to it

Note that in identifying problems no suggestions concerning types of problems have been made. The entire range of medical care activities should be considered. For example, it may not seem that there is much point in considering nontreatable conditions or those in which therapy is not apt to be of great significance. However, just as many errors may be made here as in the conditions most amenable to therapy. The errors in these nontreatable conditions will cover the entire spectrum from underutilization (or lack of care), to overutilization, to improper therapy. The example of prescribing an antibiotic for a simple upper respiratory infection is such an example. Lack of response or lack of adequate response to a patient terminally ill with cancer is another. Many records have been seen wherein the ambulatory chart properly indicates that the prognosis is hopeless, with a life expectancy of a few weeks, but sufficient analgesic is withheld because of fear of addiction. Overutilization is often encountered in terminal cases with extensive diagnostic testing even though it is clear no therapeutic action could or should possibly follow, regardless of results. It is clear then that consideration should not be limited to conditions wherein therapeutic efficacy is known to exist. Similarly, consideration should not be limited to "scientifically proved" concepts. Many currently accepted aspects of care have not and likely will not be sci-

entifically tested to assure their validity. It is not anticipated that a controlled clinical trial will be performed on the need to respond to telephone calls regarding temperatures over 104 F or the need to observe patients who report melena and fainting. "Scientifically proved" beliefs seem to change with time just about as much as those based on the "common wisdom." Tunnel vision in searching out specified conditions has no place in problem identification. If it's wrong, and the reviewer is fairly certain his or her peers will agree, it should be identified as a potential problem.

During the process of serial unanimity, several different decisions can be made in regard to any specific problem identified. These may be categorized in three ways.

First, all agree that the element of care is one that deserves attention. This can then proceed to the next step of the CQAS, which is criteria or standard setting.

Second, all agree that the incident noted is an important and significant deviation from desirable care but that further action is not in order because it was "just an anecdote" or "one in a million, will never happen again." The group will be unwilling to proceed to establish a criterion in regard to that element of care because it is felt it would be wasteful. It is management's responsibility at this time to point out that the frequency of this problem is not known and that before dismissing it the frequency of the problem should be known. Moreover, if it has a frequency other than zero, the distribution among practitioners should be determined. If the total frequency of a serious departure from desirable practice is only 5%, but that 5% represents 100% of one physician's performance, a significant problem has been discovered. The way to determine the frequency and distribution of a problem is to set a criterion and objectively measure performance in regard to it. In the early days of the CQAS, it was assumed that the "one in a million'' transgression would be a common result of microsampling. As time has gone by, it has become apparent that "the unthinkable error" is usually not an isolated instance. In addition, usually several practitioners are responsible. Management should be warned not to succumb to brushing these oddities under the rug. Frequently they are not rare. Management must realize that it cannot even claim good care until it has measured the frequency of these oddities and has shown that, in fact, they are rare.

Third, heated argument may develop in regard to a microsample finding, with one faction believing the problem to be deplorable and not wishing to accept the veto of the other faction that claims that the performance in the particular case at hand is acceptable. It is clearly not possible to move from this point to that of setting a criterion for measurement. The situation in regard to a specific case has

not been clearly established as a problem, and therefore the general statement of the problem cannot be formulated. When this situation arises, it is necessary to defer the problem to an educational meeting, conceivably with appropriate consultative help. Time should not be wasted during a quality assurance session attempting to determine the right or wrong of a highly contested event. Similarly, research projects should not evolve from such disagreements at the quality assurance meeting. These should be appropriately referred. Figure 27-6 diagramatically shows the flow proceeding from identifying a problem in a specific case through serial unanimity to setting a criterion for the general situation. This is an important sequence of the overall quality assurance scheme as shown on p. 280. Figure 27-7 shows with an example how an actual specific problem can lead to a more general statement of a standard.

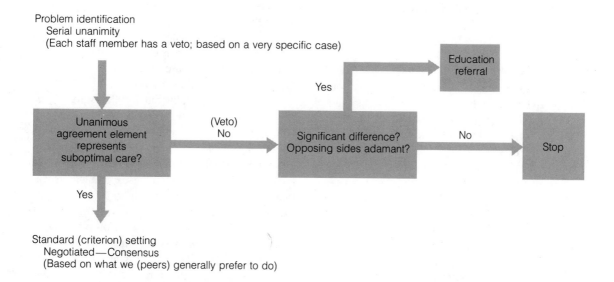

FIGURE 27-6.   Flow chart illustrating the sequence from problem identification to criterion setting.

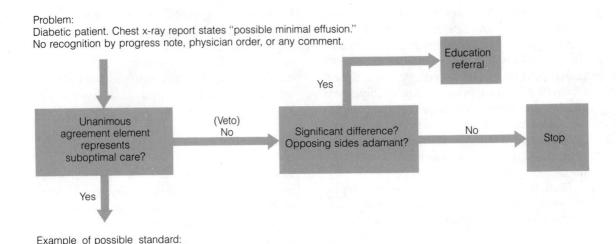

Problem:
Diabetic patient. Chest x-ray report states "possible minimal effusion."
No recognition by progress note, physician order, or any comment.

Example of possible standard:
All chest x-ray films revealing an abnormality not specified as old
will have some follow-up action or a note referring to x-ray film or report.

FIGURE 27-7. Specific problem can be a catalyst for the establishment of a general standard.

Criterion (Standard) Setting

Basic Considerations

In the CQAS the terms "criterion" and "standard" are used interchangeably in a synonymous fashion and are used that way throughout this chapter. The concept of "an allowable deviation from the criterion," or "action level," or "threshold value," or "expected compliance" with reference to not meeting a criterion is not used at all. A discussion of the reasons for this departure from the definitions established by the BQA follows. The explanation is in considerable detail, because major concepts in quality assurance are involved, not just a semantic debate.

The terms "standards, norms, and criteria" were defined by the PSRO program when it first began and have since become part of the lexicon of regulations and jargon. Unfortunately, although the BQA and the National PSR Council labored long and hard to make these definitions helpful to the PSROs, many problems in their use have surfaced. Additonal consideration of these definitions reveals that more confusion will develop as the PSROs develop data bases and attempt to deal with these terms in actual operation.

Several reports delivered by the staff of the DHEW at the National PSR Council meetings contained comments in which it was stated that for a variety of reasons the strict definitions of norms, criteria, and standards were not used. It seems that the common thread through these explanations was that the definitions did not seem to fit the intended use or that it was more natural to use the terms as used in common parlance. Recent proposed regulations in the *Federal Register* have defined "norms" as "standards, norms and criteria." In common parlance the terms "standards" and "criteria" are often interchanged. The third edition of Webster's international unabridged dictionary defines a criterion as a standard. Other government agencies outside the BQA use the terms interchangeably and much more loosely. In addition, examination of the PSRO definitions reveals internal inconsistencies that will prove troublesome.

Subscripting is necessary to avoid confusion. Note the following PSRO definitions:

norms (medical care appraisal norms) numerical or statistical measures of usual observed performance.

standards Professionally developed expressions of the range of acceptable variation from a norm or criterion.

criteria (Medical care criteria) predetermined elements against which aspects of the quality of a medical service may be compared; developed by professionals relying on professional expertise and on the professional literature.

If one were to use these PSRO definitions, the following would occur. If only one variable (length of stay) is considered for one condition (diagnosis X):

Norm at Hospital B = 15 days	$N_{HB} = 15$
Norm for PSRO = 14 days	$N_P = 14$
Criterion for Hospital B = 14 days	$C_{HB} = 14$
Criterion for PSRO = 12 days	$C_P = 12$

With these data, there is a variety of standards for this one variable for this one condition. In addition, the norms for other hospitals will vary, and the criteria for other hospitals may vary. The standard can be a range of acceptable variation from a *norm* or *criterion,* therefore:

$S_{NHB} =$	14–16
$S_{NP} =$	13–15
$S_{CHP} =$	13–15
$S_{CP} =$	11–13

Each time a standard is used it must be subscripted even in a report or discussion limited to uniform PSRO-wide data (eliminating consideration of variation between hospitals) because it is necessary to note whether the standard is a variation of a norm or a criterion.

Since a standard is a *range* of acceptable variation, one would think it has an upper and lower limit. This is probably always true when one is dealing with the standard of a norm (which by definition is numerical or statistical). However, if one is dealing with a criterion that is not numerical, such as preferred use of penicillin for diagnosis X or surgical intervention for condition Y, what is the meaning of a "range"? Even in the case of a numerical variable whether it is a norm or a criterion, confusion will exist in that the variation may apply to the variable itself or to the frequency of the variable. For example, for the criterion "all patients will be discharged with a temperature under 100.1 F, the standard could allow 90% of patients to be discharged with a temperature 100.3 F (the 0.2 degrees being the acceptable variation).

The previous discussion had to do only with the complexities and confusing aspects of standards and the fact that much greater definition would be needed if they are to be used. For example, it would be necessary to specify whether the acceptable variation of a variable is in regard to the frequency of the variation or to the variation of the variable itself. The following arguments are even stronger arguments against the use of "acceptable variations" based on medical considerations.

If the intent of the standard, in the nonnumerical example just given is that the standard modifies the "all," and it would be acceptable for, say, 5% of patients with diagnosis X not to receive penicillin, how would one know that these are not the ones in greatest need? In fact, medical care evaluations reveal that the exceptions to the criteria often occur when the need is greatest. A common example is the criterion that "all patients with fluid balance

condition X be weighed daily.'' The usual deficiencies are in those patients ''too sick to be
weighed'' even though bed scales are available.
This also occurs in the ambulatory setting as demonstrated by the fact that debilitated children or
those with chronic asthma, for example, usually
have not had routine pediatric immunizations. If
these are the ''5% acceptable variation'' they are
the ones who might be considered to need it most.
A ''standard'' or acceptable variation is an indis-
criminate waiver, often antithetic to the intent of
the criterion.

Similar problems exist concerning the responsible agent. For example, if there is a 5% acceptable
variation in regard to a particular aspect of care,
how can one be sure this is not 100% of the activity
of one physician on the staff (or one nurse, one
ward, or one shift)? This is another example of the
antithetic nature of acceptable variations. To manage this, the procedure advocated by the California
Medical Association (CMA) has had to be modified. The CMA program uses ''thresholds,''
which are acceptable variations beyond which the
staff is committed to taking corrective action. The
term ''thresholds,'' therefore, is identical to the
term ''standards'' as defined by PSRO. Because of
the inherent problem in the concept, it is necessary
in the CMA system for peers to review all variant
charts, anyway, even if the action threshold has not
been reached. The reason for this, of course, is the
distribution problem just described. This inherent
fault in ''allowable variation'' makes the entire
concept of an ''allowable variation'' unacceptable
in quality assurance or quality improvement, because unless these ''allowable variations'' are
scrutinized as carefully as ''unallowable variations,'' certain segments of the population may be
disenfranchised with regard to good care.

Some advocates adhere to the ''threshold'' concept primarily because it is believed to contain
some immunity from medicolegal hazard. That is,

100% compliance with anything is not really
achievable. Legal cases are apt to be judged on different grounds, however, and there seems little likelihood that avoiding 100% as a ''standard'' is actually a safeguard against unwarranted malpractice
action.

Another consideration that has to do with medical care and audit argues against the use of allowable variations. As previously mentioned, there is
an almost infinite number of significant elements
of care to consider in quality assurance. It is necessary to confine the discussion to a select group of
the most important elements. Even this number is
considerable. Attention should be focused on the
problems that are of the ''res ipsa loquitur'' variety. Anything less than total compliance with regard to such serious matters would truly speak for
itself.

When one deals with significant and important
criteria, the concept of an acceptable variation
ceases to exist. It is for this reason that the JCAH
in its PEP program has abolished the concept of a
standard by stating that criteria are all either 0% or
100%, that is, there are no ''allowable variations.''

In actual practice, ''action levels'' are determined by the other crises and problems facing the
institution at that point. The intensity and speed of
corrective action will depend on the gravity of the
problem discovered, the resources of the institution, and the other problems facing the institution
at that time, not some *a priori* percentage set at a
committee meeting. Even in systems where action
levels have been set, the lack of validity of the
concept of a standard is demonstrated by the fact
that action is taken even when the standard has
been met. Such an example is evident in the middle
paragraph of Elwood's book describing Williamson's work with auditing those with hypertension.[4]

Standards, thresholds, actions levels, and so
forth are not only costly to determine and without
inherent validity but also are totally superfluous to

an effective quality improvement system. It is for these reasons that the concept is not used in the CQAS.

The CQAS uses the concept of "clinical significance" rather than "statistical significance." Because of the very large number of elements of care that may be performed suboptimally, it is necessary to be very selective and pick only those that are critical. When this is done properly, an unjustified deviation from the standard is significant, and some corrective activity should be instituted. These deviations may be too small in number ever to show true statistical improvement, but a decreasing incidence of a truly critical error in care is always clinically significant.

In spite of many earnest attempts by voluntary agencies, government bureaus, and independent workers in quality assurance to explain the purpose of standards in medical audit, they are still considered directives for care by most practitioners. Many consider them analogous to hospital bylaws that must be followed and that must be studied by new members of the staff. Some want to post them in emergency rooms and other locations "so they may be followed." This unfortunate misconception that a standard is a rule or instruction has contributed significantly to negativism toward quality assurance in general and has resulted in the construction of many standards of no value.

In an earlier description of the CQAS, it is stated that criteria or standards are necessary "to save professional time by using nonprofessionals to screen activities or records and to evaluate corrective measures." Experience gained since then requires some modification. Just as standards for medical care are true only today, it is appropriate that what now turns out to be an error be corrected at this time.

The main purpose for writing a criterion or standard is to enable the frequency and distribution of a suspected problem to be determined. A second

reason is so that medical record professionals can do their job on the health care team by making these measurements without having to resort to professional judgments beyond their discipline. (The change from the older use of "nonprofessional" is another example of change and should not go unnoticed). A third reason for writing standards is so that corrective measures may be evaluated. With time it has become apparent that this reason is least valid, because with almost every iterative measurement of a standard there are sufficient changes (as is described shortly) so that simple comparisons of actual numerical values of achievement of the standard must be made with considerable reservation. (This is discussed more fully later.) Conspicuous by its absence is the purpose of a standard as a directive or instruction in providing care.

Process of Setting Criteria or Standards

The process of problem identification is in essence stating "what's wrong" in a specific instance. The essence of standard writing is to state in effect what is generally felt to be right today in a more general sense *under ordinary circumstances* (for example, not limiting it to a 42-year-old white male).

A number of aspects of standard writing have been considered in detail elsewhere and will not be repeated here.[3] These relate primarily to the art of negotiating, the seat of responsibility and authority for setting a standard, and characteristics of standards. Again, it is necessary to correct what has turned out to be an error, this time in regard to gaining agreement on a standard.

Agreement on standards is reached by negotiation and consensus. Voting has no place in standard setting for reasons described in detail previously.[3] At one time it was felt that standards had to be adopted unanimously by those involved in the standard, because if practitioners openly stated that they did not agree with the standard and did not practice in that way, there seemed little point in measuring the known variations. It has been found that there is sufficient opposition to the entire concept of quality assurance as well as standards among physicians that frequently there will be one or two holdouts who will oppose every standard until it is watered down to an absolutely meaningless level. They do this by quoting the rare exception or the remote possibility. They will not accept the definition that a standard is what peers generally prefer to do under normal circumstances. At times this opposition comes from antagonism to the entire quality assurance activity; there is still a feeling that the old informal methods worked best. At other times the opposition to setting standards comes from fear of setting standards. The fear may be caused by the feeling that these are directives for care (notwithstanding all the assurances to the contrary), and conscientious physicians may not want to obligate themselves to follow a rule they know may have to be modified under appropriate circumstances. At other times the fear may be due to concern that a medicolegal hazard will be created if the standard is not followed even for good reason.

Usually these fears are expressed by one or two individuals and preclude achieving unanimity in regard to the standard. It is clear, however, during the discussion that the proposed statement of the standard does describe how they usually practice. When this occurs, rather than have the procedure become useless and a waste of resources, it is necessary to state that "the consensus seems to indicate this is what is generally done" and proceed to measure the performance. The opposing physicians usually are found not to practice any differently from the others. Should the circumstance occur that these practitioners do have an unusual practice and have justified variations from the standard, the system will allow for that as described later.

In summary, although it is necessary to have unanimity in establishing that a particular event was undesirable in a specific situation or case, it is not necessary to have unanimity for the proposed standard, a statement pertaining to the more general situation. This in no way indicates that ratification of a standard is either unnecessary or undesirable. Ratification of the standard before measurement of performance is necessary and desirable but does not have to be unanimous.

Data Management

To expedite the data handling and to provide a mechanism for tracking of the quality assurance activities by staff or management, three forms have evolved over time and are shown in the CQAS work sheets I, II, and III (see Figure 27-8). Just as it is obvious that parts of the CQAS system can be used independently of others (such as microsampling), the basic system could work quite well without these forms. However, these forms were developed to provide easy tracking, minimize data collection, avoid duplication, and most important, attempt to assure avoidance of some major pitfalls. Probably the greatest pitfall is carefully hammering out a standard in regard to a serious deficit in care, laboriously collecting the data and subjecting it to peer analysis, and then discovering that the wrong data was collected because of an imprecise term in the standard. This is a particularly serious error, because it is a major disincentive to staff, decreases attendance at subsequent quality assurance meetings, and results in high costs and low cost effectiveness, which causes lack of motivation in management, and thus sets in motion a vicious circle resulting in cessation of any effective quality assurance activities.

Since these forms evolved for use in a large system consisting of many hospitals and clinics, not every bit of data is necessary in every application. The following instructions for use of these forms identify some entries merely for informational purposes, but for others greater detail is given so that the importance of some of the entries can be understood. These work sheets were designed to minimize the total record keeping necessary for management of a quality assurance program. They allow each responsible individual to know at a glance that information he or she needs to know. In essence, they report what standards are being measured, with any changes from audit to audit, how they are being measured (in very specific terms), the proportion of practice noncompliant with the standard, the recommendations that have been made to correct the problems, and when and how the recommendations were implemented. Because of the data on the work sheets, quality assurance committee minutes may be extremely brief.

A major difference between the CQAS and other quality assurance systems is that in the CQAS each element of care to be considered is handled separately. This was noted in microsampling, was carried through to standard setting, and is continued through data collection and implementation of remedial action. The importance of this cannot be overstated. To mix different elements of care serves no good purpose and creates unnecessary problems. Pooling standards does not give one an overall sense of care in any area because there are too many elements to consider. It does create the problem that changes in the statement of one standard of a set are difficult to manage when the others remain the same on subsequent measurements. Different standards have different turnaround times for institution of remedial action and different times for remeasurement. The results of measurement of one standard in regard to a specific clinical situation may require almost emergency corrective steps. The results of measurement of another standard in regard to the same clinical condition may require 6 months for any modification of behavior to be perceptible. Similarly, one element in a specific clinical situation may require re-

ferral to the pathologist, and another element in the same clinical situation may have to do with nursing.

The single element approach to quality assurance thus maintains this element-by-element characteristic through all steps of the process. This is not to say, of course, that if two or more standards on different subjects can be measured on the same set of charts that this economy of operation should be ignored. It just means that the data should not be commingled on the same sheets.

An example of a completed set of CQAS worksheets through several audits is shown in Figure 27-8. This is synthetic to demonstrate a number of features. Note that each audit cycle is tracked horizontally across the various columns. A line is drawn under the entries on a work sheet when the entries are completed for a given audit. Entries for subsequent audits of the standard continue on the same sheet below the line in a manner similar to that of progress notes in a patient's chart.

Specific instructions and descriptions for each item in CQAS work sheet I, of audit standard and measurement instruction follows:

Audit standard number is self-explanatory. Note the repeated use of the combined term ''audit standard'' in an effort constantly to remind the staff that these are not practice standards but are written purely for purposes of audit. Unfortunately, the belief that these are directives for care still abounds, and no assurance regarding the success of this effort in terminology can be given. *Medical center* is also self-explanatory.

Origin of standard is not important, and is primarily for large institutions. It is the problem leading to the standard and the reference (such as postoperative infection, case review, surgery 8/19/76; discussion of increased mortality, pediatrics 1/7/76; medicolegal notes 5/6/76; missed cancer, microsampling medical department, 2/4/76).

The *first CQAS agenda date* is not important and is primarily for large institutions. It refers to

AUDIT STANDARD AND MEASUREMENT INSTRUCTION CQAS WORKSHEET I

| | STANDARD NUMBER | PAGE 1 |

MEDICAL CENTER	ORIGIN OF STANDARD	1ST CQAS AGENDA DATE	DATE STANDARD SET
Shore Medical Offices	Medical Department CQAS 1/17/74	February 25, 1974	March 15, 1974

AUDIT STANDARD
All patients over age 40 seen in office will have blood pressure recorded biannually if seen biannually.

MEASUREMENT INSTRUCTIONS

1. DEPT(S) PARTICIPATING AND CONTACT PERSON(S) 2. LOCATION(S) OF CARE (e.g. Hosp., OPD, SNF, Home) 3. INTERPRETATION OF TERMS 4. MODIFICATIONS/EXCLUSIONS TO STANDARD (1)	Case (record, activity etc.) Selection Procedure (2)	Specific Screening and Testing Procedure Within Case (3)	Max. No. (4)	DATE REF. FOR MEAS. (5)
1. Department Medicine 2. Clinic 3. Seen = by appointment or "walk-in." Over age 40 = birth year before 1934. 4. None	Office records from registration slips to medical department after 3:00 P.M. starting on 3/21/74.	Recording of blood pressure in any progress notes, or copies of physical examination for hospital admission or emergency room visits, only since March 1972.	100	3/20/74
Same	Same selection, start 5/17/74.	Also check EKG report and insurance forms if blood pressure not found elsewhere. All sources listed check only to May 1972.	30	5/15/74
1. Add accepted by Ob/Gyn Department for patients seen in Gyn (Minutes 7/5/74)	Add registration to Gyn Department also – same instructions as for Medicine. Total number 1/4 Gyn, 3/4 Medicine.	Same	60	9/11/74

A

Figure 27-8. CQAS work sheets. **A,** Audit standard and measurement instruction. **B,** Clerical measurement results, **C,** Recommendations and action.

B

CQAS WORKSHEET II   STANDARD NUMBER   PAGE

CLERICAL MEASUREMENT RESULTS | CLINICAL/ADMINISTRATIVE REVIEW OF VARIATIONS

No. Scr. (6)	No. Tested (7)	No. of Var. (8)	% of Tested (9)	Patterns Noted/Other Comments (10)	ID of Variation (chart or pt. no. or other ID) (11)	Date Meas. Rep. (12)	Just.? yes/no (13)	% of tested not justified (14)	Clinical/Administrative Review Findings and Date Reviewed (15)
20	20	10	50	None. Distributed among appointments and "walk-in" and many physicians.	183-040	3/29/74	No	40	---
					729-176		No		---
					221-011		No		B.P. 180/110 in E.R. in 1971. No F.U. Patient 221-011 has been called in by his physician.
				Many patients without blood pressure seen in several departments.	146-784		Yes		B.P. on EKG requis.
					132-749		No		---
					144-666		No		---
					311-042		No		---
					221-011		Yes		B.P. on insurance form.
					343-212		No		---
					224-689		No		---
30	29	7	24	4 of 7 were registered at 5:00 P.M.	342-901	5/27/74	No	23	---
					211-089		No		---
					411-800		No		B.P. 190/110 in Gyn in 1970. No F.U. Patient has been called in by her physician.
				One new patient registered as a "walk-in" but left after 5 minutes without being seen, "couldn't wait."	334-627		No		---
					284-357		No		---
					331-112		No		---
					176-429		No		---
60	60	2	3	None	384-715	9/20/74	Yes	2	Seen only once for marked despair concerning unexpected death in family.
					198-299		No		---

Figure 27-8   *(continued).*

RECOMMENDATIONS AND ACTION

COAS WORKSHEET III   STANDARD NUMBER   PAGE   C

ANALYSIS CONCLUSION	ACTION RECOMMENDED			ACTION TAKEN	
TYPE OF NEED IDENTIFIED/SOURCE(S) OF PROB. (ID of dept., indiv., etc.) (16)	ACTION &/OR NEXT AUDIT (17)	TO (18)	DATE (19)	ACTION - WHAT, TIME, PLACE (20)	DATE (21)
Awareness of importance of hypertension identification needs improvement. Follow-up of identified may be a problem.	Consider education program regarding identification and follow-up of hypertensives.	Director Medical Education	4/10/74	Interdepartmental Conference. See education minutes.	4/26/74
	Re-audit May 1974	CQAS		Re-audit done.	5/15/74
Same as above.	Consider place on agenda of Department Chiefs meeting.	Chief of Staff	6/5/74	Discussed at Dept. Chiefs meeting. Subsequent decision: Medical Dept. Office Assistants to be instructed on taking blood pressure and are to do so as time permits. Also adopted new standard (#81) regarding follow-up of hypertensives. (Med. Dept. Minutes 7/2/74.) Ob Dept. Minutes 7/5/74 in addition wrote standard (#86) regarding blood pressure measurement in patients on oral contraceptives.	7/2/74 7/5/74
	Re-audit Sept. 1974	CQAS	7/10/74	Re-audited.	9/20/74
Improvement satisfactory.	Re-audit March 1975	CQAS	10/2/74		

Figure 27-8 *(continued).*

the date of the first quality assurance meeting where this was discussed.

The *date standard set* is important primarily in large institutions but may be important in all situations. It is the date when the appropriate body (such as medical department or whole medical center) ratified the standard or the dates when additional departments ratify the standard indicated in the column under department(s) participating.

The *audit standard* is very important in any quality assurance activity. These are the exact words of the audit standard as formulated for the initial measurement. The statement should be simple, not compounded with multiple requirements, and should be a positive "all" or "none" statement. It does not contain a range of acceptability. It is stated in precise enough terms to allow measurement by nonpractitioner personnel. It is never a question since it must state what is currently generally thought to be desired performance or result of care.

The *first column* contains four different types of information: (1) department(s) participating and contact person(s), (2) location(s) of care, (3) interpretation of terms, and (4) modifications or exclusions to standard. For each audit cycle, changes or additions in any of these items are recorded.

The *department(s) participating and contact person(s)* are important to know to be sure right charts or activities are audited. They include the departments that are participating in the audit and the person in each department who is responsible. Parties other than departmental divisions should be named when applicable (such as receptionists, all surgical services, fourth floor hospital, and entire medical center).

As time goes on if other parties adopt the audit standard, it is recorded here. The *date* the change occurred should be included with such an entry. This is quite important, because it is necessary to know who was involved in any particular audit to be able to interpret changes over time. For example, suppose a problem was discovered in a medical department, and after a criterion was set and measured, compliance rates were determined. If the surgery department subsequently developed or discovered the same problem and accepted the same criterion, a marked change in compliance rate in either direction could be due to variation in denominator rather than numerator, and totally wrong conclusions could be reached unless retrospectively the date the surgery department was added to the audit was known. This is not a serious problem at all if the data described on the work sheet are kept. This same problem will be faced by PSROs as institutions start or stop activities within the PSRO area.

The *location of care* (such as hospital, outpatient department, skilled nursing facility, and home) is a concern primarily for large systems. *Where* the care being audited takes place should be indicated. If both hospital and outpatient care are being audited, both are specified. If both hospital and clinic care are listed here, the measurement instructions will ordinarily reflect audit of both the clinic and hospital records. As for all other entries, this may change from audit to audit for the same audit standard as other areas of care delivery are incorporated into the audit.

The *interpretation of terms* is very important in any quality assurance activity. Everything in the audit standard that is not completely precise should be defined in specific terms. The purpose of this entry is to be sure the data collector knows exactly what to look for without using judgment beyond his or her knowledge. It also allows the audit to be repeated months later in an identical manner if desired. Proper use of this column will avoid confusion and wasted time during quality committee discussions. Interpretations often provide synonyms and describe inclusion or exclusion of specific terms applicable to the standard. For example, an audit of the use of long-term anticoagulants would include in this column not only a definition of "long term" (such as 6 months or longer) but a list of the specific anticoagulants, such as warfarin sodium (Coumadin, Panwarfin), dicumarol, not aspirin, to be included in the study.

The words "normal" or "abnormal," for example, must be defined. If the audit standard refers to "without temperature elevation," it is imperative for the staff, not the audit chairperson, data collector, or any other individual, to agree that in this circumstance it means "over 101 F." If no specification is made, the data retriever is very apt to use 98.6 F as normal. Enormous waste of time, effort, and temper can be saved by not reporting spurious results based on such simple communication errors.

Modifications or exclusions to standards are very important in any quality assurance activity. From audit to audit, the standard may be modified by addition of terms, exclusions or inclusions of age groups, change of meaning of "temperature," and so forth. These modifications should be specified here. The intent of the CQAS is not rigidly to maintain uniformity from audit to audit for the purpose of having comparable results suitable for publication. The intent of the CQAS is to change the audit as necessary to address areas of operation requiring attention and result in sensible improvement.

The second, third, and fourth columns contain *measurement instructions.* Under the *second column* is the *CASE (record, activity, and so forth) selection procedure,* which is very important in any quality assurance activity. The procedure for choosing the cases (records, patients, and so forth) to be studied including the *time* and *place* such information is to be sought is entered.

It is important not to confuse this record selection procedure with that described on p. 280 for microsampling. Some of the considerations are the same, but some are quite different. In microsam-

pling, selection is made in a very specific way to cut across all medical conditions, medications, locale of care delivery, time of day, practitioners, and so forth. It is specifically designed not to be biased by medical considerations. In record selection described here for measurement of performance with regard to an audit standard it is still important to involve all practitioners, all shifts of the work schedule, weekends and weekdays, and so forth, but now only records based on certain medical considerations are wanted. This may be all patients getting intravenous solutions, being treated for hypertension, complaining of headache, or having abnormal Pap smears, and so forth.

One bias that should be applied to both record selection procedures is to favor the times when care is apt to be bad. It does no good to be satisfied with fine care at 2:00 P.M. if the 2:00 A.M. care is poor. In ambulatory care if the audit standard calls for a blood pressure determination every 2 years for any patient seen for any reason within the time frame, the 30 records should have a heavy concentration of walk-in patients at closing time rather than 10:30 A.M. office visits when everything is much more apt to be running smoothly. The compliance rate in no way should ever be used as an assessment of care at an institution. To do so would require much more rigorous sampling of a different sort and would not give information useful for an improvement process. For example, if the true incidence (based on proper sampling) was that 98% of patients seen had a blood pressure determination every 2 years, this could lull one into a sense of security that no improvement is needed. The actual fact may be that the 2% may represent essentially all last walk-ins of the day, and this may consist primarily of school teachers or carpenters whose work schedules result in almost all their care being delivered as last minute walk-ins.

If the instructions for record selection are not precise, unknown bias will inevitably be introduced and often totally spoil the study. Intentional bias looking for the worst case is desirable in an improvement process. Unknown bias may hide poor care. The word ''random'' should never be used, because it is not apt to be ''random'' (it is usually interpreted as ''any''), and in analysis of data it will be impossible to determine what charts were selected. The degree of specificity necessary is shown by the following examples:

1. Select every third medical record number from walk-in log for afternoon and evening shifts of the Monday and Thursday before measurement of performance.

2. Select seventh and twelfth charts in rack from each hospital nursing station at 4:00 P.M. on day of measurement of performance.

3. From operating room log, select medical record numbers of last 15 patients receiving halothane anesthesia.

4. Select diet trays at the bedside in every fifth room (room number ending in two and seven) in the hospital at lunch time on the day of audit.

The *third column* contains *specific screening and testing procedure within a case*. In regard to testing procedure these items are fairly important. The items in regard to ''screening'' data are not absolutely necessary and have to do with less important aspects of economy of operating the system.

The procedure for examining the cases (usually medical records) once in hand after selection by the procedure in the second column is described. This should include which specific pages or documents within the record are to be examined as well as what to look for in these documents. This saves considerable time for both the data retriever and peer justification later. It also gives much better data. For example, if an audit standard calls for checking ''tetanus toxoid within the last 10 years,'' a great deal of time will be lost if medical records

personnel have to hunt all over the charts for this information. On the other hand, if the instruction is given to search just billing records and injection record, many variations will later be found to be justified by peer review, because many such injections will have been entered only on the emergency room progress sheet and either paid in cash or not paid at all.

If applicable, the entry in the third column should be divided into two parts. Most standards imply a set of circumstances, or ''givens.'' For example, if ''A'' is present, then ''B'' should have occurred. More specifically, ''if the patient was seen because of a headache, then the blood pressure should have been recorded.'' The ''if'' part (the presence of a headache) is the ''screen.'' The ''then'' part (the recording of the blood pressure) is the ''test.'' The ''screen,'' therefore, is the procedure for further selecting only those cases to be ''tested'' against the standard. Three more examples follow.

1. Examine progress sheet for date selected (second column). Screen—if visit is for headache: Test—is blood pressure recorded?

2. Examine physician order sheet for date selected (second column). Screen—if oxygen ordered: Test—does order contain instructions for specific volume per unit of time?

3. Examine anesthesia reports in records for each anesthesia. Screen—if patient had halothane more than once: Test—was second anesthesiologist consultation obtained?

The fourth *column* contains the *maximum number* of cases. This is necessary only to avoid waste and is not essential. The number of cases estimated as desirable to *test* against the standard is entered. The number is viewed as a *maximum*, because it is not always known how often an event occurs (for example, all ''stats'' on Saturdays between 4:00 and 6:00 P.M.) and the instructions in the second column may yield considerably more than necessary. Also, at times the compliance rate is so poor that it is not necessary to complete the anticipated number. This may be due to true noncompliance reflecting undesirable performance. In this case the existence of the problem has been demonstrated, and further testing is unnecessary. However, at times the apparently poor compliance is due to an error in writing the standard or an error in the measurement instruction. Again, continued testing to the preset maximum number is wasteful. (For example, if 50 is the "maximum number" to be tested but of the first 15 tested ten do not meet the standard, it is not necessary to go on without having the standard or its measurement process reexamined.)

The fifth *column* contains the *date referred for measurement,* which is self-evident. It is the date that all the measurement instructions have been completed and approved, and the standard is ready for measurement of performance.

Specific instructions and descriptions for each item in CQAS work sheet II concerning clerical measurement results and clinical administrative review of variations (Figure 27-8, *B*) follow.

The sixth through the twelfth columns involve the *clerical measurement results*. The *sixth column* contains the *number of cases screened* and is not essential but is helpful in determining how laborious the measurement is. It includes the number of cases (records, individuals, and so forth) that had to be examined after the initial case selection process for "qualifying data." For example, 125 records may have had to be searched to find 50 in which an intravenous order could be tested to see if a specific rate of administration was given, or 42 fractures had to be screened to identify 40 with casts that could be tested.

The *seventh column* contains the *number tested.* It is important and is needed in all cases. It includes the number of cases (records, individuals,

and so forth) that were actually tested for the standard. In the first example just mentioned this would be 50; in the second it would be 40. The number tested is the denominator in determining percent variation from a standard.

The eighth and ninth columns involve variation. The *eighth column* is the *number of variations* and is self-explanatory. It refers to the number of cases (records, individuals, and so forth) that did not meet the standard (that is, did not pass the "testing"). The *ninth column* is the *percent of cases tested* and is not important at all. It is the number of variations divided by the number tested. This gives the percent of cases not meeting the standard according to the *clerical measurement*. The important percentage is in the fourteenth column.

The *tenth column* includes the *patterns noted and other comments*. It is not essential but helpful. These are observations made by the data gatherer that were not necessarily requested but that may help to elucidate the problem. This person may have noted that the variation occurs only in certain departments, certain shifts, or on certain days. This does not mean that the data gatherer should routinely keep track of these variables on paper; this results in unnecessary and wasteful activity. At times the patterns noted may be totally unanticipated and not related to usual factors, such as shift, days, or weekends. The column is intended for "patterns" that the person happens to notice and that may be helpful. The data gatherer may also have other comments relating to other aspects of the standard, such as confusing aspects of the standard itself, better data sources, observations about the data found, or reasons that measurements could not be made. One example is finding that intravenous solutions are given without any order at all, let alone without the rate of administration (as in the example previously discussed).

The *eleventh column* contains the *identification of variation* and is important in all cases. This is the medical record or patient number or other identification of specific cases not meeting the standard. It might be dates and medical record numbers for x-ray reports, or names, dates, and places of patients not wearing identification bracelets, or personnel not wearing radiation film badges, and so forth. These data are necessary so that each variation may be further investigated for clinical or administrative justification.

The *twelfth column* contains the *date the measurement was reported* and is self-evident. It is the date the measurement results of an audit are reported back to the quality committee.

The thirteenth, fourteenth, and fifteenth columns contain *clinical administrative review of variations*. The *thirteenth column* refers to whether the decision was *justified (yes/no)*. It is very important in all quality activities. It is a yes/no decision concerning whether the variation was clinically or administratively justified as determined by peers or those administratively responsible. A "no" response indicates that the variation is not justified; the finding is a real deviation from desired performance or represents a complication that could be prevented. A "yes" response indicates that the variation was justified and under the particular circumstances of that case was desirable; this case is then dropped from further consideration.

The *fourteenth column* is the *percentage of those tested not justified*. It is very important in all quality assurance activities and is the "bottom line." The percent of true deficiencies or noncompliance is entered as determined after peer analysis. This equals the total of the "no" responses from the thirteenth column divided by the number tested in the seventh column for the current audit cycle. Because it represents a summary of results, there is only one entry in this column for each audit cycle. *This is the most important column on all of the work sheets, because it will reveal the actual status of compliance with regard to any*

standard. Watching the changes in this column for each audit cycle may reveal whether progress is being made in improving compliance over time.

The *fifteenth column* is the *clinical/administrative review findings and date reviewed*. It is important in all quality assurance activities. Brief comments concerning why each variation was clinically justified are entered for each "yes" in the thirteenth column. These reasons for justification specify the extenuating circumstances (such as preexisting medical conditions) that preclude the standard from being met. The entries should be sufficiently clear so that other members of the audit committee will understand without reviewing the records. This information often contributes to modification of the wording of the standard or the measurement instructions so that similar cases will not fall out as variations in subsequent audits, thus saving additional practitioner time.

Entries of "no" in the thirteenth column do not need to have an entry in the fifteenth column for each record or case. A composite entry should be made during this peer review step if reasons why the standard was not met are apparent. This will assist in directing corrective action properly.

Specific instructions and descriptions for each item in CQAS work sheet III of recommendations and actions (Figure 27-8, *C*) follow.

The *sixteenth column* is the *analysis conclusion*. It includes the *type of need identified and/or source(s) of problems (and identification of department, individual, and so on)*. The conclusion resulting from the types of problems found in nonjustified cases is entered here. A succinct comment summarizing the type of problem(s) found and what apparent needs were identified is made here. In addition, any localization of the problem in an individual, a set of individuals, a department, and so forth, is made to allow for more targeted problem solving to be instituted. The conclusion may indicate a knowledge deficit, a systems problem, the absence of a particular piece of equipment, and so forth.

The seventeenth through the nineteenth columns contain the *action recommended*. The *seventeenth column* is the *action and/or next audit*. Actions recommended as a result of the analysis conclusion are entered here. When the need is very clear, and the responsible individuals are already on the audit committee (or have been consulted in connection with the analysis conclusion), the recommendation may be very specific. Examples might be "get a baby scale for the emergency room" or "education program for nurses on blood pressure measurement skills." At other times the action recommended may be less specific, and details will have to be developed and implemented by those responsible. An example here might be "need more cardiac monitors for observation area at night (through purchase, redistribution of those on hand, and so on)" or "plan (education or systems development) to make physicians more conscious of medications patients are taking from other practitioners either by education or system change, such as having nurse get medication history." At times the recommendation is even less specific and requires an individual or a task force to study further the conclusions and findings. For example, an action recommended might be to determine if the incidence of a complication could feasibly be reduced by any means.

Each entry in this column sets up a "tickler file" concerning the status of recommendations regarding this standard. Dates on which the recommendations should be implemented or a progress report expected should be listed here as part of the recommendation. Details of discussions or findings resulting in these recommendations may be found in appropriate department or committee minutes, and appropriate references to these sources should be listed in this column to avoid repetition.

In all cases, a recommendation concerning the approximate date of the next audit for this standard should be entered.

The *eighteenth column* heading is *to*, which records entries that indicate to whom the recommendation is made and who is to be held responsible for carrying out the recommendation. Examples include administrator, chief of education, nursing director, chief of pediatrics, and laboratory supervisor.

The *nineteenth column* is the *date* the recommendation was sent to the responsible agent, as specified in the eighteenth column.

The twentieth and twenty-first columns involve *action taken*. The *twentieth column* includes *action—what, time, and place*. This column documents the completion of an audit cycle. Entries should be made here *only after* the recommended action has actually been taken. A specified statement of what actually happened and where it took place should be listed. Appropriate references to educational programs, memos, departmental minutes, and so forth should be included. *If no action is taken, the entire process is apt to be just talk, and the likelihood of improvement is decreased.* The *twenty-first column* is the *date* the action was taken.

EVALUATION

Evaluation is addressed briefly from two points of view, internal by the organization or individuals involved and external by extramural agencies, such as accreditation bodies or the PSROs.

Internal evaluation of a quality assurance system by management for purposes of determining whether the system should continue will be done, as are almost all other operational components of a health care delivery system, that is, without predetermined objective criteria. Internal evaluation will be made on a judgmental basis depending on such factors as effect on morale of staff, demonstrated improvements and their apparent value, costs, and how much it helps or hinders direct care delivery operations. It would be folly to set up an internal evaluation system as is done in most research activities, because management decisions will not and should not follow the carefully laid out but theoretic plans. However, one criterion of a quality assurance system that is essential in almost every situation is that the system must meet external evaluation requirements. Neither staff nor management will support a system that lacks necessary approvals. They will not bother with two systems, and since external approval is usually necessary for the economic viability of the institution, whatever is necessary for external approval will be done, no matter how little is the effect on quality of care by the approved system.

Evaluation by external agencies thus assumes very great significance. If absence of external approvals does not threaten economic viability, it frequently disrupts activities that the institution values, such as teaching programs, the value of prestige in recruitment of professional personnel, or the ability to conduct one's own professional review without the onerous presence of the ubiquitous "outsider."

Another factor that gives external approval great significance is that institutions have limited economic and motivational resources for performing quality assurance activities and for the most part cannot sustain two systems. The externally required system survives, and because there is no ownership, it is performed in a pro forma manner without accrual of any benefit. In essence, it stops any effective quality assurance activity, and this perhaps is the greatest loss to provision of good care.

It is extremely important, therefore, for internal quality assurance activities themselves to be per-

formed in a high-quality fashion and to have the required features so that external approval is achieved.

External agencies have a major responsibility to conduct reasonable evaluation programs lest all be lost. Unrealistic requirements could well result in cessation of any meaningful quality assurance activities, notwithstanding the mountain of obfuscating documents that will accumulate and that will be offered to satisfy those who are demanding accountability. It is unfortunate that Congress has placed impossible evaluation demands on the PSRO system. The impact of these in turn filter down to the small health care delivery units. For example, it will not be possible to isolate and demonstrate the effect of PSRO on the health status of the population. This is an extremely complex variable recently influenced enormously by events varying from the unfortunate occurrence of a breast malignancy in the wife of a President (which made more women pay attention to their health in this regard than most other health education programs) to a governmental activity having to do with influenza vaccine that has had major impact on health costs and medical conditions far removed from influenza. It will not be possible to determine the effect of PSRO on health status of the population.

Similarly, with its effect on cost containment as well as quality, it will be impossible to determine the cost effectiveness of PSRO. Who is to put a dollar value on improved quality for each of the infinite elements of care or for even one of them?

As can be seen from the characteristics of a quality assurance program for either voluntary or governmental agencies on pp. 277–279, quality assurance activities are perceived as mechanisms for change or improvement. Many of the essential characteristics need not exist if audit is primarily to demonstrate good care. As has been discussed, it is not feasible to demonstrate "good care" in either a comprehensive or valid manner because of the infinite number of aspects of care. Furthermore, if mere demonstration of good care were feasible, it would hardly make the PSRO program cost effective to maintain the status quo. The latter can be done without any activity. Since improvement is the objective of quality assurance activities, it seems quite appropriate to use achievement of improvement as the criterion for evaluation.

Current requirements of voluntary and governmental agencies require that a certain number of audits be done dependent on degree of medical care activity. The element of improvement is not a component of the assessment of the adequacy of the audit activity. By far the most common current medical audit activity consists of measuring a variety of factors relative to a diagnostic category during which good care is documented and change is not indicated. These audits clearly do not meet the objective of the basic process. Certainly any audit activity will occasionally pursue a suspicious area of activity and find that the suspicion is not substantiated. However, this should occur infrequently and should not count toward meeting requirements.

It is suggested that the major consideration that management or external agencies (voluntary or governmental) should use in evaluation is evidence of improved performance in regard to elements of care being performed suboptimally. To merely require that a certain number of audits be done without respect to improvement seems wasteful. Obviously other factors such as costs must be considered in evaluation, but the essential factor is improvement.

A few examples of improvement as a result of the CQAS are shown in the following list.

1. Infectious disease (genitourinary, pneumonia, syphilis, ear)*
2. Hypertension detection*
3. Use of patient identification bracelets
4. Vital sign measurement
5. Use of infant seat belts*
6. Radiation protection in pregnancy*
7. Preoperative management*
8. Breast examination frequency*
9. Pelvic examinations with Pap smears and follow-up*
10. Glaucoma screening*
11. Intravenous fluid management
12. Dietary services
13. Neonatal management
14. Appointment handling and record keeping*
15. Speed of consultation, antibiotic medication administration and laboratory work
16. Management in extended-care facilities
17. Inhalation therapy
18. Use of oral contraceptives*
19. Surgical operative procedures
20. Rh problems
21. Patient counseling and management of neoplasm

These were selected primarily to show the wide range of activities addressed. They include ambulatory as well as hospital activities and practitioner as well as patient responsibilities.

SUMMARY

An existing quality assurance program that has been functioning in the ambulatory as well as the hospital area for almost a decade has been described. It requires only some interested practitioners and is not (and should not be) dependent on style of practice (prepaid or fee-for-service practice), form of record keeping (3 × 5 inch cards to

*Ambulatory.

typed problem-oriented records), or any other accouterment of modern practice, such as abstracts or coding schemes. The described program was funded entirely internally as part of normal operations and as a result costs only 25¢ per health plan member per year. It is further characterized as having an extremely short lead time, and improvements in care could be demonstrable in less than a month after a decision is made to start the program. (See the previous list for examples of improvement in various elements of health care.)

REFERENCES

1. Ellwood P., Jr., et al. 1973. *Assuring the quality of health care,* p. 41.

2. Rubin, L. 1975. *Comprehensive quality assurance system: the Kaiser-Permanente approach.* Alexandria, Va.: American Group Practice Association.

3. Sanazaro, P.J. 1976. *Medical audit, continuing medical education and quality assurance,* West. J. Med.

4. Nelson, A.R. 1976. *Orphan data and the unclosed loop: a dilemma in PSRO and medical audit.* N. Engl. J. Med. 295:617–619.

28

Ancillary Services Review

Len Rubin

Exactly when and for what purpose ancillary services were designated as a separate part of medical care delivery is not clear. Although the BQA in a recent draft transmittal[1] tied the definition to services that appear on a hospital bill as separate line items, others have used the term to designate services provided by other than physician health care practitioners. It is clear that there is no common definition. There is good reason to question whether or not review of ancillary services, whatever they are, can or should be separated from other parts of health care delivery review. The recent BQA draft transmittal just mentioned makes reference to this fundamental consideration by noting that the PSRO's responsibility for ancillary services review is not in addition to its responsibility for hospital review but is part of it. Ancillary services are such an integral part of health care delivery that separate consideration may well result in fragmentation with no constructive component.

This discussion addresses issues concerning review of what is generally considered related to "ancillary services," including whether multiple review systems are advantageous or whether a single comprehensive review has greater virtues.

DEFINITION, SCOPE, AND PURPOSE OF ANCILLARY SERVICES REVIEW

It is easy to agree with the BQA that there is no common definition of ancillary service. It is just as easy to take exception to the proposed definition that "refers to those hospital services for which separate payment is requested. Such services appear on a hospital bill as separate line items." The draft transmittal goes on to state that "they are those services exclusive of routine services such as room and board, dietary and nursing services and routine services and routine supplies."

Limiting ancillary services to hospital care would exclude consideration of such services in the ambulatory setting or in extended-care facilities. Experience indicates that there is considerable overutilization and underutilization of ancillary services in these settings.

Associating ancillary services with those for which separate charges are made creates immediate problems for certain kinds of institutions, such as HMO organizations or federal hospitals in which such distinction is not made. It is obvious that the BQA was not intending to eliminate ancillary services review from these institutions. It is equally obvious that it was not intended that these institutions should start an elaborate pseudobilling system to keep track of these services for purposes of review.

Tying these services to hospital billing systems and payment schemes has other disadvantages. It tends to set planning of ancillary services review systems off on the wrong path by confining it to billing systems that, as previously stated, will not work in many organizations (such as HMOs) or settings (such as ambulatory). Also, what is included as "routine services" changes regularly and may not even be the same from hospital to hospital. Excluding "routine services" eliminates areas in which significant excesses have been observed, such as the wanton use of expensive medically unsupportable special diets, the "ubiquitous intravenous infusion,"[2] or nurse-administered but ill-advised respiratory therapy. Some areas of separate payment are constantly under debate and undergoing change, such as services by house staff and physician surrogates. Some institutions have specialized services separately billed that are performed by regular staff in other institutions. It would not be desirable to have activities included in or excluded from the ancillary review process because of the allowable payment practice at the moment.

These considerations give one pause in attempting to define ancillary services. In fact, it makes one wonder about whether they should be considered separately at all from other activities in the review process. It is clear that the charge given to the PSRO is not to consider this area apart from other review. Why separate it functionally? Is any useful purpose served?

The intent of adding ancillary services review as a specific component of the review process seems to have been to address overutilization of activities associated with health care delivery in addition to the already targeted unnecessary hospital admission and excessive length of stay. The urging of the National PSR Council, quite appropriately, to address underutilization as well gives further argument against fragmentation. It is hard to imagine what underutilization could address that is not an outright quality issue (as opposed to cost containment) and therefore already addressed by current PSRO activities, such as MCEs. The boundaries of ancillary service review and general quality assurance seem to cease to exist as attempts are made to identify them.

As stated in Chapter 27, the intent of review ought to be to address anything wrong in health care delivery, regardless of what the error was or who was responsible. Apart from the differences in corrective action, it does not seem that it should make much difference whether one is addressing a problem in overutilization or underutilization or whether the wrong medication was ordered by a physician or given by a nurse. Classification of these problems in an *a priori* fashion serves no purpose. Obviously, after analysis of the problem, a target for correction must be set, but this is apt to cross any arbitrary division set up in advance, such as independent or dependent practitioner, nursing or physical therapy, general surgery or gynecology. The scope of review should not be truncated by arbitrary classification schemes serving no beneficial purpose. It should not matter whether the excess blood chemistry determinations are billed separately or are included in the capitation fee, or were generated by an ill-advised physician order or by the failure of the laboratory technologist to stop the determination after 2 days as appropriately ordered by the physician.

The scope of ancillary service review is also widened by extension into quality considerations. Underutilization is almost always a matter of poor quality rather than economic waste. Overutilization also may represent poor quality as well as waste. Inundating the laboratory with unnecessary tests is apt to have a negative effect on the quality of work done in the laboratory. In addition, it diverts resources (personnel, equipment) from areas in which a need is greater. Many observations have been made of nursing time misspent on measuring unnecessary fluid intake and urinary output to the detriment of other important nursing needs of patients. These second-order effects on quality are in addition to first-order effects, which also result in lower quality. Examples of these first-order effects include the pain, suffering, and hazard caused by an unnecessary lumbar puncture, the radiation of an unnecessary gastrointestinal series, and the infection caused by the third unnecessary venipuncture.

In summary, it seems that isolating ancillary services for review purposes is highly artificial and serves no desired function. Although ancillary services review is inextricably interwoven into quality assurance activities, discussion is warranted since a number of issues normally associated with ancillary service review ought to be reexamined. In spite of the absence of a definition of ancillary services for purposes of the subsequent discussion, one can assume that it is defined as any service offered to a patient beyond a history or physical examination whether he is admitted to a hospital or is seen in a medical office. As is mentioned in the draft transmittal, current quality assurance activities should include ancillary services review and new systems need not be devised.

TECHNOLOGIC ASPECTS AND PITFALLS

A comprehensive review of technologic aspects of ancillary services review is not attempted in this section, but a few comments are made because of the many pitfalls that exist in current approaches. In addition, some techniques have the promise of fulfilling the intent of such review while avoiding many of these problems.

Because of a variety of characteristics of ancillary services, most review programs tend to depend on profile analysis. This is a consequence of the fact that many ancillary services are charged separately, and therefore, in some systems billing provides such a profile. Also, in many institutions "utilization statistics" have to do with ancillary services in large part, and therefore another profile is provided. The customary and historic approach by diagnostic categories used in most quality assurance systems was not used in ancillary services

review because these services didn't lend themselves to such categorization.

Just as the diagnostic approach in quality assurance is fraught with problems that are becoming more evident as time passes, the profile analysis approach also has problems serious enough that its usefulness may be more apparent than real. Quality assurance activities as yet have not accumulated sufficient uniform data to allow the mandated profile analyses. This early examination could be very helpful in avoiding blindly venturing further into the morass of profile analysis.

A discussion that seems to advocate less reliance on profile analysis should not lead to the inference that individual case by case analysis is the only alternative. Measurement of group performance in regard to specific items of care is still the primary tool advocated, but profile analysis usually refers to other examinations. Utilization review by profile analysis customarily relates to examining data that have been collected for other purposes. Prospective data collection for utilization review purposes is less frequent.

The high cost, relative lack of interest, and problems associated with effective use of the data contribute to the paucity of prospective profile data collection. Profile analysis has many inherent problems regardless of whether data are collected prospectively for review or have been collected for other primary purposes. Since these analyses are being advocated as the mainstay of ancillary service review, it is appropriate to examine some of the pitfalls.

Profile analysis by definition seeks out the performance that deviates from the pattern. The intent is to discover the lower end of the "goodness" curve, as described in Chapter 27. Although this may reveal poor practice, it is usually a matter of missing the forest for the trees. Improvement in the tail end alone will hardly improve medical care delivery materially. A recent example is demonstrated by the finding by profile review of about 100 practitioners who seemed to have earnings in excess of expectations. Even if all these were to prove to be truly undesirable and inexcusable practice patterns and somehow were completely stopped, the total savings to the community would be insignificant compared with a single common-place excess performed by most practitioners and therefore invisible by profile analysis.

What is more important than the argument just given concerning the relatively small impact of correcting the deviant from the norm is the fact that deviations from the desirable (when performed by the majority) go unnoticed when there is dependency on profile analysis. There are many examples of such excesses. Because these are perpetrated by the vast majority of practitioners, they constitute a very considerable amount of waste, much more than that caused by the 5% of practitioners exceeding two standard deviations. Examples include routine tests of a wide variety, such as unnecessarily repeated preoperative tests immediately before and also at the time of admission, repeat serologies on every admission (including the fourth admission in 6 months for congestive heart failure), the routine ordering of both calcium and phosphorus in parathyroid screening (when the calcium is adequate), the routine intravenous solution for patients without any threat of fluid imbalance or need for emergency medication, and routine printed standing orders. In one institution this attempt at attention to good care led to the routine ordering and performing of two sedimentation rates, two white blood cell differentials, and a variety of enzyme determinations within the first 36 hours for every patient with myocardial infarction, regardless of the patient's condition, diagnostic certainty, or any other consideration.

The counterargument is likely to be offered that when most physicians in an institution overutilize,

cross institutional profile analysis would discover such transgressions from desired performance. Although this is true on occasion, corrective action is not likely to follow such disclosure. Routine orders as in the examples just given are often copied by departments at other institutions as examples of "assuring good care," and therefore interinstitutional differences cease to exist. When the differences are not obliterated, improvement frequently still does not follow, and practice patterns do not change because the staff at each institution staunchly defends its mode of practice as either being less wasteful or of higher quality. These variations in very similarly sized institutions with relatively similar patient populations reach proportions exceeding multifold differences. Many such examples can be given, from the use of relatively esoteric chemistry determinations (but performed by the thousands) to nuclear medicine diagnostic procedures. An example of the surprisingly slow change that occurs when profiles indicate significant differences between institutions is demonstrated on a national scale in regard to the marked differences between the East and West in length of stay for common diseases.

Changes have been achieved in institutional performance but usually not as a result of the use of profile analysis either for discovery or as evidence of undesirable performance. Analysis of utilization data has been used to demonstrate the magnitude of a problem discovered through and acknowledged to be undesirable by other means. Such utilization statistics have also been used to measure changes after institution of actions for improvement.

One of the very first problems of concern in regard to ancillary services review utilizing statistics accumulated for other purposes is the validity of the data themselves. Specific data collection rules pertinent to the ultimate use of the data are usually not established. If established, they are often not followed because they are part of large ongoing data collection procedures for many different purposes. As a result, the data contain serious inconsistencies. This problem is apparent when such profiles are analyzed for the purposes of quality considerations and general utilization review, such as length of stay. A few examples can explain this concern. Diagnostic categories are severely affected because of significant vagaries and deficiencies in and in the use of existing classification systems. For example, in spite of much discussion concerning the definition of the primary diagnosis at the time of discharge, there is no uniformity as revealed by record review and inquiry of medical record personnel in a wide variety of settings. Although many institutions specify that the primary diagnosis is the major reason for admission to the hospital, record review indicates that the diagnosis listed as primary may be the major complication that occurred. The condition responsible for the major portion of the stay or at times the condition listed as primary seems to have no distinguishing characteristics from other conditions treated during that same stay, and a random assignment seems to have been made. Some conditions requiring hospitalization are not codable, and for the purpose of "closing out the record" a diagnosis known to be incorrect is listed. This occurs, for example, when patients are appropriately admitted to the hospital because of justifiable suspicion that they are having gastrointestinal bleeding that is not substantiated during the 1-, 2-, or 3-day hospitalization. These patients are frequently discharged as "gastrointestinal bleeding" because there is no diagnostic category with a code for "suspicion of gastrointestinal bleeding not substantiated." The effect of such invalid data on interpretations concerning length of stay, number of procedures done, or kinds of procedures done is obviously substantial. For a significant fraction of patients with the diagnosis of gastrointestinal bleeding, data concerning length of stay and the use of ancillary services are decreased by those patients requiring absolutely no

therapy because, in fact, they do not have the condition.

Similar considerations regarding severity of disease cause further degradation of the data. For example, one hospital medical staff may have a policy of admitting patients with diabetes in earlier stages of the disease for the purpose of acquainting the patients with diet or insulin or to get some physiologic measurements performed. These hospitals will have relatively short lengths of stay and low ancillary services use for diabetes and very low mortality. Other hospitals in the same community, dealing with the same type of patient population, may have a medical staff that belongs to another school of thought and who admits patients with diabetes only when they are in ketoacidosis. This hospital will have a long length of stay and high ancillary service utilization for diabetes and may well have a high mortality. In no way are these data comparable. The short length of stay does not imply good utilization practice. The low utilization of ancillary services does not imply frugal operation. The long length of stay and the high mortality in the other hospital does not necessarily indicate bad practice. In short, the data signify nothing.

Other problems in validity of profile data have to do with failure to record known data or failure to recognize a clinical condition. It is not unusual to discover records in which such events as cardiac arrests have occurred for reasons either related to or not related to the reason for admission and in which these major events are not coded. Records have been observed with "code blue" emergencies because of grand mal seizures postoperatively, myocardial infarction occurring postoperatively, or myocardial infarctions occurring after insulin reactions. In all of these cases—and they are not isolated—neither the code blue, the myocardial infarction, nor the epilepsy were coded or listed in any statistical compilation, notwithstanding the presence of fairly sophisticated coding and data retrieval systems. The following is a real example of one patient who was hospitalized over a period of time by two different physicians for what is obviously a chronic lung condition.

FRONT SHEET SUMMARY

Hyptertension (190/110) Missing 1/17/72

First admission 11/68:   Acute bronchitis, asthma, MS, MD (500, 241)

Second admission 5/69:   Acute bronchial asthma, chronic bronchitis, RK, MD (493, 491)

Third admission 11/69:   Bronchial asthma, chronic obstructive lung disease, eczema, RK, MD (493.9, 492, 696.9)

Fourth admission 3/70:   Chronic obstructive lung disease, acute bronchitis with bronchospasm, chronic bronchitis and emphysema, RK, MD (492, 489, 519.5, 491)

Fifth admission 8/70:   Chronic lung disease, chronic bronchitis, bronchial asthma, emphysema, MS, MD (519.4, 491, 490, 492)

The multiplicity of diagnostic codes assigned indicates some of the difficulty that might be encountered in an attempt to select charts based on this system and the subsequent effects on a "profile." What is even worse, of course, is the fact that this patient had hypertension, but in none of the five admissions was this identified or coded and therefore never would appear in any profile.

The situation in which a condition is known and managed but not properly recorded and therefore escapes entry into the profile is obviously a major fault and a very frequent one. Examples are seen involving major conditions in essentially every record review of just a handful of records. What is even more serious, however, is the failure of information to enter the profile because the clinical condition was not even recognized. Thus surgeons whose profiles indicate they have never seen a depressed patient are probably missing the diagnosis frequently. Internists whose profiles indicate that they do not see rheumatoid arthritis or sexual dysfunction are probably missing these diagnoses. Similarly, physicians who have a high percentage of congestive heart failure but have no entries of hyperventilation in their practice profiles are probably missing the latter diagnosis. The implications for this problem in ancillary services review are enormous, because such diagnostic profiles would inappropriately justify high usage of electrocardiograms, electrolyte balance studies, and use of digitalis and diuretics, among other activities.

The use of such practice profiles to determine educational needs of physicians is likewise frequently pointed in the wrong direction. For example, hematologists who may appropriately have many entries for hematologic diseases of one sort or another but no diagnoses of psychophysiologic gastrointestinal reaction or congestive heart failure probably do not need more education in regard to pernicious anemia and leukemia but do need education in those conditions that must exist in their patient population but that they are not identifying.

Although the validity of the data in many profiles is open to question, as shown by the previous discussion, the profiles nonetheless do exist and are used for a wide variety of review purposes. Apart from the validity of the data, serious problems in the use of such profiles exist, and a discussion of these follows.

One of the problems with the use of profile analysis is that the norm (in the PSRO sense of the word) tends to become the criterion, and the status quo is perpetuated. This is antithetic to an improvement process. It is especially evident as a system problem when the customary and usual practice involves significant overutilization by essentially all physicians for no other reason than "we've always done it that way." Even when physicians recognize the waste and futility of a procedure that is commonly performed and prefer to discontinue the practice, they are fearful of wandering from the practice profile of their peers for medicolegal as well as peer pressure reasons. This is one of the ways that concentration on profile analysis and searching for the deviation tends to perpetuate the waste that has grown into the system. Examples include ordering both blood urea nitrogen and creatinine for routine screening purposes when either would do, ordering calcium and phosphorous as a hyperparathyroidism screen when the calcium is sufficient, pursuing excessive bacteriologic studies in simple nonrecurring acute lower urinary tract infections in adult women, or performing the innumerable radiologic procedures for what has become known as "defensive medicine." The list of such excesses is lengthy and includes many situations that cross diagnostic and other classification lines. Because some of these patterns of practice are communitywide as a result of peer pressure or medicolegal fears, pattern analysis is not apt to identify problems as cost effectively as one would like to believe. Overutilization can be detected more easily by thoughtful review of extremely small samples of medical records as part of the total quality assurance activity. In this way problems of misuse of ancillary services will be discovered even though the overuse is caused by essentially all of the physicians in the community. In addition, items not normally entered into the usual profiles collected or into claims-based data collection systems will be recognized. Examples of this include substantive overuse of parenteral fluids, the use of outmoded special diets, and the routine use of expensive medicinal preparations when less expensive preparations of the highest quality and identical clinical pharmaceutical activity are available.

On the other hand, search of small numbers of records may reveal that different undesirable practice patterns exist in various institutions or communities. It is for this reason that ancillary services review should be focused on known or suspected problems just as is recommended for other quality assurance activities. For example, it would be wasteful (and therefore counterproductive) for an institution or a community to perform ancillary services review in regard to excess ordering of all electrolytes in those situations in which a potassium is all that is needed just because the custom is prevalent in a neighboring area. Searching for such differences by profile analysis has been found to be akin to looking for a "needle in a haystack." It is unrewarding when compared with in-depth review of small numbers of medical records.

Claims and billing review obviously can contribute to detection and monitoring of overutilization, but it must be remembered that this will detect only aberrations from the norm, not from the desirable, and only for those aspects of care for which separate billing is made. The virtue of claims review is the fact that it is an ongoing system, has no start-up costs, and under any circumstances must be continued for other purposes. It must be realized, however, that it focuses on an extremely small segment of operations and is not problem oriented. It has none of its advantages in capitation systems.

Cost effectiveness will be increased by incorporating ancillary services review into a problem-related focused, element-by-element system of quality assurance. In addition, the fact that the review can then be done either retrospectively or concurrently, whichever is appropriate, has significant merit because of the potential for intervention to assure improvement. Moreover, overutilization by any member of the medical care delivery team can then be assessed without limiting the activities to those originating with physicians.

In addition to the pitfalls just discussed regarding some of the technologic aspects (such as heavy reliance on profile analysis), it is worth pointing out one other important aspect that must be considered in performing ancillary services review. A major problem for which there does not appear to be an obvious solution is the fact that curtailment of overutilization of ancillary services often has an unwelcome economic impact on some members of the medical care system. This is not true of pure quality considerations. The implications on motivation for this type of review are obvious. Conflict of interest is not apt to be a factor in pure quality considerations. Generally no one benefits from poor quality. One must be alert to the fact that there are definite disincentives for ancillary services review not present in other aspects of quality assurance.

POTENTIAL

Notwithstanding the negative aura that may have characterized much of the preceding, the potential for ancillary services review is enormous. The fear is not that ancillary services review cannot be done but rather that it may be done in a way that is self-defeating because the system itself may be expensive, cost ineffective, and act as a disincentive to quality assurance activities in general. The proper approach to ancillary services review as an integral part of quality assurance activities, focusing on problems, objectively measuring performance in regard to these problems, and taking effective improvement action has substantial potential in regard to aspects beyond medical care improvement. Performed effectively, such an approach may modify a current significant threat to the enjoyable practice of medicine and the desired quality of professional life.

Recent fears exhibited by several segments of society, such as consumer groups and government agencies, have resulted in responses to the high cost of medical care that may be inappropriate and ill advised. The high cost of medical care in itself is not necessarily undesirable, but inappropriately high cost due to waste or necessary activities is indefensible. Such reflex reactions to high cost may serve further to reduce the quality of care. The fact that some of the waste is understandable and a di-

rect response to other characteristics of current societal pressures, such as defensive medicine, does not prevent countermeasures that are equally unfortunate. Effective measures for proper resource allocation may do a great deal to decrease these ill-advised but understandable countermeasures by governmental agencies. The greatest potential for effective ancillary services review may be in decreasing these unfortunate reactions to high cost with their accompanying potential for decreasing quality of care.

Ancillary service review may also serve to focus attention on other areas not routinely addressed by quality assurance activities. An example is the need for physician education in regard to methods of decreasing costs. It has been found that physicians are frequently misinformed concerning significant cost differences in essentially identical medications. In the same manner, many physicians have the misconception that it is less expensive to order certain batteries of tests rather than the individual test desired. Clinical pathology is fairly dynamic. Combinations of tests might be less expensive under certain circumstances and at certain times, but this is not uniformly true. In addition, more often than not the costs generated in turn by such unnecessary testing are entirely avoidable.

Although what is considered high quality in regard to an element of care may vary from day to day as medical advances are made, waste is always undesirable. This fact alone indicates that the greatest potential for quality assurance activities may lie in the area of curtailment of overutilization that is so frequently manifest in the area of ancillary services.

SUMMARY

The potential for ancillary services review exerting a beneficial effect on health care delivery is considerable. One of the pitfalls to be avoided includes avoiding waste within the ancillary services review process itself by the collection, analysis, and storage of large amounts of invalid data. Review focused on known or suspected local problems as part of the quality assurance activities has promise of considerable cost effectiveness. Such systems have been worked out and are not experimental. The potential for review in this area to exert a beneficial effect on resource allocation with resultant diminution of the need for ill-advised governmental attempts at cost containment is great and may be the major benefit of quality assurance activities.

REFERENCES

1. U.S. Department of Health, Education, and Welfare. May 10, 1977. *Ancillary services review.* Draft transmittal. Bureau of Quality Assurance.

2. Viljoen, J.F. 1977. The ubiquitous (and extravagant) intravenous infusion. *JAMA.* 237:18.

29

PSRO and HSAs—Shall the Twain Meet?

Jonathan E. Fielding

Both Professional Standards Review Organizations (PSROs) and Health Systems Agencies (HSAs) are new to the health care block. The blueprints for the PSROs were finalized in 1972, but despite some preexisting Foundations for Medical Care, not all PSRO areas are inhabited. Of those that are occupied, the majority are still conditional; permanency is promised but not yet secured. Although PSROs are authorized to work in hospitals and nursing homes and are encouraged to initiate review in physicians' offices, to date most have had time only for those patients staying overnight in hospitals.

HSAs were invited onto the scene early in 1975, but many areas contained the prior generation of comprehensive health planning ''b'' agencies. Some of these agencies have changed so much in organizational structure and board membership that they hardly recognize themselves. Some have changed little but feel they have grown up so much since their CHP days that they prefer to be considered new in the neighborhood. The HSAs are supposed to make everyone in the neighborhood keep themselves well and when sick to be cared for efficiently and effectively. Although the HSAs are to make all health care resources fit into a grand plan, they have hardly had time to survey their responsibilities and have spent a large part of their time deciding what the federal government is de-

manding of them to achieve full designation and how to organize their complex tasks.

In this early stage of development for both types of organizations, it is unrealistic to expect that they have carefully worked out how they should relate to each other. The first question each type of organization with resources much more limited than its mandates must ask is, ''How much can the other help me accomplish my highest priority projects?'' Nonetheless, there is governmental pressure for the two agencies to develop comprehensive and detailed memoranda of understanding that spell out respective roles, responsibilities and mutual assistance. One reason for this pressure is the related objectives of PSROs and HSAs as agents of federal health policy. The *PSRO Fact Book,* published by the Health Care Financing Administration, lists the major PSRO program goals as:*

1. Assuring that health care services are of acceptable professional quality.
2. Assuring appropriate utilization of health care facilities at the most economical level consistent with professional standards.
3. Identifying quality and utilization prob-

*From U.S. Department of Health, Education, and Welfare. 1977. *PSRO fact book.* Health Care Financing Administration, p. 1.

lems in health care practices and working toward their improvement.

4. Attempting to obtain voluntary correction of inappropriate or unnecessary practitioner and facility practices and, where unable to do so, recommending sanctions against such practitioners and facilities.

Compare these with the priorities to be considered in the operation of federal, state, and area health planning and resources development programs:*

1. The provision of primary care services for medically underserved populations, especially those which are located in rural or economically depressed areas.

2. The development of multi-institutional systems for coordination or consolidation of institutional health services (including obstetric, pediatric, emergency medical, intensive and coronary care, and radiation therapy services).

3. The development of medical group practices (especially those whose services are appropriately coordinated or integrated with institutional health services), health maintenance organizations, and other organized systems for the provision of health care.

4. The training and increased utilization of physician assistants, especially nurse clinicians.

5. The development of multi-institutional arrangements for the sharing of support services necessary to all health service institutions.

6. The promotion of activities to achieve needed improvements in the quality of health services, including needs identified by the review activities of Professional Standards Review Organizations under part B of Title XI of the Social Security Act.

7. The development by health service institutions of the capacity to provide various levels of care (including intensive care, acute general care, and extended care) on a geographically integrated basis.

8. The promotion of activities for the prevention of disease, including studies of nutritional and environmental factors affecting health and the provision of preventive health care services.

9. The adoption of uniform cost accounting, simplified reimbursement and utilization reporting systems, and improved management procedures for health service institutions.

10. The development of effective methods of educating the general public concerning proper personal (including preventive) health care and methods for effective use of available health services.

PSROs and HSAs share the twin objectives of high-quality care and efficiency of health care delivery. Many critics have charged that the overlap of goals and objectives made it very wasteful to develop two wholly independent area-based networks of quasi-public entities. Although the sponsors and administrators of both programs have responded that the functions are complementary and not competing, they also acknowledge the need for close cooperation to avoid duplication of effort. An added reason to push cooperative efforts is the formidable expense of both programs. In the fiscal year 1977, $61 million was appropriated for PSRO activities, with an additional $41 million budgeted from the Social Security Trust Fund for reimbursement of hospitals for all reviews. For the same year, Congress appropriated $121.5 million for administration and implementation of PL 93-641. The high level of expenditures ensure continu-

*From National Health Planning and Resources Development Act. 1974. PL 93-641, Section 1502.

ing and careful scrutiny from the Congress and the General Accounting Office. The 1977 level of expenditure, however, is insufficient for PSROs and HSAs to perform all their mandated duties. This places added pressure on PSROs and HSAs to cooperate in a manner that permits their collective budgets to enhance each other's productivity. Such cooperation permits more acceptable replies to congressional and Office of Management and Budget questions on what an HSA or PSRO has accomplished with its appropriation. A stronger case can be made for any proposed PSRO appropriation level if data essential to HSA planning or review functions became a no-extra-cost byproduct of performing several mandated functions.

HSA AND PSRO AREAS

Section 1152 of the Social Security Act authorized the secretary of DHEW to designate PSRO areas throughout the country. The areas were to be large enough to ensure a broad, diverse, and objective representation of physicians, yet small enough to allow efficient and manageable operation. Specific criteria for designation were published as regulations in March 1974, and included the following:*

1. In general, a PSRO should not cross state lines.
2. In general, a PSRO should not divide a county.
3. Existing boundaries of local medical review organizations *and health planning areas* should be considered (emphasis added).
4. A PSRO area should generally include a minimum of approximately 300 licensed practicing physicians. Although the maximum can

be expected to vary with local circumstance, generally the designated area should not exceed 2,500 licensed practicing physicians.
5. A PSRO area should, to the extent possible, coincide with a medical service area and ensure broad, diverse representation of all medical specialties. The PSRO area should be drawn to include to the extent possible the existing medical service or medical trade areas.
6. The designation of a PSRO area should take into account the need to allow effective coordination with Medicare/Medicaid fiscal agents.

Designation under PL 93-641 was to be based on four principal criteria:*

1. The area should be a geographic region appropriate for the effective planning and development of health services.
2. The area should include at least one center for the provision of highly specialized health services.
3. The population of each area should be one-half to three million, although waivers can be granted for both smaller and larger population areas. In general, each standard metropolitan statistical area (SMSA) should be within the boundaries of a single health service area.
4. To the maximum extent feasible, the boundaries are to be coordinated with those of PSRO areas, existing state planning, and administrative areas.

Since both HSAs and PSROs are, to some degree, meant to perform functions for the federal government, financed by federal funds, and with

*From U.S. Department of Health, Education, and Welfare. April 5, 1976. PSRO Transmittal No. 33. Health Services Administration.

*From U.S. Department of Health, Education, and Welfare. April 5, 1976. PSRO Transmittal No. 33. Health Services Administration, p. 2.

overlapping purposes, would it not facilitate public purposes to have uniform coterminous boundaries? The easy answer is that congruence would facilitate efficient operation, maximize interactions between HSAs and PSROs, and facilitate monitoring by HEW and states. There are, however, defensible rationales for having different boundaries. A medical service area may in some cases be smaller than the size needed to provide for objective PSRO review, that is, the number of physicians in many specialties may not be large enough to assure that personal and professional friendships do not make impartial peer judgments difficult. Conversely, an SMSA may have too many physicians for efficient organization and fulfillment of required PSRO functions, such as New York City or Los Angeles. Yet in some of these cases, it is essential that the SMSA be in one HSA, because decisions regarding appropriateness of services and unnecessary duplication of specialized services can best be made in the context of an entire metropolitan area.

The rational arguments for different boundaries, however, have been generally less important in the area designation process than has the political process. When area designations were being considered under the PSRO statute, organized medicine in many parts of the country did not support PSROs. The criteria that PSROs should not cross state lines or divide counties were developed to help gain support of state and local medical societies. In some cases, political decisions were made to accept areas recommended by the medical hierarchy even if these areas were not the preferred designations based on the guidelines. Since PL 93-641 was not passed until December 1974, and neither its passage nor some of its provisions were assured until after PSRO area designations had been made, it was difficult to specify criteria assuring congruence with the areas required by that statute. Since the PSRO areas were first designated, the option existed to make the same areas

stand for planning purposes. Militating against complete consistency was the role of governors in the HSA designation process. There was reluctance to reverse the recommendations forwarded from governors to HEW, especially since the state chief executives were upset that PL 93-641 had bypassed them by allowing them only a minimal role in planning.

A third problem was the multiple possibilities for HSA area designation based on the criteria. In many cases, defining health service areas is difficult and amenable to several interpretations. A major reason for lack of congruence was the failure of the PSRO area designations to meet the criteria for HSA designation specified in the law, especially with respect to medical service areas. At times the PSRO area seemed less appropriate than that proposed for the HSA. Whereas PSROs had precursors in only a handful of cases, the Comprehensive Health Planning ''b'' agencies had blanketed the country and had conducted considerable planning activity within their defined areas. Therefore there was local pressure, especially in areas with strong ''b'' agencies, to maintain preexisting boundaries to provide continuity and build on past efforts. A final reason for lack of coterminous boundaries was the absence of a suitably placed HEW official to push hard to force congruence. The PSRO program was administered by the BQA and health planning by the Bureau of Health Resources Development in the Health Resource Administration. Although responsibility for both programs converged in the office of the assistant secretary of HEW for health, no strong and consistent HEW support existed for both agencies to minimize area boundary differences.

Given these impediments to designating the same areas under both statutes, the result is not surprising. One hundred and eight PSRO areas of the 194 PSRO areas designated are congruent with HSA areas when congruent is defined as identical with, totally subsuming an HSA, or totally sub-sumed within HSA boundaries.* The HSA area and PSRO area are identical in 37 cases, including 11 states where the statewide PSRO is identical with a statewide HSA. In 71 cases, the PSRO is totally contained within an HSA area, but the HSA area is large. Fifteen PSROs deal with multiple HSAs. In ten of those cases, a statewide PSRO encompasses multiple HSAs, but at least one of the HSAs is divided between the state and one or more other states. In five states, the statewide PSRO totally encompasses several HSA areas. As a result of designations, 108 PSROs will deal with only one HSA, 52 PSROs with two HSAs, and 30 PSROs with three or more HSAs. In four cases, PSROs do not deal with any HSAs, because HSAs have not been designated in those states.[1]

In April 1976, the BQA sent a transmittal to all PSROs in which it listed the designated health service areas and provided information on "how PSROs may . . . request redesignation of a PSRO area if they wish to initiate a change to bring the PSRO area into greater congruence with the health service area."[2]

The transmittal states further:**

While DHEW does not anticipate that these respective boundaries can in all cases be congruent, an attempt to maximize congruency, where legally feasible, at this early stage in the implementation of the PSRO and the HSA programs may significantly improve their opportunities for HSAs and PSROs to work together in the future to perform their respective functions more effectively.

The same transmittal, however, points out that

*Texas currently does not have any PSROs while court action is pending on designation issues.

**From U.S. Department of Health, Education, and Welfare. April 5, 1976. PSRO Transmittal No. 33. Health Services Administration, p. 1.

changes in areas to correspond to those of HSAs are not required. Since the transmittal was issued in April 1976, four or five applications for redesignation of PSRO areas were filed with the BQA. None of the applicants, however, sought redesignation for the purpose of maximizing congruency with HSAs, although that effect may be a result of redesignation activities.

HEALTH PLANNING AND RESOURCES DEVELOPMENT ACT (PL 93-641)

PL 93-641 is even longer and more detailed than those sections of PL 92-603 that established the PSROs. The official act fills 52 pages and reads as though the drafters wanted to leave as little as possible to the discretion of the executive branch of the federal government. In the initial section of the act, entitled *Findings and Purpose,* the Congress states: "The massive infusion of Federal funds into the existing health care system has contributed to inflationary increases in the cost of health care and failed to produce an adequate supply or distribution of health resources, and consequently has not made possible equal access for everyone to such resources."[3] Also noted are "inadequate incentives for the use of appropriate alternative levels of health care, and for the substitution of ambulatory and intermediate care for inpatient hospital care." Lack of knowledge of large segments of the public regarding proper personal health care is also cited as well as the importance of participation of providers in developing solutions to these problems. Table 29-1 compares the structures and functions established under the old Comprehensive Planning Law and PL 93-641.

Four cardinal functions are mandatory under the law. In every case, the requirements build on preexisting federal legislation but provide greater specificity.

TABLE 29-1.   Comparison of Health Planning Structures Under Section 314 of the Public Health Act
With PL 93-641*

	PL 93-641	SECTION 314
A. *Regional Planning Agency*		
1. Structure	a. A Health System Agency may be a nonprofit private or public body.	a. A 314 (b) agency may be a nonprofit private or public body.
	b. The governing body must be composed of a majority, but no more than 60%, of consumers.	b. The governing body must be composed of a majority of consumers.
	c. No Health Systems Agency can accept funds or contributions from individuals or organizations that have a direct interest in the development, expansion, or support of health resources.	c. A 314 (b) agency may accept provider contributions.
2. Functions	a. Establish, annually review, and amend as necessary a health systems plan (HSP) and an annual implementation plan (AIP).	a. Develop comprehensive regional, metropolitan area, or other local area health plans.
	b. Make grants and contracts from Area Health Services Development Fund to assist the agency in planning and developing projects and programs to achieve the health systems described in the HSP.	b. No such provisions.
	c. Review and approve or disapprove applications for assistance under the Public Health Service Act, the Community Mental Health Centers Act, the Alcohol Abuse and Alcoholism Act, and grants under Titles IV, VII, or VIII (NIH health manpower and nurse training) for the development of health resources in the concerned area.	c. No such provision in Section 314, but federal guidelines give "b" agencies the authority to review the use of federal funds.
	d. Review and make recommendations to the appropriate state agency respecting the need for proposed new institutional health services to be offered or developed in its area.	d. No such provision in Section 314.
	e. Review on a periodic basis all institutional health services offered in the area and make recommendations to the designated state agency respecting the appropriateness of such services.	e. No such provision.
	f. Annually recommend to the state agency projects for construction or modernization of health facilities.	
3. Designation	After consultation with the governor of each state, the secretary of HEW enters into agreements for designating health systems agencies.	The Surgeon General is authorized to make grants under Section 314(b) after receiving approval from the state agency that administers the state plan.

TABLE 29-1.   Comparison of Health Planning Structures Under Section 314 of the Public Health Act With PL 93-641* *(continued)*

	PL 93-641	SECTION 314
4. Funding	Planning grants will be awarded on the basis of the lesser of 50¢ per capita or $3750000 per year. Also, a grant may be increased by the lesser of 25¢ per capita or an amount equal to nonfederal funds contributed to the agency.	Federal grants are awarded on a matching basis for up to 75% of an agency's costs.
5. Boundaries of planning areas	The governor of each state designates health service areas to be approved by the secretary of HEW. The areas must meet minimum and maximum population requirements. Preference is given to existing 314(b) areas.	The state agency that administers the state plan determines regional planning areas in conformance with federal guidelines.

B. State Health Planning Agency

1. Designation of state agency	The governor of each state selects an agency of the state government to serve as the State Health Planning and Development Agency.	Each state submits plans for comprehensive health planning that designate a single state agency, the 314 (a) agency, to administer the state's health planning.
2. Functions	a. Prepare, review, and revise, at least annually, a preliminary state health plan made up of the HSPs of the Health Systems Agencies. Such preliminary plan shall be submitted to the Statewide Health Coordinating Council for approval or disapproval.	a. Prepare and annually review a state health plan.
	b. Assist the Statewide Health Coordinating Council in the reviews of the State Medical Facilities Plan (Hill-Burton) and in the performance of its functions generally.	b. No such provision.
	c. Serve as the agency of the state for the purpose of Section 1122 of the Social Security Act and administer the state's certificate-of-need program. States are required to have a certificate-of-need program by the end of the first regular session of the state legislature that begins after the bill's enactment.	c. Serve as the agency of the state for the purpose of Section 1122 of the Social Security Act.
	d. Review on a periodic basis all institutional health services offered in the state and make public its findings as to their appropriateness.	d. No such provision.
3. Funding	The secretary shall make grants to State Health Planning and Development Agencies to assist them in meeting the costs of their operation, but no grant may exceed 75% of operation costs.	Grants are made to the states on the basis of population and per capita income.

TABLE 29-1.   Comparison of Health Planning Structures Under Section 314 of the Public Health Act With PL 93-641* *(continued)*

	PL 93-641	SECTION 314
C. *State Council*		
1. Composition	a. The governor appoints members of a Statewide Health Coordinating Council.	a. The governor appoints members of a State Health Planning Council.
	b. At least 16 representatives appointed by the governor are from lists of at least five nominees submitted by each Health Systems Agency. At least 60% of the membership must be nominees of the Health Systems Agencies.	b. No such provision.
	c. Each Health Systems Agency is entitled to the same number of representatives (at least two).	c. No such provision.
	d. A majority of persons appointed by the governor must be consumers (definition of consumer has been changed).	d. A majority of persons appointed by the governor must be consumers.
	e. The council shall select a chairman from among its members.	e. No such provision.
	f. The council must meet at least once in each calendar quarter.	f. The council must meet at least twice a year.
2. Functions	a. Review annually and coordinate HSP and AIP of each Health Systems Agency.	a. No such provision.
	b. Prepare annually a state health plan made up of HSPs after review and consideration of preliminary health plan submitted by the state agency.	b. No such provision.
	c. Review budget of each Health Systems Agency.	c. Require review of work plan but not of the budget.
	d. Advise the state agency generally on the performance of its functions.	d. Advise the state agency.
	e. Review and approve or disapprove plans or applications for federal funds.	e. No such provision; however, some state laws confer this authority.

*Modified from Office of State Health Planning, 1977, Massachusetts Department of Public Health.

DEVELOPMENT OF PLAN

Based on the priorities for health planning policy, a Health Systems Plan (HSP) must be developed. This plan spells out goals for health systems development within each HSA. Directed at the sometimes conflicting objectives of improving the health of the residents, increasing accessibility, preventing unnecessary service duplication, and restraining increases in costs, the goal statement must:*

*From National Health a Planning and Resources Development Act. 1974. PL 93-741, Section 1513 (b) (2).

1. Describe a healthful environment and health systems in the area that, when developed, will assure that quality health services will be available and accessible in a manner that assures continuity of care at reasonable cost for all residents of the area.

2. Be responsive to the unique needs and resources of the area.

3. Take into account and be consistent with the national guidelines for health planning policy issued by HEW covering supply, distribution, and organization of health resources and services.

In the development of a plan, an HSA is to assemble and analyze data concerning: (1) the status (and its determinants) of the health of the residents of its health service area; (2) the status of the health-care delivery system in the area and the use of that system by residents of the area; (3) the effect of the area's health care delivery system on the health of the residents of the area; (4) the number, type, and location of the area's health resources, including health services, manpower, and facilities; (5) the patterns of utilization of the area's health resources; and (6) the environmental and occupational exposure factors affecting immediate and long-term health conditions.[4]

The approach is global, conceived in the hope that the plan can cover all facets of health care delivery in the health service area, and is based on the assumption of the presence of many types of information not now available. The guidelines on how the HSP is to be constructed, however, make clear that it is difficult for the HSP to cover all areas in its initial plan and suggest a focus on priority areas such as medical care.[5] Both the guidelines and the preamble to the guidelines, issued separately, emphasize the need for specificity of plan objectives and anticipated activities to meet these objectives.

HSPs, for example, are to include particular levels of expected achievements in health status in health systems by a specific time. Examples provided are "to reduce infant deaths per 1,000 live births to 12 by 1981" or "to stabilize the increase in per diem acute inpatient charges at 7% by 1980."[6] HSAs are to incorporate into these plans the broad actions they are to take to achieve their goals and objectives, what alternatives were considered and why these were rejected, the anticipated impact of the actions, the locus of responsibility for carrying out actions, and the services, types of facilities, and population groups or areas affected by them.[7] For example, to achieve a reduction in perinatal mortality, an HSP might list as priority activities the development of objective criteria for determining which hospitals should have maternity units, the development of a network for referral of pregnant women at high risk for delivery of a low birth weight or ill neonate to a hospital with a neonatal intensive care nursery, and increasing the percentage of economically disadvantaged women who receive first trimester care. The HSA might also convene a task force composed of HSAs, appropriate state agencies, interested professional organizations, and regional and nearby tertiary care institutions to develop a referral network. The HSA might list a cooperative venture with school systems in its area to increase sensitivity to the problem of adolescent pregnancy and to develop mechanisms to facilitate early referral to prenatal care.

The HSP is to identify manpower and financing resource requirements to take the recommended actions. In developing the plan, the HSA is expected to consult widely organizations in its area with an interest in health and health care and to hold public hearings on its draft plans. Annual review including a public hearing on proposed changes is required.

Each HSA is required to establish, review annually, and amend as necessary an annual implementation plan (AIP) that identifies the priority short-range objectives on which the community wishes to act during the next 12 months. Selection of priorities is to be based on feasibility, costs, impact on the area of concern and the special needs that have been identified in the area. The AIP is to assign responsibility for accomplishing each of the short-term goals and to point out benchmarks that the HSA and outside agencies can use as guides in determining how effective the agency has been in working toward its goals and objectives.

The act establishes three new organizations to carry out the required responsibilities: HSAs, SHPDAs, and SHCCs.

Health Systems Agencies (HSAs)

(1) An HSA is either an independent nonprofit private corporation that is neither a subsidiary of nor otherwise controlled by any other private or public corporation and that engages only in health planning and development function; or is (2) a public regional planning body if its planning area is identical to the health service area and has a governing board composed of a majority of elected officials of units of general local government or is authorized by state law to carry out health planning and review functions; or is (3) a single unit of general local government if the area of jurisdiction is identical to the health service area.

The governing body is to be composed of between ten and 30 members. Between 51% and 60% of the board members are to be consumers (and nonproviders according to a narrow definition) broadly representative of the social, economic, linguistic, and racial populations, geographic areas of the health service area and major purchasers of health care; a maximum of one third direct providers of service, and the balance indirect "providers" (such as representatives of Blue Cross or of a medical school). If one or more Veterans Administration hospitals is located in the health service area, the chief medical director of the Veter-

ans Administration shall designate an ex-officio member. The HSA may establish advisory subarea councils with the same membership composition as the parent body.

Unlike their predecessor health planning agencies, HSAs are forbidden to accept any funds or contributions from any person or entity who has a "financial, fiduciary or other direct interest in the development, expansion or support of health resources,"[8] unless it is recognized by the Internal Revenue Service as exempt from federal taxes under Section 501 of its code.

The secretary of HEW is empowered to enter into agreements with HSAs on a conditional basis in similar fashion to the conditional PSRO designations. During the not longer than 24-month period of conditional designation, the secretary is to assess the capability of HSAs to perform mandated functions on a permanent basis and also to allow the HSA to assume progressive increases in the functions an HSA is permitted to carry out on a conditional basis. Final designation requires the filing of acceptable HSPs and annual implementation plans (AIPs).

HSAs have three major types of responsibilities. First is the development of formal plans—the HSP, an AIP, and specific project implementation plans. The first two are described on pp. 337–340. Project implementation plans are not well defined but take the plans of the AIP and apply them to specific institutions or types of services. A second major responsibility area is specific review functions, certification of need, Section 1122, and appropriateness review, described on pp. 333–337. A related task is the review of proposals advanced by agencies within the health service area for federal funds under a number of Public Health Service Acts for development, expansion, or support for public health resources.

The third area of HSA responsibility is the provision of technical assistance and development dollars to help providers bring their facilities and services into conformance with the state and HSA plans. HSAs are required to establish Area Health Services Development Funds and to help providers develop proposals to tap this funding source. Although these funds cannot be used for new construction or modernization, they can be used to pay capital-related obligations to permit phasing out of a facility or service or to help organize a regional network of services to meet a listed need.

State Health Planning and Development Agencies (SHPDAs)

The secretary of DHEW is required to enter into agreements with the governor of each state for the designation of an agency selected by the governor as the SHPDA to administer the state program required under PL 93-641. Designation is conditional on a satisfactory plan submitted by the state. A conditional period shall not exceed 24 months. If such an agreement is not in effect by the end of October 1980:*

The Secretary may not make any allotment, grant, loan, or loan guarantee, or enter into any contract, under this Act, the Community Mental Health Centers Act, or the Comprehensive Alcohol Abuse and Alcoholism Prevention, Treatment, and Rehabilitation Act of 1970 for the development, expansion, or support of health resources in such State until such time as such an agreement is in effect.

A requirement for final designation is a state administrative program that includes not only an acceptable substantive plan for carrying out the act's requirements but also satisfactory evidence that the SHPDA has adequate authority under state law to fulfill its functions and state financial support in the form of a budget appropriation from

the state legislature. State authority for the operation of the Statewide Health Coordinating Council (SHCC) is also required.

The major functions of the SHPDA are to:*

1. Prepare a State Health Plan and revise it annually. This plan is to be based on the Health System Plans of all the HSAs in the state but revised "to achieve their appropriate coordination or to deal more effectively with statewide health need." The plan is to be submitted to the Statewide Health Coordinating Council for final approval.

2. Administer a Certificate of Need program (consistent with HEW regulations), which, after receiving HSA recommendations, reviews and either approves or disapproves all proposed new institutional health services to be offered in the state.

3. Serve as the designated agency under optional Section 1122 agreements with HEW. After receiving recommendations from the HSA, the state agency reviews proposed capital expenditures for consistency with state plans. If the state agency disapproves a proposed expenditure, it then recommends to HEW that related interest and depreciation costs be withheld from reimbursement under Medicare, Medicaid and Title V programs.

4. Conduct, at no greater than five year intervals, reviews of the appropriateness of all existing institutional health care services. Again, HSA recommendations are to be considered in these reviews and the findings made public.

5. Develop a State Medical Facility Plan based on a statewide inventory of existing medical facilities, and on a survey of health care

*From the National Health Planning and Resources Development Act. 1974. PL 93-741, Section 1521 (d).

*From U.S. Department of Health, Education, and Welfare. July 28, 1977. Draft guidelines for the development of the state medical facilities plan. Health Resources Administration.

needs throughout the state and the recommendations of the HSAs. The plan indicates the distribution of type and number of beds in medical facilities as well as outpatient and other services needed to provide adequate care to the people in the state. The plan must also indicate the need for modernization of existing facilities or their conversion to new uses. A more careful appraisal of how the State Medical Facility Plan will emerge provides insight into how the inherent conflicting objectives embodied in the legislation will enfold in the administration of the program.

State Medical Facilities Plan (SMFP)

Draft guidelines for the development of a state medical facilities plan (SMFP) appeared in the *Federal Register* in August 1977. In the preface, the need to use the development of the SMFP as a method of setting ceilings of capital resource allocations within the overall planning framework of PL 93-641 is articulated. The regulations express the preeminence of the cost issue and the hope that planning by states and HSAs will focus on this issue as well as on quality and accessibility. The proposed regulations also call for planning to curb the increasing costs of acute-care inpatient medical facilities care through encouraging less costly alternative modes of delivering needed services.[9] The statement of goals and objectives lists as national goals for inpatient medical facilities an average bed per 1,000 population ratio of less than 4.0, a minimum occupancy rate of 80%, and a national use rate not to exceed 1000 patient days per 1000 population per year.[10] The SMFP is to incorporate the planning targets and methodologies necessary to achieve these goals within a 5-year period. States are asked to enumerate specific policies that will build less expensive delivery systems, foster consolidations and mergers, increase shared clinical and support services, convert facilities to less intensive uses, and close facilities based on findings of appropriateness reviews.[11]

There is an implied schizophrenia in the way state agencies are to develop these plans. On the one hand, the plan is to be based on a survey of need. The state agencies are to review the HSA plans for service needs and "to the extent possible . . . maintain the integrity of the HSA plans with respect to number, type and location of their medical facilities project recommendations".[12] The state agencies are also to consider "the extent to which the lack of services, which would be provided by the recommended projects, is detrimental to the health and health status of the residents of the areas to be served by the recommended projects".[13] In many cases an HSA survey of need will uncover strong perceptions of increased service needs due both to projected population changes and to the desire for all hospitals in their communities to be "full service," including the latest and most advanced technologic equipment, the need for additional space to perform functions mandated by federal and state regulations, and primary and secondary care needs unmet by the existing complement of physicians.

On the other hand, the survey is to produce results consistent with the national goals of no more than 1000 patient days per 1000 population and no more than 4.0 beds per 1000 population. This means only 17 HSA areas will be allowed to construct new beds. In addition, the survey is to take into account the results of reviews of the appropriateness of all existing institutional services. Furthermore, the state agency is to consider the appropriateness of ambulatory care facilities, long-term care facilities, and home health services as alternatives to acute-care inpatient facilities for providing adequate health services. Another brake on accepting local recommendations requires the state agency in determining need to consider "the availability and accessibility, to the residents of the areas to be served by the recommended projects, of services provided by existing medical facilities''.[12] Overall, the law refers more to access and quality than to reducing capacity. But the imperative of controlling health care costs, of which the federal government pays a growing share (46% in fiscal year 1976) and that are increasing at the rate of $20 billion per year, necessitates a process that is geared to reducing acute-care hospital capacity and stimulating less costly alternatives. As an example, any recommendations in the SMFP for new inpatient facilities must describe the basis on which the determination was made that less costly alternative modes of health care delivery could not provide the required services.[14]

Two remaining general responsibilities of the state agency are to implement those parts of the SHP that require action by the executive branch of state government and to assist the Statewide Health Coordinating Council in the performance of its functions.

Statewide Health Coordinating Councils (SHCCs)

The SHCC, which combines an advisory rule with some clear-cut, independent functions, is comprised of at least 60% representatives of HSAs chosen by the governor from HSA lists of nominees and the remainder freely chosen by the governor. A majority of the members, however, must be consumers, as required by the narrow definition of the act. No more than one third of the members can be direct providers. All HSAs must have equal representation on the SHCC. The functions of the SHCC are to:*

*From U.S. Department of Health, Education, and Welfare. July 28, 1977. Draft guidelines for the development of the state medical facilities plan. Health Resources Administration, p. 6.

1. Review and comment on the HSP and AIP of each HSA, including annual revisions that are then forwarded to HEW. It has the authority to revise the HSPs to achieve necessary coordination among the various plans and to deal more effectively with statewide health needs.

2. Prepare the SHP, considering both the plans submitted by the HSAs and the revisions made by the state health planning agency.

3. Approve or disapprove any state plan or application for federal funding of specific health programs. Negative decisions can be appealed through the governor to the secretary of HEW.

4. Review HSA applications for planning grants, annual budgets, and applications for area development programs and comment on these to HEW.

5. Review the SMFP prepared by the state agency for consistency with the SHP. SHCC approval is a necessary prerequisite for HEW approval.

SHCC functions do not include involvement in reviews of HSA or state agency functions with respect to certification of need, Section 1122, and appropriateness review. Nor is the SHCC required to review specific HSA implementation strategies. Unlike HSAs and SHPDA, the SHCC does not receive independent funding. All SHCC meetings are open to the public.[15]

PSRO/HSA INTERACTIONS

PSROs are likely to provide more assistance to the HSAs in helping the latter agencies fulfill their responsibilities than vice versa. The three major areas in which PSROs can help HSAs are data collection and compilation, development of criteria and standards, and provision of professional technical assistance and expert advice.

Data

Data are an essential ingredient in the planning process. The highest priority for all HSAs in the short run is the development of regional plans for the provision of care in and by acute-care hospitals. No HSA has sufficient funds to collect from primary sources the data they need on hospital costs and utilization. Information on the use (and associated costs) of these facilities is, however, routinely available from at least three major sources. The hospital is usually able to provide aggregate information on utilization, including occupancy rates. The hospital is also frequently the only source of information on its outpatient department and educational programs. Hospitals are also the best source of detailed cost information through their charge schedules, detailed cost reports required by third-party payors, and in a few cases, careful analyses of the true costs of providing each service. However, hospitals rarely run an internal system that provides accurate information on the origin of patients who use the facilities, the frequency of different types of problems for which the facility is used, the types of surgical and special procedures performed, the use of ancillary services, length of stay by diagnosis, and trends in all these areas.

A more frequent source of inpatient utilization information is a hospital discharge abstract service. The largest service is the Professional Activity Survey (PAS). There are in addition a number of regional, statewide, or hospital-type specific (such as children's hospitals) smaller counterparts. These services provide aggregate patient information (length of stay by diagnosis, age breakdowns, sources of third-party coverage, major procedures), and most have the capacity to add data elements of particular interest to the hospital or required to fulfill PSRO review functions. From the HSA viewpoint, these services have two main drawbacks. First, there is considerable error in completing discharge abstract forms, thus reducing their reliability and making harder the appreciation of trends.[16] Second, many pieces of information an HSA wants are not routinely collected. For example, HSAs must be concerned with the growth of ancillary services, both in intensity (number of ancillary tests per patient day, per diagnosis or per spell of illness) and in scope (what new tests or procedures are hospitals adding?). HSAs have a strong interest in outpatient care and ambulatory surgery. No abstract service, however, collects the information on these service components necessary for analytic purposes.

The final usual source of information is the PSROs. Because the PSRO data collection system is primarily concurrent, the system can provide information relatively free from error on federally financed patients. Although these patients generally comprise only 40% to 50% of the total patients admitted into PSRO area hospitals, the reliability of the information makes this data base essential for planning. It helps the HSA counter usual criticisms that data collected through discharge abstracts are unrealistic. Especially important is the collection through PSROs of nonroutine data elements needed to perform special studies. The PSRO coordinator can, as an example, collect information on the lag between tests and procedures ordered and their completion, how early potential postdischarge placement problems are identified, the use of ancillary procedures by diagnosis and degree of illness, the number of elective surgical procedures that might have been done on an ambulatory basis, or the number of reducible preoperative hospital days. Other sources of both utilization and cost data include private insurers, the federal government (especially Medicare), state governments (primarily Medicaid, health departments, and rate-setting agencies), and HMOs.

One important problem that every HSA confronts is the compatibility of data from several sources. To merge information bases requires uniformity of definitions both for what constitutes each element of information and for the system used to classify the range of possible answers. The adoption by HEW agencies of a uniform hospital discharge data system will facilitate standardization. A related problem is how to merge computerized data bases. In seven states the organizations interested in hospital utilization and cost information have formed consortia to pull together existing data bases into one system and to act as a service bureau to both members and nonmembers who want aggregate information retrievable from that system. For example, in Massachusetts a

2-year effort to establish an independent data consortium was supported by the National Center for Health Statistics under a CHSS grant. The constitution of the board of directors of six of the seven different state consortia is shown in Table 29-2. Information available from this centralized source will be valuable to PSROs and HSAs alike. PSROs can compare their diagnoses, procedure rates, and other parameters against information on private patients. HSAs can get a composite picture of care in short-stay hospitals and compare institutional performance both within their health service area and

TABLE 29-2.   Consortium Composition in Massachusetts and Other States

ORGANIZATIONS	REPRESENTATION					
	Mass.	Vermont (CHICV)	Maryland	Missouri	New York	Rhode Island
Blue Cross/Blue Shield	1		1*	1		2
HIAA	1		1*			
Nongovernment third-party payors				1	14	
HSAs	3		1		14	
SHCC	1					
State hospital associations	4	Not	1	7		2
Hospital administrators		structured				
PSROs	3	by	7	1 (out of 5)	14	2
State medical societies	1	organization.	3	5		2
Osteopathic physicians and surgeons		Board is		2		
Department of Public Health	1	comprised		1		2*
Department of Public Welfare	1	of ⅔		1		
Rate Setting Commission	1	consumers				
Department of Mental Health		and ⅓				2
State board of education		providers				2
Undifferentiated state agencies			1		14	
SHPDA				1		
Long-term care	1					
Health Planning Council (not an HSA)						2
Universities						
Academic Medical Institution (Mass.)	1					2
Medical Records Association				1		
At large	2					
Total	21	13	22	21	70	18

*Nonvoting members.

with other areas. The growth of consortia is difficult to predict, but the independent needs of the participating agencies as well as the high cost of duplicate data collection and processing point to sharing and consolidation as cost effective trends.

Criteria and Standards

The planning and regulatory functions given to HSAs and their counterpart state planning agencies require the application of well-articulated and consistent decision rules. These agencies have frequently been attacked because their decisions appear to lack consistency. Institutions whose expansion they partly control feel that they face erratic and unpredictable decisions. Objective measures to apply to necessity, appropriateness, and quality of care are important to ensure consistency and equity. But both true costs and quality trade-offs are difficult to calculate, because underlying definition problems are not solved. Few criteria are available to guide planners or regulators in reviewing the adequacy of outcome for a cohort of patients with even a well-defined problem. Nonetheless, PSROs, alone or with other organizations, are an excellent potential source of preliminary standards on efficacy and efficiency of medical intervention. A typical question might be, "If all cases of otitis media are treated properly, what should be the prevalence of hearing loss as a sequela of this condition in a community?" Another is "What should be the mortality for complications of hypertension if all patients adhere to physicians' regimens, are appropriately treated, educated about their illness, and vigorously followed-up?" Scientifically developed criteria and standards are needed that answer these types of questions. A coalition of PSROs can be effective in promoting the research necessary to build a data base on these issues and to incorporate information from MCEs into objective indices.

First-generation criteria and standards are already available that cover acceptable complication rates of various medical and surgical procedures, mortality rates for serious operable conditions, and other outcomes of care that can be assessed while a patient is still in the hospital. Armed with these measures, HSAs can at a gross level compare results in different institutions and HSA areas. The results can be factored into the planning process as different institutions compete for additional space, services, and technology. Areawide MCEs that use publicly available criteria can also provide gross information on the quality of care.

The most prevalent criteria and standards relate to the process of care. Although these are clearly not adequate proxies for acceptable outcomes, they can be employed to detect patterns of care that are so deficient in process that they seem unlikely to be associated with acceptable outcomes. Criteria and standards for the use of ancillary procedures are especially needed by HSAs. Ancillaries have been responsible for a significant share of total cost increases in the operation of many hospitals. In 1976, for example, 43.7% of the total increase in hospital costs per patient day came from increases in services rather than from wage and price increases.[17] PSRO criteria and standards that concentrate on when use of specific x-ray procedures and laboratory tests is clearly indicated would be enormously beneficial in HSA reviews of proposed construction to increase laboratory and x-ray capacity.

One of the difficulties for state and regional planning agencies is to convince each subarea that these agencies are concerned with its unique problems and are using assessment tools derived from local settings. Since the PSROs are free to adopt their own criteria and standards (and many have spent considerable effort in their development), HSAs using these guidelines can enhance their credibility by pointing out that their methods reflect the concerns of local medical leaders.

Over time, PSROs can be expected to develop criteria and standards for long-term care (both institutional and home care), ambulatory surgery, and hospital-based ambulatory care, all of which are legitimate concerns of HSAs and SHPDAs. The importance of criteria and standards will increase significantly if the basis for planning shifts from demonstration of need to a rationing approach. In such an event, they will be used to help determine priorities among competing projects on the basis of the record of each applicant in delivering efficient and high-quality care.

Professional Expertise

A major part of HSA activities involves assessment of various professional services. In evaluating the health care needs of their health service areas, the HSAs require some technical assistance from experts in various specialty areas. An important element in this assistance is an areawide perspective that is not biased in favor of an individual institution or group of institutions. The PSRO as an areawide group of physicians can provide this perspective. In addition, the PSRO, whose primary responsibilities include looking at both cost and quality, is in a good position to provide advice on alternative methods of delivery of a particular service and to help rank medical needs in terms of relative impacts of new services on patient outcomes. The PSRO can also provide assistance for the HSA by reviewing the general quality of care in an institution that is the subject of a complaint or of general community concern. Use of a local medical organization to provide technical assistance can help build HSA credibility and enhance the ability of PSROs to help forge the system of health care that will prevail in their areas for many years. A creditable job in helping HSAs will also be a counterforce to any community beliefs that PSROs are interested only in protecting traditional physician

prerogatives and supporting the status quo for their self-interest.

PSRO ASSISTANCE TO HSAs IN FULFILLING REQUIRED FUNCTIONS

Although the literature contains considerable discussion of the general ways in which PSROs and HSAs can interact, specifics are usually lacking. A discussion of the four major required HSA functions as well as suggestions for how PSROs can directly assist HSAs in performing their duties follows. Following this discussion is a summary of possibilities for PSRO-HSA cooperation as developed by a group at the University of California under an HEW contract (Table 29-3)

Certification of Need and Section 1122 Reviews

As previously described, PL 93-641 as further defined by regulation requires that by 1980 all states have in place a Certification of Need statute that requires approval by the SHPDA for any institutional capital construction project over $150,000, a change of ten beds or 10% of the facility's inpatient beds (whichever is less), or new services. The SHPDA is required to consider recommendations from the HSA in performing this function. As of August 1977, 35 states had enacted certification of need laws, although not all are consistent with federal requirements. Thirty-seven states have Section 1122 programs under which states enter into contracts with the federal government to review health care capital expenditures. These programs overlap because they are both directed at avoiding duplication of services or services in excess of what is needed. Under Section 1122 agreements, the responsible state agency must review projects over $100,000 for hospitals, nursing homes, and ambula-

TABLE 29-3.   Summary of Possibilities for PSRO-HSA Cooperation*

PSRO CAPABILITIES	PLAN DEVELOPMENT	PLAN IMPLEMENTATION	
		Review	Other Implementation Act
Routine Data Data currently collected for federal requirements; describe patient, diagnoses, facility, care, disposition, payment.	To identify underserved groups, demographic and geographic, and problems, such as accessibility. To project need for services, manpower, and facilities on the basis of trends in utilization patterns. To plan for observed shifts in epidemiologic factors.	To assist in selecting areas for appropriateness review. To assist in selecting parameters and setting criteria for review of applications for certificate of need, Section 1122 reimbursement, and certain federal grant applicants about community need for proposed services.	To monitor and evaluate the impact of new services on health status and service utilization patterns.
Special Studies Data that can be collected by PSRO methods and personnel, in addition to routine data, from charts, physicians, discharge planners, patients.	To supplement other PSRO or non-PSRO inputs to plan development or to provide data in areas where none is available.	To supplement other PSRO or non-PSRO inputs in any phase of the review process or to provide data in areas where none is available.	To supplement other PSRO or non-PSRO inputs used to monitor impacts of new programs.
Information on Institutional Quality Data and other information on quality of care in individual facilities or classes of facilities, based on MCEs.	To identify quality deficiencies related to resource or organizational problems that can be addressed in the planning process. To refine estimates of "available" services in light of quality-related barriers to utilization of specific facilities.	To include quality as a parameter of review of proposed changes in existing institutions, especially in cases of competing applicants. To include quality as a parameter in appropriateness review.	To indicate when HSA supply-limiting actions or innovations are lowering quality.
Criteria for Patient Care Norms, criteria, and standards for hospital admission, length of stay, diagnostic and therapeutic procedures; also information on their validation status, anticipated obsolescence and underlying consideration.	To modify projections for needs based on past utilization. To make policy decisions to increase or decrease community services on the basis of an understanding of factors underlying criterion-based demand.	To assess proposed changes in services or facilities in view of influences on demand of revisions in criteria. To estimate need for new types of services for which no utilization data exist. To identify areas for which exceptions to the plan should be made in review decisions, as reflected by variation in criteria among facilities. To use as a basis for HSA requests for quality-related information from applicant institutions.	To negotiate with PSRO for criteria modifications that would help HSA implement plans.

TABLE 29-3. Summary of Possibilities for PSRO-HSA Cooperation* *(continued)*

PSRO CAPABILITIES	PLAN DEVELOPMENT	PLAN IMPLEMENTATION	
		Review	*Other* *Implementation Act*
Standards for Facilities Standards for equipment, space, manpower, volume of services, extrapolated from patient care criteria and outcome findings.	To provide guidelines for categorizing facilities by level of care in regionalization of services.	To judge qualifications of institutions in review decisions, especially in cases where applicants have no previous track record for a proposed service. To develop standards for types of facilities and services for use in appropriateness review.	
Expert Opinion Judgment (based on PSRO experience and data) on factors affecting quality of care or appropriate utilization.	To incorporate the perspective of the practitioner community into the priority-setting process. To aid in analyzing descriptive data on trends and patterns, and possible consequences of various planning decisions on quality of care and appropriateness. To assist in identifying medically interrelated services that should be planned together.	To estimate expected demand for proposed services not covered by the plan and predict consequences for quality and utilization patterns. To aid in choosing areas and parameters for appropriateness review, and in setting guidelines.	To aid in estimating possible consequences of certain implementation strategies on the quality of care and appropriateness of utilization.
Remedial Action Programs PSRO actions that enforce utilization or quality control decisions, including provider education, peer pressures, and legal sanctions.		To coordinate PSRO remedial action strategies and HSA review decisions for maximal effectiveness of both.	To coordinate HSA and PSRO strategies in promoting remedial actions for quality deficiencies and utilization problems.

*Modified from Health System Agencies and Professional Standards Review Organizations, report prepared under contract No. HRA-230-75-00-71.

tory care facilities to determine if a prorated share of these should be eligible under reimbursement by Medicare, Medicaid, and Title V (Maternal and Child Health and Crippled Children) programs. The review covers expenditures for plant or equipment, whether new or renovated, and any bed complement or service change if capital expenditure is required. Under Section 1122, principal, interest, and depreciation from projects not approved by the designated agency cannot be reimbursed by the federal program. Determinations made by state certification of need programs are enforced by court injunctions and threat of license revocation.

PSROs can help both the HSAs and SPHDAs administer these programs by providing information relevant to their review functions. Information derived from an institution-by-institution compilation of discharge abstracts can help determine whether utilization of existing facilities is appropriate when measured by average length of stay, diagnosis, and age. Longer than average length of stay is one indication of possible overutilization. PSROs can also provide information on the frequency with which the physician advisor had to confront the attending physician to discharge a patient no longer needing hospital care as well as the frequency of admissions not certified. PSRO coordinators can collect information that would help determine if tests were conducted promptly after being ordered, if preoperative length of stay was as short as possible, and if postdischarge planning was initiated at the earliest possible time. Although the required activities of a PSRO cover only federally funded patients, problems discovered that relate to the organization of the institution or the practices of a particular physician are likely to have more general applicability. If nonfederal patients, as reviewed by a composite of discharge summaries through a discharge abstract service, have a longer length of stay or have a high incidence of certain diagnoses, the HSA could ask the hospital to allow the PSRO to do a special study of nonfederal patient admissions over a specific period of time to determine whether a problem exists. Refusal by the hospital to participate in such a review might be established as justification for denial of the certificate of need. For both federal and nonfederal patients, the presence of physician advisors and nurse coordinators not employed by the hospital to perform these special studies could be re-

quired to ensure objective review. Asking personnel from the institution itself to perform these studies for the HSA could create a conflict of interest.

An untapped but promising area for PSRO participation in review of capital construction projects relates to ancillary services. A large percentage of applications proposes expansion of radiology, clinical and special laboratories, or additional space for physical or respiratory therapy. The PSROs are probably in the best position to develop the capacity to audit the appropriate utilization of existing services in these areas. They could, for example, sample 100 radiologic procedures in a hospital and by referring back to the charts try to answer questions such as: Was there clear documentation in the chart of the need for the x-ray at that time? Could the x-ray have been performed before the patient entered the hospital? If a repeat x-ray, was there a need to repeat the x-ray at that time? Is the percentage of repeat radiologic studies in line with current standards? Would a different procedure have provided more useful information than the test requested? Although this type of review will require subjective judgments, an indication from a group of impartial PSRO physicians, including, for example, a radiologist, an internist, a surgeon, and a pediatrician, regarding the percentages of procedures clearly appropriate, questionable, and inappropriate, would help both the institution and the HSA.

Another area in which assistance is needed relates to quality of care. PSROs are currently not allowed to provide information from MCEs that reflect directly on an identified physician. The PSROs, however, should be able to provide information on the overall quality of care in an institution on the basis of the results of all studies performed by the institution and of a comparison of this institution with others in PSRO-conducted areawide studies. In general, an HSA will want to give priority consideration to those certification of need applications from institutions with highest marks for both appropriateness and high quality. Although the danger exists that unvalidated process criteria can lead to confusion between care that includes all components *thought* to be associated with good outcome and care that *is associated* with good outcome, attention to validating criteria and standards and an increased emphasis on outcome should reduce this tendency.

Appropriateness Review

PL 93-641 is the first federal statute to address the question of need for all existing institutional services. Both the state and HSAs are required to "review on a periodic basis (but at least every 5 years) all institutional health services . . . respecting the appropriateness of such services." HSAs first make a recommendation to the SHPDA regarding the appropriateness of services within their areas. The SHPDA then has a year to act on the HSA's recommendations and to make its findings public. Although no sanction is attached, a public finding on inappropriateness would generate significant pressure from third-party payors and the public to discontinue that service. In addition, over the next several years, pressure will increase to link appropriateness reviews with reimbursement mechanisms and licensure.

Some of the PSRO activities that aid in reviewing applications for new services or construction could be equally helpful to the planning agencies in performance of review of appropriateness. In addition, the PSROs could provide both advice on what types of services should take priority in this review process and necessary professional assistance in HSA development of criteria for the review of specific services. For example, professional advice is needed on the minimum volume a particular service requires to ensure maintenance of the necessary skills and experience by those performing that service. This approach can be applied to such services as open heart surgery, special radiologic procedures (such as angiography), chemotherapy and radiotherapy for oncology patients, and maternity units. Finally, HSAs need professional advice to assist them in developing minimum requirements for staffing and organization of specific services. For example, what medical specialists, other trained personnel, equipment, and support services are necessary to run a neonatal intensive care unit or a burn unit? Whereas standards for many services are available from some source, most of these measures are disputed and require careful review, including physician participation.

Development of a Health Systems Plan (HSP)

Each HSA must develop and annually update an HSP, which is a "statement of desired achievements for improvement in the health status of area residents and in the health systems serving that population."[18] The requirements in the law for this plan are so broad as to be beyond the capacity of any planning agency at this time. An acceptable plan, however, is a prerequisite to the secretary of HEW's entering into a full designation agreement with any HSA. At a minimum, the plan must contain health status and health systems goals that describe desired achievements in health status and health systems serving the area's population. The first HSP must give in-depth attention to the diagnostic and therapeutic services delivered in each of the health settings of the area. Most of the attention is to be devoted to cost, availability, and accessibility. For each goal, the HSP must contain related objectives, recommended action, and resource requirements for high priority areas, including those with deficiencies or inefficiencies.

Since the requirements of the plan exceed the resources of the agency involved, many agencies are segmenting their planning by devoting their attention to a few high-priority areas at one time. In a number of cases a group of HSAs has formed a task force or committee to analyze specific service areas. In Massachusetts, for example, all HSAs have joined with the SHPDA in forming task forces to develop objective measures of need for: (1) acute-care hospital beds (except as addressed in No. 2 and No. 3), (2) general psychiatric beds in acute-care hospitals, (3) neonatal intensive care beds, and (4) long-term care beds and complementary community services. Other task forces are reviewing the requirements in terms of capacity and support services for specialized units, burn care, and spinal cord injuries. Physicians and other interested parties participate in these task forces.

Much of the data routinely collected by PSROs can help in developing HSPs and deciding on priorities for in-depth planning activities. For example, information on case mix at each hospital can be matched with existing services and equipment, and assessments can be made as to where the plan should include increases and decreases in services. Patient-origin data can help HSAs review the availability and accessibility of services in every part of their area. Diagnostic mix by institution can provide information essential to deciding on sites for regionalization of specialized services. Trends in incidence of particular diagnoses and patterns of illness can be derived from PSRO information and used both to monitor the effectiveness of programs designed to reduce hospitalization and to help update the needs enumerated in the HSP. An increase in the hospital incidence of a serious problem may indicate that increased services and an improved system for caring for that problem are necessary. If that problem is preventable, such an increase can signal the usefulness of increased efforts in primary or secondary prevention.

PSROs can also collect data on the staging of major illnesses on hospital entry or procedure.[19] A high proportion of patients with hypertension who entered with hypertensive crisis, appendectomy patients with perforated appendices at the time of operation, or patients with cancer who entered the hospital long after having been seen as an outpatient with signs or symptoms strongly suspicious for cancer all indicate problems in the organization and delivery of care appropriate for consideration in the development of the HSP. Also useful could be information on readmission rates by institution for problems that might not reoccur if adequate community support services existed (for example, an efficient system of mental health clinics, social workers, and others can help to prevent recurrent problems of child abuse). PSRO information can also document the difficulty in finding placement in long-term care facilities for both private and Medicaid patients and provide one index of the need for more long-term care services, both home based and institutional. PSRO data on quality and criteria and standards for use of specialized procedures can together help HSPs reflect where consolidation or phasing out of low-quality or inefficient services is advisable. If a service is clearly needed in an area but the existing service suffers from insufficient resources to provide high-quality care, the HSA could recommend that the provider file for a certification of need to remedy the situation and include provision for this in the HSP. Where PSRO information suggests poor-quality care in a marginal institution, the HSP may disregard that facility in planning for increased capacity to respond to identified unmet needs.

Finally, PSRO expert opinion in terms of priority needs can ensure the inclusion of the physician perspective in the development of the HSP. This perspective is essential to HSAs and will help build support for the changes necessary to transform the HSP into a plan of reallocation and reorganization of health care resources in its area.

Development of an Annual Implementation Plan (AIP)

Each HSA must establish, review annually, and disseminate widely an AIP that translates the HSP short-term goals into well-defined objectives that can be fulfilled within a 12-month period. As stated in the HEW guidelines:*

The AIP identifies the specific priority short-range objectives upon which the community wishes to act during the ensuing year. While the objectives need not be achievable in one year, the AIP should also identify the actions the community intends to take, and the effects of the actions, to achieve those objectives.

The AIP is also to include other mandated functions, such as certification of need review, provision of technical assistance to help develop a list of projects, appropriateness review, and review of federal funds to come into the area. Approval of this plan by the HSA governing body is a prerequisite to full designation agreements with the secretary of DHEW. The role of PSROs in assisting HSAs with their AIPs is largely consultative. PSRO information can help HSAs decide on high-priority action items for the coming year. For example, a PSRO might indicate that it has reviewed many cancer patients inappropriately treated and believes that a well-delineated referral system for cancer diagnosis, chemotherapy, and

*From U.S. Department of Health, Education, and Welfare. Dec. 23, 1976. *Guidelines concerning the development of health systems plans and annual implementation plans.* Health Resources Administration, p. 47.

radiotherapy is a pressing need. The PSRO might advise that on the basis of its reviews care of the elderly in skilled nursing facilities is poor, and improvements in this area are a high priority. Unlike some of the other parties who will be part of the decisions regarding priorities, PSROs will have a data base to buttress their formal opinions. They also have the ability over time to collect data that can show a change in the quality or appropriateness of care based on the actions taken.

Another role of PSROs is participation in the implementation of the actions described in the AIP. Many of these actions are politically sensitive. For example, the closing of an obstetric ward because of a very small number of births and questionable support services may involve stiff opposition from the hospital's board of trustees, the elected officials of the city or town in which the facility is located, and the physicians and other health care professionals who provide the service. The participation of a physician group in the development of criteria and standards that are not met by that service will make it easier for the HSA to overcome the opposition and to educate the public that its actions are in their interest. PSROs can also assist in helping plan for urgent unmet needs. For example, if the need for primary care is not being met because of inadequate physicians in the area, the PSRO could help document this to the community and help the HSA and institutions in the area plan how to fill the service gap most efficiently.

Another PSRO role related to the AIP is to provide feedback on how the actions taken in accordance with the plan have affected the quality of services in the area. For example, PSRO information (either alone or in combination with data from other sources) can help answer whether interhospital referral arrangements for cancer treatment are being observed; whether community hypertension screening and follow-up programs have decreased hospital admission rates for hypertension, its related problems, and mortality; and whether improved community mental health services are associated with a decrease in readmission rates to state mental health institutions or psychiatric wards of general hospitals. Special PSRO studies could show whether consolidation of services had improved outcomes of care or whether the availability of a new specialized service in the HSA area had decreased the number of area patients who travel to get the same service at a distant site.

MAKING PSRO/HSA COORDINATION WORK

The federal government is making strong efforts to have PSROs and HSAs coordinate their activities. Regulations covering the operations of conditionally designated HSAs state: "The agency shall coordinate its activities and seek to enter into a written agreement with each PSRO whose PSRO area is in whole or in part in the agency's service area, for the purpose of achieving coordination of their respective activities.[20] These regulations also require an HSA to report to HEW if it has not been able to finalize an agreement with the involved PSROs, the reasons for lack of such agreements, and what further actions they plan to take to finalize them.

Among the suggestions for ongoing coordination is the formation of an HSA/PSRO coordinating council, whose responsibilities are to foster mechanisms for data exchange, provide an avenue for input into each other's related activities, resolve any differences and promote more extensive cooperation. One report of HSA/PSRO relations suggests such a committee be composed of members of the respective governing bodies as well as experts in prime areas of concern not strictly representative of either group.[21]

Another potential mechanism to bring the or-

ganizations closer together is to have overlapping representation on each other's governing body. Although this will ensure that each organization has full knowledge of the other's final decisions, the governing body, especially of the HSA, will rely heavily on the reports and recommendations of technical committees. Therefore, it is important that representatives from each organization sit either as appointed members, ex-officio members, or as technical consultants on the relevant committees of their companion organization. For example, a PSRO representative might sit on HSA committees that are developing standards for review of facilities and services, developing approaches to resource distribution, formulating draft HSPs based on areawide health care needs, and performing reviews of specific projects. HSA representatives might sit on PSRO committees that are reviewing available standards and criteria or reviewing the efficacy of expensive procedures.

A joint committee to deal with a subject of great importance to both agencies, such as data, might help specify the data needs of each organization that could be met by the other, promote coordinated data collection through a statewide data consortium, and address problems with accuracy and timeliness of data sharing.

The written agreement between HSAs and PSROs should contain specific information on how data and information will be exchanged. A PSRO must release information collected on the basis of the Uniform Hospital Discharge Data System when such data cannot lead to identification of individual patients or practitioners. The organization supplying the data can request nominal payment on a cost basis for copying, compiling, or reorganizing data. Each HSA and PSRO is required to interpret the data and information it provides and to make available its methodology for analyzing the data.[22]

Agreements are to provide for PSRO input into the development of the HSP and AIP, and PSRO review and comments before final adoption by the HSA governing body. The topics on which the need for PSRO comment is greatest include quality of care, utilization of services and facilities, availability of alternative, less costly or more effective methods of providing services, and the need for new resources. In turn, PSROs should provide HSAs with the opportunity to identify priority areas for PSRO review as well as to suggest topics for future areawide MCEs.

Part of an agreement is to cover PSRO advice and comment during the development of HSA standards and criteria for certification of need and Section 1122 reviews, appropriateness reviews, and review and approval of federal grants, especially as these have an effect on federally funded patients. PSROs are also to help select areas for appropriateness review (such as particular services, type of facility, or specific facility). In addition, PSROs are encouraged to provide HSA review panels with all relevant information (consistent with confidentiality constraints) on specific institutions undergoing project or service review.

The required memoranda of agreement are to be reviewed periodically, with review triggered by particular calendar interval, changes of status (such as a PSRO or HSA acquiring full designation status), or a milestone in terms of functions (such as completion of an HSP by the HSA).

REFERENCES

1. U.S. Department of Health, Education, and Welfare. April 5, 1976. PSRO Transmittal No. 33. Health Services Administration, p. 7.

2. U.S. Department of Health, Education, and Welfare. April 5, 1976. PSRO Transmittal No. 33. Health Services Administration, p. 1.

3. National Health Planning and Resources Development Act. 1974. PL 93-741, Section 1513, p. 2.

4. National Health Planning and Resources Development Act. 1974. PL 93-741, Section 1513 (b) (1).

5. U.S. Department of Health, Education, and Welfare. Dec. 23, 1976. Guidelines concerning the development of health systems plans and annual implementation plans. Health Resources Administration, p. 10.

6. U.S. Department of Health, Education, and Welfare. Dec. 23, 1976. Guidelines concerning the development of health systems plans and annual implementation plans. Health Resources Administration, pp. 26–27.

7. U.S. Department of Health, Education, and Welfare. Dec. 23, 1976. Guidelines concerning the development of health systems plans and annual implementation plans. Health Resources Administration, pp. 27–28.

8. National Health Planning and Resources Act. 1974. PL 93-741, Section 1512 (5).

9. U.S. Department of Health, Education, and Welfare. July 28, 1977. Draft guidelines for the development of the state medical facilities plan. Health Resources Administration.

10. U.S. Department of Health, Education, and Welfare. July 28, 1977. Draft guidelines for the development of the state medical facilities plan. Health Resources Administration, p. 6.

11. U.S. Department of Health, Education, and Welfare. July 28, 1977. Draft guidelines for the development of the state medical facilities plan. Health Resources Administration, pp. 11–12.

12. U.S. Department of Health, Education, and Welfare. July 28, 1977. Draft guidelines for the development of the state medical facilities plan. Health Resources Administration, p. 19.

13. U.S. Department of Health, Education, and Welfare. July 28, 1977. Draft guidelines for the development of the state medical facilities plan. Health Resources Administration, pp. 19–20.

14. U.S. Department of Health, Education, and Welfare. July 28, 1977. Draft guidelines for the development of the state medical facilities plan. Health Resources Administration, p. 20.

15. National Health Planning and Resources Development Act. 1974. PL 93-641, Section 1524 (c).

16. Reliability of hospital discharge abstracts. Feb. 1977. Washington, D.C.: Institute of Medicine, National Academy of Sciences.

17. Congressional Budget Office. 1977. Expenditures for health care: federal programs and their effects. Washington, D.C.: U.S. Government Printing Office.

18. U.S. Department of Health, Education, and Welfare. Dec. 23, 1976. Guidelines concerning the development of health systems plans and annual implementation plans. Health Resources Administration.

19. Goran, M., and Gonella, J. 1975. Quality of patient care: a measurement of change—the staging concept. *Med. Care* 13:467.

20. Final HSA legislation. *Federal register.* March 1, 1976. Washington D.C.: U.S. Government Printing Office.

21. Program of Continuing Education. June 15, 1976. Report of the Region II Task Force of HSA and PSRO relationships. New York: Columbia University School of Public Health, pp. 14–15.

22. U.S. Department of Health, Education, and Welfare. Dec. 1976. Draft guidelines concerning cooperation between health systems agencies and professional standards review organizations. Health Resources Administration.

30

Quality Assurance and the PSRO

Paul J. Sanzaro

The PSRO program has survived a slow and shaky start, underfunding by Congress, major court tests, sustained bureaucratic in-fighting in Washington, and persisting opposition in principle if not in fact by large numbers of physicians and consumer interest groups. Support for PSRO among physicians has been enhanced by the present policy statements in DHEW that the main function of the PSRO is to assure the quality of care, not merely control unnecessary hospital use.[1,2]

The conviction that PSROs should concern themselves primarily with the quality of care was the motivation for *Private Initiative in PSRO* (PIPSRO).[3] This project, funded entirely by the W. K. Kellogg Foundation, was sponsored by the American Association of Foundations for Medical Care, American College of Physicians, American Hospital Association, American Society of Internal Medicine, and initially, the American Medical Association. Under the direction of a management committee composed of representatives of these organizations and two other members representing the public interest generally, PIPSRO carried out a series of studies between 1973 and 1976. Included in these was an experiment in concurrent quality assurance (CQA), conducted through formal agreement with five PSROs. These were the Colorado and Multnomah Foundations for Medical Care, Pine Tree Organization for PSR, Inc. (Maine), Area IX PSRO of New York, and the Bal-

timore City PSRO, Inc. PIPSRO provided an opportunity to examine the current state of the art of quality assessment and quality assurance in numerous hospitals and in many PSROs. This chapter presents the recommendations emerging from PIPSRO as well as findings and observations that help point the way for those PSROs that wish to make quality of care their primary concern. Certainly for this aspect of the PSRO program, the words "promise, perspective, pitfalls and potential" have a special meaning.

THE PROMISE

The intent of Congress in enacting PL 92-603 was clearly stated in the report of the Senate Finance Committee: "There is no question, however, that the Government has a responsibility to establish mechanisms capable of assuring effective utilization review." "In light of the shortcomings outlined above [reference to the token nature and ineffectiveness of retrospective utilization review], the Committee believes that the critically important utilization review process must be restructured and made more effective through substantially increased professional participation." "Medicine as a profession should accept the task of advising the individual physician where his pattern of practice indicates that he is overutilizing hospital or nursing home services, overtreating his patients, or performing unnecessary surgery." "Existing medical organizations, such as the San Joaquin and Sacramento Foundations in California, and others have developed . . . review methods which may provide the bases for development of uniform data gathering and review procedures capable of being employed in many areas of the Nation."[4]

The BQA implemented this intent literally by issuing a *PSRO Program Manual* that required that PSROs establish concurrent admission certification and review of hospital stay procedures as had been carried out in Sacramento, Utah, and New Mexico.[5] Chapter 7 of the manual defined the components of the PSRO review system as interrelated and as comprising a comprehensive quality assurance system "that will improve quality, assure appropriate utilization of health care services and provide ongoing feedback about the effectiveness of the entire system." The only required procedure that directly and immediately related to the quality of care was the medical care evaluation study. MCEs were intended "to improve quality through an organized and systematic process designed to (a) identify deficiencies in the quality of health care and in the organization and administration of its delivery, (b) correct such deficiencies through education and administrative change and, (c) periodically reassess performance to assure that improvements have been maintained." The results of MCEs, if they revealed deficiencies in quality, were to be used "by a hospital or PSRO in the development of curriculum for and in the monitoring of the effectiveness of its continuing education efforts."

It was the policy of the BQA that the PSRO rely primarily on the bi-cycle model of quality assurance, in which medical audit and continuing medical education together are the principal means of identifying deficiencies and removing them.[6] The BQA also enforced the legal requirement that the PSROs delegate to a hospital responsibility for review, including MCEs, when that hospital demonstrated it could effectively carry out these functions in a timely manner.

If one summarizes these considerations (primary focus on utilization control, reliance on medical audit and continuing medical education for quality improvement, and delegation of these functions to hospitals whenever indicated), it becomes evident that the initial promise of PSROs as a strong force for quality assurance was not bright. Indeed, throughout 1974 and 1975 the total resources of the bureau were consumed by the overwhelming task of implementing the PSRO program on a national scale. By early 1976, however, it began to be evident that PSROs could not continue to justify their existence on the basis of "cost containment" or even "utilization control." It had been anticipated at the outset that initiation of PSRO reviews would restrain utilization in those areas where the Professional Activities Study (PAS) and other data sources revealed that lengths of stay and admission practices were more generous than the average in that region. But once these had been controlled, it was evident that PSROs could not continue to "squeeze down" total utilization of hospitals.[7,9]

In recognition of the need to advocate continuation and expansion of the PSRO program on a firmer political base, testimony before the Subcommittee on Oversight, Committee on Ways and Means, House of Representatives on May 21, 1976 described the mission of the PSRO program as follows:

The PSRO program represents a significant effort by Congress and the Department of Health, Education and Welfare to assure that the medical care provided to beneficiaries and recipients of Medicare, Medicaid, and Maternal and Child Health and Crippled Children's Services programs is of high quality and that such care is provided in a manner that reflects the most appropriate and efficient utilization of our Nation's health care resources.

The statement closed with "a word of caution on expectations of a PSRO's ability to control expenditures. A PSRO is primarily a mechanism for assessing the quality and appropriateness of medical care services which are delivered." This definition of the mission of the PSRO as primarily a quality assurance organization was reinforced by statements appearing in the DHEW Forward Plans for Health for 1976–1981 and 1977–1982. In these statements, the function of PSRO in quality was defined as "assuring the highest quality of care."

In the span of 2 years, the federal mission of PSROs in quality was lifted from its distinctly secondary position of importance initially to the rank of first priority. Further, the language conveyed the expectation that PSROs would assure the highest quality of care.

PERSPECTIVE

The PSRO provisions of PL 92-603 do not require anything more in relation to utilization review (UR) and quality assurance than was contained in the original Medicare law (1965) and its amendments in 1967 that extended the UR functions to Medicaid. The Social Security Amendments of 1965 in Title XVIII of PL 89-97 required that hospitals and extended care facilities undertake "utilization review" as a condition of participation in the program, that is, to be eligible for reimbursement. A UR committee composed of physicians was to be established in each hospital to ensure that medical services covered under the program (1) were necessary, (2) were provided in the appropriate facility, and (3) met professionally acceptable standards of quality. The Social Security Amendments of 1967 (PL 90-249, Title XIX) extended these requirements to the Medicaid program, describing them as a "safeguard against unnecessary utilization" and as assurance that reimbursements would not be "in excess of reasonable charges consistent with efficiency, economy, and quality of care."

Comparison of the stated intent of Title XVIII with the statement of purposes of PSROs in PL 92-603 makes it clear that Congress simply reaffirmed existing national policy. The original provisions of Title XVIII were administered by the Bureau of Health Insurance in the Social Security Administration. The prevailing philosophy of that administration was recently described by its former commissioner:

The government has taken the view that it owed the people on whose behalf it was acting an assurance that the care being furnished met specified minimal standards of quality—in other words, it defined what it would buy—and increasingly it has taken the view that it has an obligation to try to hold down the cost for the defined product to reasonable amounts.*

This states explicitly the inherent limitations on enforcement of national standards: inevitably the federal government can require conformity only to a minimal standard. Even though the more recent descriptions of PSRO functions may indicate higher aspirations, the economic, political, and day-to-day reality is that the government cannot enforce or indeed require that any program assure "the highest quality of care."

A second factor that should shape one's perspective on quality assurance is the type of PSRO organization that has been required by the BQA. The BQA has promoted the adoption of the organizational model developed by foundations for medical care. These foundations were originally created specifically for the purpose of monitoring overutilization of services in the office and the hospital. Recognizing the limitations of the foun-

*From Ball, R.M. 1975. Background of regulation in health care. In *Controls on Health Care*. Washington, D.C.: Institute of Medicine, National Academy of Sciences, p. 12.

dation model for quality assurance, the Experimental Medical Care Review Organization (EMCRO) program was begun in 1971 to determine how best to organize an areawide system for examining and improving the quality of medical care.[10] Most of the initial grants were made to foundations because of their prior experience, staff, and knowledgeable leadership. Unfortunately, the PSRO law was enacted scarcely 1 year after the EMCRO program began. Consequently, the experience from the latter was too limited to provide any alternate model to the Congress. By conveying the impression that Congress mandated the foundation model, the BQA required virtually all PSROs in the United States to adopt a structure best calculated to deal with peer review in relation to inappropriate utilization of services. It is still not known how compatible this form of organization is with a primary mission of assuring a basic standard of quality.

PIPSRO dealt with this problem at length. In developing its conclusions and recommendations, it was mindful of the pessimistic report of the Institute of Medicine regarding the generally substandard performance by PSROs in quality assurance.[11] The conclusion endorsed by the Management Committee of PIPSRO was as follows:*

The Management Committee believes that there remains a good and sufficient basis for concluding that PSROs are necessary as a professionally controlled mechanism of quality assurance, interposed between the purchasers of services and the providers (physicians and hospitals) on the one side and patients on the other. The basis of this conclusion resides in the current political, social and economic conflicts surrounding the issue of how to justify the continuously escalating expenditures for medical care in a way that satisfies those who demand and are entitled to greater accountability. Given the ever mounting pressures to restrain utilization (in the

*From *Private initiative in PSRO*. Dec. 16, 1976. Draft report and recommendations.

mistaken notion that this can substantially restrain overall costs), an organization like PSRO, composed of physicians capable of setting reasonable standards and promoting their attainment, is a necessary concomitant of any program, public or private, directed to containing costs. The PSRO program is potentially the best mechanism so far devised to assure that reasonable standards of care are upheld uniformly throughout the country.

However, it is unrealistic to assume that PSROs could become the principal vehicle by which physicians and health care institutions will continually raise the quality of care toward the highest practicable levels. PSROs are legally institutionalized mechanisms for protecting patients from inappropriate and unwarranted restrictions on needed services, and as such can provide a reasonable guarantee of a basic level of quality. But the generic function of assuring the highest quality of hospital care requires far greater professional support and resources than can be mobilized through the PSRO program.

Given the confluence of forces pushing for more and more "quality assurance," it is indeed remarkable that Congress should have passed a law that permits only physicians to organize local efforts for examining and improving the quality of care received by Medicare and Medicaid patients. In essence, Congress granted the medical profession an extension of its traditional heritage of self-regulation in quality. But those concerned with the future of quality assurance by organized medicine to forestall regulation by the government must remain acutely aware of the fact that PSRO is no more than an opportunity and perhaps a temporary one. The PSRO, at least as conceived and operated in its present form, could be judged politically embarrassing by the Congress any time the "medical care cost crisis" is shown to be immune to PSRO activities. The only unassailable defense of the PSRO program will be unequivocal demonstration that PSROs themselves have objectively improved the quality of care given Medicare and Medicaid patients.

It is evident on examination of PSRO efforts nationwide that physicians controlling PSROs have rarely acted aggressively with this rationale in mind. Many boards of PSROs have adopted a passive relationship with DHEW, often explicitly enunciating the philosophy that they will do only what DHEW pays for and only insofar as DHEW can enforce its requirements. This attitude is understandable, but it is not realistic and does not serve the interest of the public or the profession. If PSROs make progress in quality assurance only by virtue of additional funding and technical assistance directly from DHEW, they are in essence admitting that the federal government has the right to require whatever quality assurance activities it stipulates and pays for. In pursuing a policy of passive defiance, these physicians might well surrender their most important professional heritage—the right to self-regulation in the quality of medical care. The guiding perspective should be one within which the private sector strives to satisfy society's new expectations of quality assurance and more explicit public accountability without at the same time demanding that these new or expanded functions be reimbursed fully out of public funds.

PITFALLS

The BQA gave early guidance to the PSROs in setting up programs of assessing and improving the quality of care. In so doing, it inadvertently created two pitfalls. The first is reliance on MCEs, responsibility for which is delegated to hospitals that meet the JCAH requirements for medical audits. The second is the unfortunate choice of terms—norms, standards, and criteria—and their definitions. Each of these two circumstances put the PSROs at risk of frustration in achieving their goal of "objectively documenting improvement of the quality of care given Medicare and Medicaid patients." The several reasons for this deserve discussion.

At present, medical auditing is probably carried out in substandard fashion in the majority of hospitals, large and small. The explanation is straightforward. The general model for an audit is simply the generic model for evaluation of procedures or products in any field of endeavor—engineering, business, banking, plumbing, or medicine. The basic audit model promoted by the BQA conveys the impression that merely by following those steps, a clear-cut determination can be made that the particular aspect of care being studied does or does not conform to a specified criterion of quality.[12] In short, the audit model is portrayed as a simple formula.

Logically, many PSROs concluded that by adopting this model they would automatically meet the requirements for "quality assurance." This was thought to be the case even when hospitals were delegated responsibility for conducting MCEs. But careful review of audit programs in a number of hospitals reveals that there is generally much more form than substance in Performance Evaluation Procedure (PEP) and MCEs regardless of the considerable investment of time and dollars. Three major factors account for this. First, most hospitals do not have a formally organized quality assurance program that clearly assigns responsibilities and authorities to the board of trustees, administration, and medical staff. When the motivation in conducting such studies is to fulfill an external requirement, they are more likely to be done pro forma. This was true of retrospective utilization review, as required by the original Medicare law. Because it was pro forma, it did not demonstrate consistent impact on admissions and lengths of stay in hospitals. It may be that the reason concurrent review shows an initial impact is not because the review is concurrent; it has been made clear by Congress and by the intermediaries that there is serious intent to deny payment for hospital admissions and lengths of stay that are clearly unnecessary. It is the *intent* and not the *method* of review that probably has brought about the results.

The same principle applies to quality assurance. If the intent is merely to comply with external standards, then the method of auditing probably will produce completed forms that will satisfy the technical requirements for a specified number of audits per given time.

Second, most medical staffs do not realize that *the limits of quality assurance are set by the capability for objectively assessing the technical quality of care in important areas.* "Quality assurance" cannot proceed in a vacuum. It can be directed only to documented, important deficiencies. Yet consideration of the published literature and the much more extensive unpublished experience in hospitals strongly support the conclusion that most audits are not directed to important deficiencies, that is, problems that on their face would convince physicians that they should no longer be permitted to continue. The disease or condition chosen for study via medical audit should be one whose consequences for the patients, if left untreated or treated improperly, are serious.

If medical audits are not designed to yield unequivocal data that document the existence of important deficiencies in care, the medical staff exhibits the well-known "so what?" attitude.[13] No improvement in care can be expected. The main results are (1) pro forma but acceptable satisfaction of the JCAH or PSRO requirements, (2) waste of resources, and (3) cynicism by staff over "futile efforts to measure quality."

The main pitfalls encountered by medical staffs attempting to assess the quality of care through medical audit are the type of criteria and the methods of adopting them. Many physicians across the country still object deeply to the use of explicit written criteria. Their allegations of "cookbook medicine" and "strait jacket medicine" are less audible today, but they are expressed passively in quiet and even in determined resistance to the evaluation of care by means of explicit criteria.

The attitudes of these physicians are justified when their initial experience in audits has been to use "optimal care criteria." These were first extensively developed by Payne and Lyons.[14-15] They were widely copied initially by foundations for medical care and then by other peer review groups. These criteria are called "optimal care" criteria because they stipulate in detail the factual information derived from the history and physical examination that *should be recorded* in the chart. They list all laboratory, x-ray, and special diagnostic procedures that *might be indicated* in a patient with a particular diagnosis. They also list all the treatments and procedures that might be indicated in a given patient.

These laundry lists of optimal care criteria are not suitable for objectively assessing the technical quality of care. In their requirements for extensive documentation of findings under history and physical examination, they call for a degree of detail much greater than is habitual for the average physician. Most physicians resent being told how much they should record in their charts, and they are quite correct in stating that there is no necessary relationship between the degree of documentation in the history and physical and the technical quality of care.

But the second limitation of optimal care criteria, that which earns them the epithet "cookbook medicine" and leads to the accusation that adherence to these will simply drive up the costs of care, is traceable to their origin in Michigan. The reason optimal care criteria contain all possible procedures and treatments that might be indicated in a patient is that they were originally devised by practicing physicians as guidelines for the Michigan Blue Cross Plan. Physician committees were convened to define the *range* of acceptable diagnostic and treatment procedures for patients with common conditions that would justify admission and treatment in a hospital. These were "pay or no pay" criteria for Blue Cross: whenever a claim form was submitted that contained any of the procedures listed for a particular diagnosis, it was to be paid without further questions. The fundamental limitation of such criteria is evident if one tries to use them in objectively assessing the technical quality of care: when such lists are used in a medical audit, *there is no way of knowing which of the procedures was specifically indicated in a particular patient.*

This is the reason that the "expected level of performance" as used by some hospital staffs defeats the purpose of medical audits as objective methods of quality assessment. If an audit committee estimates that 80% of patients should have a particular diagnostic or treatment procedure, and it is then found by auditing that 80% of patients have had the procedure, the conclusion that their care was satisfactory is not warranted. The question is not what percent of patients should have a certain procedure. The question is, did all patients with condition X for which treatment Y is indicated receive treatment Y? And conversely, did any patients with condition X in which procedure Z is contraindicated receive procedure Z? The answers to these two questions are the basis of evaluating the technical quality of care and the first step toward assuring that every patient receives treatment specifically appropriate to that patient's condition with the fewest possible side effects or complications. Neither of these aims is advanced by reliance on optimal care criteria.

When the PSROs delegate responsibility for MCEs to hospitals, it behooves them to carefully examine the nature of criteria adopted by those hospitals in performing those studies. If the medical staffs persist in using the long-list approach, the PSRO should urge consultative assistance that is probably available within other hospitals in the area.

The ideal criteria for medical audits, if they were available, would be derived directly from the results of randomized clinical trials that clearly establish the causal relationship between a particular procedure (applied with particular indications to a particular type of patient at a particular stage of a disease) and desirable outcomes: avoidance of preventable risks and complications and improved clinical and functional status. Understandably, few definitive studies can be translated so directly into criteria for use in medical auditing. In the absence of such clear-cut guidelines, medical audit should be based on critical or *essential criteria.*[3,16] These criteria apply to "almost every patient" with a particular condition because they are derived from basic principles or sound clinical research that objectively establish the elements of care known to produce the desired clinical results in patients with that particular condition. Audits based on such criteria enable the medical staff to determine objectively whether the care of *individual patients,* and the results of that care, conform to "acceptable professional standards." These essential criteria are analogous to the "critical management criteria" promoted by the JCAH.

The concept of essential or critical criteria emerged from the experience of EMCRO.[10] Chapter 7 of the *PSRO Program Manual* incorporated the early formulation of essential criteria as developed in PIPSRO and other programs:

Criteria are usually developed with reference to a particular diagnosis or health problem. These criteria usually encompass the following categories and should result in the identification of those elements critical to the health care of the patient.
(A) Findings of history, physical examination or diagnostic procedures which confirm the diagnosis.
(B) Diagnostic or therapeutic services (including tim-

ing, frequency, and quantity) which should be provided to a patient with a specified diagnosis.

(C) Contraindicated diagnostic or therapeutic services.

(D) Indications for discharge from the hospital (expected health status at the time of discharge).

(E) Necessary post-hospital care.

It is instructive that despite this clear-cut statement in the *PSRO Program Manual,* the AMA Task Force on Guidelines of Care initially published an endorsement of optimal care criteria.[17] Its first report made evident the committee's difficulty in illustrating how the use of these guidelines could be helpful in assessing the quality of care. After consultation with several physicians working with PIPSRO, the AMA committee changed its position and recommended that PSROs use critical or essential critiera.[18] These two reports should be studied side by side by any individual who still doubts the advantage of essential criteria in objectively assessing the technical quality of care.

It is against this background that one can appreciate the pitfalls introduced into the PSRO program by the reference to "norms" in Section 1156(a) of the PSRO law and by the National PSR Council's endorsement of the following definitions for inclusion in the *PSRO Program Manual:*

> *norms* Medical care appraisal norms are numerical or statistical measures of usual observed performance.
>
> *standards* Standards are professionally developed expressions of the range of acceptable variation from a norm or criterion.
>
> *criteria* Medical care criteria are predetermined elements against which aspects of the quality of a medical service may be compared. They are developed by professionals relying on professional expertise and on the professional literature.

What the PSRO calls "norms" are actually statistical or empirical criteria. These statistical averages are compiled by data systems on what is actually being done. For example, it has been established that fewer than half of the patients admitted to hospitals with presumed bacterial infection have the causative organism identified by culture and the appropriate sensitivity tests performed before antibiotic treatment. This is apparently the national norm. Similarly, in office care it has been documented by statistics on actual practice that more than half the patients presenting with the common cold are given an antibacterial agent. These are also norms. If these *statistical averages* are used as criteria for judging the quality of care, then by definition, PSROs are endorsing existing practice as an adequate level of quality of care. These may or may not be equivalent. Some procedures may be done too often, others too seldom. Prevailing customary practice is not a reliable basis for judging the technical quality of care, because the key determinant of quality is the appropriateness of the procedure to the patient's conditions, and the degree of appropriateness can never be reflected in the simple numerical frequency of a procedure.

The one use of statistical averages that may be defended is the determination of the appropriate lengths of stay. Ever since records have been kept, it has been known that the average length of stay is different in the various regions of the United States. On the average, the longest stays are in New England, and the shortest stays are in the West (in California). No one has satisfactorily explained these differences, but it is manifestly clear that they must relate to local custom or practice, not to differences in quality of care. Therefore, the *PSRO Program Manual* should have stated that the use of norms based on existing regional statistical averages was acceptable for lengths of stay, but it should not have implied that norms could be used for evaluating quality.

What the *PSRO Program Manual* calls "standards" are actually professional norms or normative criteria. These criteria reflect the consensus of physicians on "what ought to be done." The items under the sections on history and physical examination in optimal care criteria are normative criteria or standards.[17] They represent the consensus of one group of physicians on what ought to be recorded to assure "optimal care." The validity of normative criteria depends on the extent to which the clinical expertise and knowledge of those setting the criteria correspond to the best available data from sound clinical and epidemiologic research. The unfortunate implication of the term "standards" in the *PSRO Program Manual* is that physicians are permitted arbitrarily to define as acceptable a level of quality that may be quite different from that defined on the basis of available scientific literature.

The definitions of "criteria" in the *PSRO Program Manual* overlap with the others. If criteria are set by general physicians and surgeons, they are no different from standards, that is, normative, consensus criteria. If the criteria are based on the professional literature, it depends on whether that literature represents a statement of opinion by a particular individual or group or sound clinical research, preferably, randomized clinical trials. In the latter, these would correspond to scientific criteria. They would embody the best that can be achieved when a given therapeutic procedure is applied in a specified manner to a specified type of patient with a specified stage of disease.

These overlapping definitions have led the committees of a number of PSROs to adopt statistical or general consensus criteria as the local guidelines for evaluating the quality of care. As a result, these PSROs are inadvertently maintaining the status quo in the quality of diagnosis and treatment in their area. It should be more widely understood that the criteria can best be devised by those physicians most expert in the actual care of patients

with the particular condition being evaluated. The group judgments of clinical subspecialists can accurately define the objective basis for validating a diagnosis, the particular treatment or procedures known to be effective on the basis of clinical research, and the reasonably attainable outcomes of such treatments. These are the principles underlying the use of essential criteria. PSROs should conduct and promote MCEs based on these principles. The guidelines contained in the *Sample Criteria for Short-Stay Hospital Review* prepared under the auspices of AMA reflect an uneven understanding of "essential criteria."[19] Despite this, the format is useful. In large PSROs, local committees of specialists corresponding to those that developed the sample criteria should revise these to conform to the principles of essential criteria. Smaller PSROs that lack such expertise can enter into cooperative arrangements with neighboring PSROs or work on this problem through their state support center.

A corollary pitfall was introduced by Section 1156(a) of the PSRO law that refers to "norms of care, diagnosis and treatment based upon typical patterns based upon its region." No doubt this concept of "local norms" has helped overcome some apprehensions that local PSROs would merely be rubber stamps. However, determination of "local criteria and standards" is considered their right by many PSROs. There are two problems with this. First, not every PSRO has within it the distribution of specialties and subspecialties capable of deciding the appropriate criteria for evaluating certain technical aspects of care, especially pertaining to certain surgical procedures performed relatively uncommonly. Second, the concept of "local standards" is at variance with a number of rulings of state courts. For example, the California Supreme Court ruled in 1956 that practice or custom does not conclusively establish the standard of care, that is, actual and current practice is not the equivalent of acceptable quality. Similarly, the landmark

Brune versus Melinkoff decision in 1968 held that care provided by specialists should conform to national, not local community, standards. This potential conflict between locally set normative criteria and national (scientific) standards may be serious. PIPSRO addressed this in its recommendations (see pp. 353–355).

Still another pitfall encountered by PSROs attempting effectively to address quality assurance has been their inability to acquire staff with the necessary technical expertise. Funding limitations and lack of external motivation for PSROs to move in this direction are partial explanations. Only a handful of PSROs are aware of the need to bring on board individuals whose background qualifies them to formulate workable programs of quality assessment and assurance throughout the PSRO area. These are the same PSROs that have given special attention to "quality" from their very beginning. Such developments are not so evident in the newer PSROs. It is unlikely that PSROs can attract the highest caliber of technical staff, that is, those with a record of contribution and now active in a professional school or organization engaged in medical care studies. Consultant agreements may make such expertise available to a PSRO's less well-trained staff, assisting them in developing greater competence in design and analysis of quality of care studies.

The contribution of PSRO to quality assurance has yet to be demonstrated. Not more than four PSROs could be considered to have strong programs in quality assessment. Demonstration of actual improvements in the technical quality of care has been limited.[9,13] Yet many of the newer PSROs appear to believe that somewhere there is a perfected model of PSRO and that their responsibility is simply to copy that model. It seems to require a considerable period of time before the leaders of these new PSROs come to realize that (1) there is no generally accepted model except the

"foundation" structure that has been promoted by the DHEW and (2) "quality assurance" cannot simply be tacked on to the other PSRO reviews.

On the basis of all experience to date, it appears that the most that can be achieved with current PSRO methods is identification of bottom-of-the-barrel performance by some hospitals. This is an important contribution, but much more is required if PSROs are to succeed in providing a unique service to the entire community: assuring a basic standard of quality in all hospitals in its area. To attempt this with realistic expectations of what can be achieved, PSROs will require the guidance and direct assistance of individuals who understand the epidemiologic approach to the analysis of medical care. Until such expertise is available on site, PSROs will make slow progress toward this goal.

A final pitfall is that inherent in the specific formula for quality assurance provided the PSROs by the BQA—MCEs combined with continuing education.[6] This is not the most effective combination for promptly removing important deficiencies. Yet PSROs are led to believe that this will satisfy the federal requirements. One could say that most PSROs are passively responding, not actively initiating new approaches. As the BQA moves more directly in support of the principle that PSROs are primarily quality assurance mechanisms, and as the pressure mounts on the BQA to transform PSROs into comprehensive review systems (hospital plus long-term care plus ambulatory care review), the BQA staff may once again issue directives intended to expedite PSRO activities in quality assurance. The direct analogy is to the steps taken initially in implementing PSRO, when the BQA took the intent of Congress literally and, like a cookie cutter, created PSROs as replicas of foundations for medical care. The same approach in the area of quality may destroy the intrinsic motivation of PSROs to devise new methods. Such initiative may be essential to the future survival of PSROs.

More passive responses to directives may accelerate the discrediting of the PSRO program's commitment and contribution to the public welfare.

PIPSRO dealt with these several issues at some length. They are explicitly dealt with in the PIPSRO's recommendations issued by the Management Committee at the conclusion of its studies in 1976.

Major Issues and Recommendations

ISSUE 1: *Federal regulation of professional mechanisms for assuring the quality of care.* The sponsors of PI were concerned that the PSRO law fundamentally changed the relationship between the private sector of medicine and the federal government in the regulation of quality. The two key questions were these: Would PSRO enable the private sector to advance its own efforts in public accountability for the quality of care? Or would PSRO merely set new precedents for federal regulation of medical care? The Management Committee agreed that the paramount issue to be addressed in its recommendations was the appropriate balance between the federal government's regulatory requirements and the private sector's voluntary activities in quality assurance.

RECOMMENDATION 1: *The following principles should guide the formulation of the respective responsibilities of DHEW and the private sector in the regulation of quality assurance:*

1. DHEW has the legal responsibility to require an accounting by physicians and hospitals that services reimbursed by the government are necessary, of acceptable quality and provided at the appropriate level of care.
2. The private sector retains its professional responsibility to devise and continually refine methods of examining and improving the quality of care for all patients, including those whose services are paid for by the federal government.
3. The legal responsibility of DHEW to require public accounting does not extend to stipulating the exact

procedures to be used in assuring that care is necessary and of acceptable quality. DHEW can meet its legal requirements in this aspect by specifying the types of data and the documentation necessary to demonstrate that the conditions of the PSRO law are being met.
4. The private sector has the obligation to establish administrative procedures and information systems through which to document the nature and effectiveness of its procedures for reviewing and improving care. By this means, quality assurance mechanisms are made publicly accountable to all parties.
5. DHEW, directly or through designated agents, must periodically determine by inspection of the review programs that the data and documentation sent forward do represent actual procedures in use and do reflect their results.

Federal requirements for quality assurance cannot exceed the capabilities of the current state-of-the-art. DHEW should not prescribe the actual methods to be used, particularly those for which effectiveness is uncertain at best. It should instead stipulate the desired end results of those methods and the reasonable documentation of those results. This documentation then becomes the basis of the federal reporting and rendering of a satisfactory public accounting. The development and application of methods for improving the quality of care remain the responsibility of the private sector. This balance of mutual yet separate responsibilities by the government and by physicians and hospitals is more likely to serve the immediate and long-term interests of the public in quality assurance.

ISSUE 3: *Federal Administration of the PSRO Program.*

B. A second administrative issue of concern is the recent redefinition by DHEW of the PSROs' mission. Their purpose as now stated is to "assure that high quality care is delivered." The emphasis on quality, rather than on controlling costs, is sound, but the explicit expectation for excellence is at variance with the language of the law and with the potential of PSROs generally.

Throughout the law, reference to "quality" is couched in such terms as "consistent with professionally recognized and accepted patterns of care." Section 1156(b)(1) states . . . "norms of care, diagnosis, and treatment are to define acceptable modes of treatment." The intent here is realistic: physicians should be able to assure a basic standard of care for all patients whose care is paid for by federal funds. Presently, PSRO activities in quality assurance are largely limited to reviewing medical care evaluation studies (MCEs) conducted by hospitals in delegated status. Few have attempted to expedite the elimination of deficiencies uncovered in these audits. Even fewer PSROs have the capability of conducting area-wide MCEs and following through on observed deficiencies. Yet this is the unique potential of PSROs for contributing to quality assurance.

RECOMMENDATION 4: *PSROs should be assisted by a systematic program of technical development in implementing effective methods of area-wide quality assurance.*

Amounting to a sharply limited developmental program, this should be supported initially in PSROs selected for stability, potential technical capability and leadership. Its purpose is to put in place and test the range of methods applicable to PSROs for designing and carrying out effective community-wide monitoring of quality. As the methods for carrying out these professional and technical functions become more clearly defined, all PSROs can then be funded to acquire the organization, staff, and expertise needed for area-wide assurance of a basic standard of quality.

C. DHEW has yet to resolve the issue raised by State court rulings which have cast doubts on the definition of "norms, standards and criteria" used by PSROs. The PSRO program has endorsed local norms and standards as the basis of guidelines for screening the appropriateness of care given Medicare and Medicaid patients. However, legal decisions in malpractice suits have established the principle that local practice is not a suitable point of reference for judging the adequacy of quality of care. Specialist level care, for certain, is being judged by national standards in the courts. The full impact of these conflicting trends—adoption of local standards by PSROs and of national standards by courts—may not be felt until PSROs are granted full operational status.

RECOMMENDATION 5: *DHEW should assign to a working group the task of compiling and interpreting the major court rulings on the question of local vs. national standards of practice.* The National PSR Council is an appropriate sponsor of such a working group.

The premise that PSROs will abide by local standards has engendered necessary physician support. If this premise were found to be contrary to prevailing trends in judicial decisions, the credibility of PSRO as a quality assurance program could be seriously undermined. It would be well to forestall this possibility.

Public Participation

One intended product of Private Initiative was a set of recommendations on how to involve the public meaningfully in PSROs. However, the participating PSROs took no steps in this direction during the study. Accordingly, in 1975, the Management Committee enlarged its concept of public participation, endorsing the view that there are three separate aspects: 1) public representation on policy making boards; 2) education of individual patients as a component of good patient care; 3) participation by carefully selected members of the public in quality assurance and cost control activities.

Acknowledging that present DHEW policy and local circumstances preclude strong public participation in PSRO, the Management Committee adopted the position that patient education is an important aspect of public contribution. In this view, criteria for quality of care should include evidence of appropriate education of the patients regarding their own illness and their responsibilities in self-management.

In the absence of formal recommendations, the Management Committee offered the observation that persisting opposition by physicians to public participation increases the burden of proof that PSRO is becoming a productive and publicly accountable approach to quality assurance in the full contemporary meaning of these terms.

Observations and Conclusions

The information obtained by PI offers no basis for predicting how well PSROs can assure the quality of care. Delegation of responsibility for MCEs in essence recognizes the primacy of hospitals and their medical staffs in this important aspect of quality assurance. No PSRO participating in PI had, by the end of the study, established a formal means of relating reported deficiencies in care to a systematic program of continuing medical education. Nor did the PSROs make much progress in organizing community-wide programs of quality surveillance and improvement. These functions must be carried out effectively if PSROs are to assure acceptable standards of care for all Medicare and Medicaid patients.

During the PI study, PSROs carried out concurrent utilization review entirely by use of guidelines for admission and length of stay. As a consequence, the potential impact of such reviews on quality of care was minimal. The question was often raised whether such intensive use of costly professional time concurrently is actually necessary to restrain unjustified admissions and lengths of stay. It was suggested many times that the effects of such reviews on the admission practices of physicians were not a direct consequence of the reviews but rather the realization by physicians that PSRO (and fiscal intermediaries) "meant business".

The Management Committee of PI believes that there remains a good and sufficient basis for concluding that PSROs are necessary as a professionally controlled mechanism for quality assurance, interposed between the purchasers of services and the providers (physicians and hospitals) on the one side and patients on the other. Given the ever mounting pressures to restrain utilization (in the mistaken notion that this can restrain overall costs) an organization like PSROs, composed of physicians capable of setting reasonable standards and promoting their attainment, is a necessary concomitant of any program, public or private, directed to containing costs. The PSRO program is potentially the best mechanism so far devised to assure that reasonable standards of care are upheld uniformly throughout the country.

POTENTIAL

The most important potential contribution of PSRO in the field of quality is to assure a basic standard of hospital care in all hospitals in its area. One avenue has already been suggested in the discussion of the role of PSROs: upgrading the design of MCEs or the PEP audits of those hospitals whose staff is not conversant with current concepts. But no matter how sophisticated and advanced the medical audit techniques and other quality assurance mechanisms used by individual hospitals are, PSRO provides the only machinery for comparing the technical quality of care in all hospitals in its geographic area. This is fertile territory, but the task is not to be undertaken lightly. As discussed earlier, the simple-appearing model for a medical audit unfortunately conveys the impression that merely following its steps will yield the desired results. The statement that "PSROs can advance quality assurance through comparative studies of performance of hospitals" similarly conveys the simplistic notion that all that is required is the collection of similar data from hospitals and then determining what needs to be done. The experience of PIPSRO in its CQA studies is the most extensive to date in exploring the potential for areawide quality assurance. It also identified potential problems that must be addressed before a formal program can be organized with reasonable prospects of success.

The principle embodied in the CQA study of PIPSRO was the ultimate meaning of quality assurance: that each hospitalized patient receive the care appropriate to his need with minimal risk while he is in the hospital. This project was in the discussion stages when Chapter 7 of the *PSRO Program Manual* was prepared, and for that reason Section 705.21 contains the following definition: "Continued stay review is a form of medical care review which occurs during a patient's hospitalization and consists of an assessment of medical necessity of a patient's need for continued confinement at a hospital level of care and *may also include a detailed assessment of the quality of care being provided*" (emphasis added). This statement was inserted to authorize experiments in which ongoing assessment of quality would be piggybacked on the admission certification and continued-stay review procedures of PSRO. But the CQA concept went beyond this, to the very definition of quality assurance, namely, that any detected deficiency would be corrected while the patient was at risk. Because of the pertinence of CQA results to the potential of PSROs as quality assurance mechanisms, a summary of the CQA procedure, results, and implications is presented here.

Design of CQA

In CQA, Medicare and Medicaid patients were to be assured of receiving essential diagnostic and therapeutic procedures, properly applied, while in the hospital. CQA was tested for periods of up to 1 year in each of five PSROs. Twenty-four randomly selected hospitals in the sites were designated as experimental hospitals, and 26 other randomly selected hospitals served as controls. Eighteen other hospitals, specifically those not engaged in PSRO reviews, were designated as matched hospitals. In these, data were collected retrospectively. In the *experimental hospitals,* the medical staffs formally agreed to abide by "essential criteria" in caring for patients with specified diagnoses, barring contraindications or other justifiable reasons. The coordinators collected information on adher-

ence to essential criteria in the course of carrying out admission certification and continued-stay review. They contacted the physician advisor for clarification of clinical information in the record and whenever it appeared that one of the essential criteria was not being met. The physician advisor decided whether there was a medical or other justification for nonadherence. It was entirely the physician advisor's decision whether to raise the question with the attending physician. Similarly, it was entirely at the option of the attending physician whether or not to comply with the criteria on the basis of his or her judgment as to what constituted proper care for that particular patient. In 22 of the 24 experimental hospitals, copies of the approved essential criteria were placed on the front of each chart included in the CQA study, usually in the form of a "dear doctor" letter.

In the *control hospitals,* no endorsement of essential criteria was requested of the medical staffs. The coordinators simply recorded whether or not the criteria were met. They contacted the physician advisor only for information or clarification, and the advisor did not contact any attending physician regarding his or her care of patients included in the CQA study. The criteria were not posted on CQA patients' charts.

CQA was based on the application of "essential criteria." These comprise elements of care that are indicated in "almost every patient" with a given diagnosis. Essential criteria comprise five categories:

1. Objective substantiation of the diagnosis
2. Documentation of presence or absence of preexisting diseases or conditions (including etiologies) that can importantly modify treatment and prognosis
3. Documentation of presence or absence of complications or conditions related to the dis-

ease that importantly influence treatment and prognosis

4. Treatment and procedures whose efficacy is scientifically established or grounded in basic principles

5. Contraindicated procedures or treatment

The second and third categories are "documentation" criteria; the fourth and fifth are "treatment" criteria.

In addition, the CQA study collected information on the immediate outcomes of hospital care that could reasonably be achieved as a result of appropriate care. These included: (1) prevention of preventable complications, (2) expected clinical status of patients at discharge, (3) expected functional status of patients at discharge, and (4) the appropriateness of discharge regimen and adequacy and stability of control.

Essential criteria and immediate outcomes were developed for seven diagnoses. A procedure manual was prepared for the guidance of each review coordinator collecting information for CQA. Each of the diagnoses had to be the primary focus of care by physicians and nurses. CQA therefore included only a highly selected group of patients with these single or primary diagnoses. The study patients were not intended to be representative of all patients with those diagnoses. PIPSRO staff in each site worked closely with the review coordinators and monitored their performance in abstracting by carrying out concurrent and retrospective reliability checks. The reliability of data was maintained between 0.94 and 0.97 as determined by independent reabstracting of a sample of records.

Summary of Results

The frequency distributions of the seven diagnoses included in the CQA study in the five PSROs are shown in Table 30-1.

TABLE 30-1.   Frequency Distributions

DIAGNOSIS	NUMBER OF ABSTRACTS
Acute myocardial infarction	2,371
Cholecystitis/cholelithiasis	1,717
Massive, acute upper gastrointestinal bleeding	936
Bacterial pneumonia	908
Bacterial urinary tract infection	397
Acute appendicitis	383
Pediatric gastroenteritis	234
Total	6,946

All case abstracts included objective substantiation of the diagnosis. For example, the diagnosis of acute appendicitis had to be confirmed on the surgical specimen before entering the patient into the CQA study.

Adherence to Essential Criteria in Experimental and Control Hospitals

When the three groups of hospitals in each site were compared on the percent of abstracts showing 100% adherence to all process criteria for all seven diagnoses, the scores for the experimental group were higher in only two sites. In two PSROs the control group had higher scores, and in the fifth site the matched hospitals had the highest percentage. The observed differences were primarily in documentation criteria. Most hospitals with residency programs had higher percentages of perfect scores, whereas hospitals without residencies had lower scores. The one large experimental hospital with residency programs that did not post the criteria on the patients' charts had lower scores than its peer group in the documentation criteria. One smaller experimental hospital that had not posted the criteria on the charts had the lowest score for documentation.

When the analysis was based on the actual percent of documentation criteria met in each site, one site emerged as showing distinctly better results in the experimental hospitals (Figure 30-1). In this site, both the PSRO medical leadership and staff gave strong support to the CQA study. The positive results are explained by the preexistence of a smoothly functioning concurrent review system and a PIPSRO staff of three talented individuals who worked in close cooperation with the PSRO to make CQA work. Equal support and dedication in other sites produced little difference in documentation because so much effort had to go into setting up the PSRO review procedures.

The three groups of hospitals were much closer together in percent of cases with perfect adherence to essential treatment criteria. These scores were higher than for documentation, and the range was

much narrower. A few hospitals were considerably below their peer group, and these hospitals were without exception in the control and matched groups. Hospitals with residencies had less clear-cut superiority on these items. The two experimental hospitals that did not post the criteria on the charts (and that had scored relatively low on documentation) scored relatively high on adherence to treatment criteria. When performance in each site was analyzed on the basis of the actual percent of treatment criteria met, the average of the experimental group was higher than the average performance of control and matched hospitals in all sites (Figure 30-2). This indicates that CQA had a uniform impact in all sites in increasing the percent of patients in the study that received appropriate treatment.

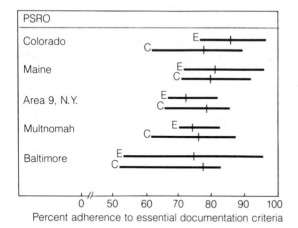

FIGURE 30-1. Range of percent adherence to documentation criteria in CQA study in participating hospitals of five PSROs, 1975–1976. (E = experimental hospitals; C = control and matched hospitals; —+— = mean value.)

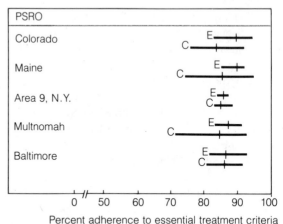

FIGURE 30-2. Range of percent adherence to essential treatment criteria in CQA study in participating hospitals of five PSROs, 1975–76. (E = experimental hospitals; C = control and matched hospitals; —+— = mean value.)

Variations in Patient Outcomes

When the three groups of hospitals were compared on patients' attainment of expected outcomes, no one group had a consistently higher score. Analysis revealed that the degree of adherence to documentation criteria was unrelated to the degree of attainment of expected outcome status. Patients who had perfect documentation scores had no better outcome status than patients whose records were deficient in documentation. However, analysis did show a significant association between adherence to treatment criteria and satisfactory outcomes in bacterial pneumonia and between inappropriate treatment and death in acute myocardial infarction.

The range in attainment of expected immediate outcomes of care was very wide. The variation among the five PSRO areas in three diagnoses is shown in Figure 30-3. The percent of cases with preventable complications or unsatisfactory clinical outcomes is significantly different in cholecystitis with cholecystectomy and in bacterial pneumonia. The number of cases of acute appendicitis in the first and third sites is too small to support statistical analysis. But if larger samples produced comparably low percentage of unsatisfactory results in these two, the results in the other three sites would be significantly worse.

Substantial variations in percent of cases with deficient outcomes were observed among hospitals in all sites (Figure 30-4). Much of the variation is attributable to small sample sizes. If hospitals with

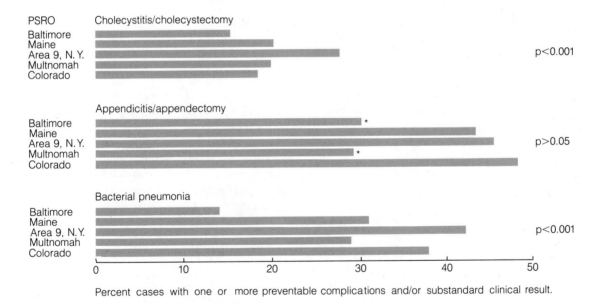

FIGURE 30-3.   Percent of cases with deficient outcomes in three diagnoses in CQA study, 1975–1976, by geographic site (pooled data from 68 hospitals). (* = fewer than 35 cases; not included in analysis.)

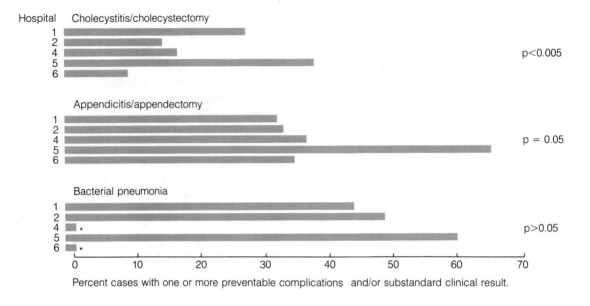

FIGURE 30-4. Percent of cases with deficient outcomes in three diagnoses in five hospitals of one PSRO. (* = fewer than 15 cases; not included in analysis.)

fewer than 20 cases are eliminated, the range of deficient outcome percentages may shrink considerably. The interhospital outcome variability may vanish, or one particular hospital may be identified as an "outlier" (Figure 30-5). The variation between hospital B and the others could represent an artifact of the radiologist or failure to adhere to essential treatment criteria. In this instance, hospital B adhered to essential criteria for use of antibiotics in 62% of its patients, as compared with hospitals A, C, and D that scored better than 85% on those criteria. Such analyses are one of PSRO's most powerful tools for screening its hospitals for potentially serious deficiencies in outcomes.

Some hospitals in the CQA study with very low outcome scores had unusually high proportions of Medicaid patients or unusually high proportions of patients over age 75, or both. This suggests that some patient factors or associated hospital factors (or both) may play a role in explaining the low outcome scores for these hospitals. Those hospitals with unusually high outcome scores, however, showed no common pattern. They were large and small, public or private, with or without residencies.

Length of Stay

Length of hospital stay was analyzed by source of payment and patient age and by diagnosis for each of the five locations (Tables 30-2 and 30-3). The length of stay increased with increasing age of patients, but no other consistent pattern was ap-

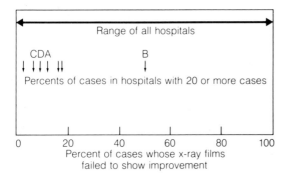

FIGURE 30-5.   Comparison of distribution of deficient clinical results in bacterial pneumonia for all
hospitals *(upper)* and for hospitals with 20 or more
cases in one PSRO.

parent. Adherence to all essential criteria did not
increase the length of stay.

Feasibility of CQA

Information collected during and after the CQA
study supports the conclusion that CQA is compatible with PSROs' concurrent reviews and that its
costs in time and money are reasonable.

In CQA, an average of 3 hours' orientation of
review coordinators followed by an average of one
half hour of biweekly monitoring by reliability
checks and discussion sufficed to maintain accuracy and completeness of CQA abstracts well
above 90%. Review coordinators devoted an average of 11 minutes to completing each abstract. The
total time devoted to abstracting was 1350 hours.
The dollar value of their services, using the average salary at each site, was $7702. Physician ad-
visors donated a total of 47 hours. At an hourly rate
of $35, the value of the time in dollars, is $1645.

The total direct dollar costs of collecting the
data—$9347—are modest, considering that the
product was seven subarea MCEs. The argument
could be advanced that piggybacking data collection for medical audits on the continued-stay
review function is less costly and yields more complete data than the usual retrospective approach.

A mail survey of review coordinators and
physician advisors who participated in the study
revealed mixed responses by the latter and strong
endorsement by the former. The reservations expressed by physicians centered on doubts concerning the efficacy of CQA; the principle behind it
was not generally challenged. The great majority
of review coordinators strongly endorsed CQA
even though they considered it an added burden on
top of an already demanding daily schedule of
duties. But nurse review coordinators with recent
clinical experience strongly supported the use of
essential criteria to monitor patient management
and status. It was evident that review coordinators
were frequently being called on to certify extensions in instances in which the clinical care of the
patient was not adequately documented. The instances of negative or pessimistic responses from
review coordinators were of two origins: belief that
review of care can best be done retrospectively (a
position taken by the few medical record personnel
serving as review coordinators) and serious doubts
that "anything would come of it" in the absence of
strong physician support.

It is reasonable to ask whether the function of
physician advisor is compatible with the role of
monitoring the quality of care. If there were disagreements with attending staff in the monitoring,
the physician advisor could lose his or her effectiveness in controlling utilization. The answer may
be twofold: (1) a clear understanding of the mutual
responsibilities and separate authorities of the
PSRO, hospital, and medical staff of the hospital,
and (2) designation of a physician consultant other
than the physician advisor when a technique like
CQA is used for concurrent monitoring and intervention for purposes of quality assurance.

TABLE 30-2. Median Length of Stay for CQA Cases Excluding Pediatric Gastroenteritis by Pay Source, Age, and Geographic Site, 1975–1976

GEOGRAPHIC SITE	MEDICARE		MEDICAID		PRIVATE	
	(45–64)	(65–84)	(15–44)	(45–64)	(15–44)	(45–64)
Area 9, N.Y.	18.0	17.3	9.9	16.0	7.6	14.2
Baltimore	15.6	16.4	9.2	12.9	—	—
Maine	13.0	13.6	7.9	13.8	—	—
Multnomah	10.2	11.7	7.6	9.5	6.7	8.2
Colorado	13.1	13.0	7.5	10.1	—	—

TABLE 30-3. Median Length of Stay by Diagnosis in CQA Study, 1975–1976, in Five PSROs

DIAGNOSIS	AREA 9, N.Y.	BALTIMORE	MAINE	MULTNOMAH	COLORADO
Acute myocardial infarction	19.4	18.8	15.9	13.5	15.5
Bacterial pneumonia	14.7	11.2	9.4	9.4	10.6
Bacterial urinary tract infection	11.0	7.3	12.0	8.1	9.3
Pediatric gastroenteritis	4.0	5.1	3.8	4.8	6.0
Acute upper gastrointestinal bleeding	11.6	12.3	12.1	10.6	9.5
Acute appendicitis	6.2	8.2	7.5	5.2	8.0
Cholecystitis	10.7	12.7	11.3	9.5	11.1

Reports of CQA Results to PSROs and Hospitals

Reports of the CQA study were furnished each participating PSRO. Each participating hospital that so requested was sent a complete summary of its data; the data were displayed so as to prevent identification of any other PSRO or any other hospital. Reports sent to each site and to each hospital requesting them included tables showing the rank order of all participating hospitals in that PSRO on the percent of abstracts with 100% adherence to the essential criteria and those with 100% attainment of expected outcomes. Using this rank ordering, each hospital can readily establish its own position relative to all other local (unidentified) participating hospitals by CQA grouping (experimental, control, or matched) and to the local and national median. By examining the actual scores on each criterion for each diagnosis in relation to relevant factors, the medical staff can ascertain whether it considers their ranking to be satisfactory or unsatisfactory.

Each site and each hospital also received graphs that provide a national perspective on the relative position of each hospital and PSRO. Using these as background, each PSRO in conjunction with the hospitals can proceed to analyze the hospitals' performance in the light of numbers of patients; patient mix, especially age; source of payment; type of hospital; and other local factors that could have a bearing on the results.

It is each PSRO's responsibility, in collaboration with the staffs of participating hospitals, to determine whether further data collection is needed or whether corrective actions are already clearly indicated. The data and these determinations for each of the seven diagnoses were to be summarized and submitted to the BQA as official reports on seven subarea MCEs.

Implications of CQA Study for PSROs

Experience acquired in the CQA study and its preliminary results have both substantive and procedural implications for the quality assurance functions of PSROs.

1. Degree of detail in the history and physical examination, that is, adherence to documentation criteria, has no demonstrable relationship to outcomes and is not a suitable topic for MCEs.

2. Treatment criteria can be validated by outcomes to only a limited extent in the PSRO population because the advanced age of patients also influences outcomes. For restrospective MCEs based on treatment criteria in the Medicare population, PSROs should use essential criteria that are externally validated, that is, by

sound clinical studies of efficacy. What should be measured is the appropriateness and correctness of application of independently validated essential criteria in establishing a correct diagnosis and instituting appropriate management.

3. The fact that adherence to essential criteria did not increase the length of stay should be reassuring to those who fear that use of criteria inevitably increases hospital stay.

4. If the board and staff of PSROs endorse and promote CQA, it will likely be acceptable to a majority of physicians if directed to important problems. The collection of accurate and reliable medical care evaluation data as part of continued-stay review by coordinators is feasible technically and appears to be cost effective.

5. The CQA technique lends itself well to objective concurrent monitoring of known or suspected deficiencies in the timing or sequence of steps necessary for the proper evaluation or management (or both) of selected classes of acutely ill patients. Examples are patients with massive acute upper gastrointestinal bleeding, severe respiratory distress, and unexplained severe chest or abdominal pain.

The CQA study has more clearly defined the task of PSROs in taking up "quality assurance" within a community perspective. The results of the study confirm what is already widely known: hospitals can vary greatly in "performance" as reflected in immediate outcomes. The PSROs are the only organizations responsible for comparing hospitals and determining whether those at the lower end of the performance scale are actually providing substandard care.

To do this, each PSRO must acquire the necessary expertise to analyze the variations objectively. As previously stated, case mix (especially the age of patients) is a vital element in the analysis. Other factors include severity of disease, effects of low socioeconomic status, and probably certain characteristics of each hospital. It is likely that after these and other local factors are corrected, variations among hospitals that can be attributed to some deficiency in performance will remain. Establishing the acceptable and effective professional machinery for performing such evaluations and instituting effective corrective measures will consume a large portion of the available resources of a PSRO and will call for additional technical help.

SUMMARY

Critics of PSRO claim that the PSRO is an unwieldy, expensive, and imprecise tool for achieving anything worthwhile in quality assurance. But the reply to such critics is the same as the reply to those who condemn the American form of government; bad as it may be, it is way ahead of whatever is in second place. The PSRO is the most valuable tool physicians presently possess to retain their historic right to self-regulation in quality. What is required is not only more enlightened redirection of effort in quality but also an acceptance of a current social and political fact of life; a more appropriate, extensive, and explicit public accounting must accompany the new effort.

The requirements for the attainment of the desired long-range goal of PSROs as a permanent quality assurance system are many. The most important is already known and demonstrated in the early history of the PSRO: local physician leadership that is capable and willing to work in the face of opposition to achieve increased support and cooperation by physicians, hospitals and all institutions that collectively contribute to quality assurance. Equally important is staff in both administrative and technical areas also capable and willing to

work for the attainment of PSRO goals. Without these two elements acting with a spirit of commitment and initiative, PSROs may well become DHEW "field offices" receiving federal money to carry out federal requirements. The PSROs that have retained the vitality that comes with local initiative demonstrate its value in the nature of their work, and in the stature they achieve in the eyes of private sector colleagues.

But despite the most capable and committed leadership, PSROs can do little in quality without the full cooperation of all hospitals, large and small, as corporate entities and of their medical staffs. The still widely prevalent "them versus us" attitude often stands in the way. Failures of honest and direct communication between the PSRO staff and hospital administrators still lead to unjustified misgivings and preventable problems in their relationships. It seems evident that hospitals stand to lose much more autonomy if PSROs go under than if PSROs survive and succeed. The motivation is surely there on both sides for a renewed pledge of sincere cooperation in "quality assurance."

Given the achievement of these fundamental prerequisites, the next requirement is highly focused technical assistance to PSROs in organizing a formal quality assurance program. The technical complexities of performing areawide MCEs have not been adequately presented to PSROs despite the otherwise excellent workshops supported by the BQA. Yet a nucleus of professional leadership inside and outside the PSRO must grasp what is involved in such efforts. This can best come about through some form of continuing education on this subject directed specifically to the average physician and average member of a hospital board of trustees.

In a parallel with this local education effort that must be sustained, there is the equal requirement of a technical staff that is competent to design and implement areawide assessments. This staff should also understand the professional constraints within which this highly sensitive activity must be carried out. An inept technical expert may do more disservice than service and may make it more difficult for successors to gain credibility and access.

In both of these undertakings (sustained programs of continuing education in communitywide quality assurance and provision through professionally oriented individuals of adequate technical assistance), private funds and contributed time and effort should comprise substantial sources of support. If these activities are supported entirely by federal funds, the medical profession and the hospital field are in essence saying that the government can indeed pay the piper and call the tune in quality assurance. This would be an unfortunate reversal of the profession's historic stance. The attempt to achieve equity in quality of care involves such high stakes for the American public that private philanthropic foundations should respond to the opportunity where the potential for creating sound models seems unusually bright.

The promise, perspective, pitfalls, and potential of the PSROs in quality assurance as discussed here amount to a brief kaleidoscopic view of some of the important considerations. They are merely prologue. To face the future prospects, one's view should be realistic and pragmatic. Simply stated, in expending their first billion dollars, PSROs must emerge as professionally competent organizations seriously pursuing and attaining the assurance of a basic standard of quality for their communities. The profession has yet to produce an alternative model with a greater potential for achieving this political and societal mandate.

REFERENCES

1. Goran, M. J. 1976. The future of quality assurance in health care: next steps from the perspective of the federal government. *Bull. N.Y. Acad. Med.* 52:177–184.

2. U.S. Department of Health, Education, and Welfare. *PSRO fact book.* May 1977. Washington, D.C.: Health Care Financing Administration, Office of Health Standards and Quality.

3. Sanazaro, P. J. 1975. Private initiative in PSRO. *New. Engl. J. Med.* 293:1023–1028.

4. Committee on Finance. U.S. Senate. Sept. 26, 1972. Report 92–1230.

5. U.S. Department of Health, Education, and Welfare. March 15, 1974. *PSRO program manual.* Rockville, Md.: Public Health Service, Health Services Administration, Bureau of Quality Assurance.

6. Jessee W. F.; Munier, W. B.; Fielding, J. F., et al. 1975. PSRO: an educational force for improving quality of care. *N. Engl. J. Med.* 292:668–671.

7. Averill, R. F., McMahon, L. F. Jr. 1977. A cost benefit analysis of continued stay certification. *Med. Care* 15:158–173.

8. Lave, L., Jr. 1976. An evaluation of a hospital stay regulatory mechanism. *Am. J. Public Health* 66:959–967.

9. Brook, R. H., Williams, K. N. 1976. Evaluation of the New Mexico peer review system, 1971–1973. *Med. Care* 14 (suppl.) 12.

10. Sanazaro, P. J.; Goldstein, R. L.; Roberts, J. S., et al. 1972. Research and development in quality assurance: the experimental medical care review organization program. *N. Engl. J. Med.* 287:1125–1131.

11. *Assessing quality in health care: an evaluation.* 1976. Washington, D.C.: Institute of Medicine, National Academy of Sciences.

12. Goran, M. J.; Roberts, J. S.; Kellogg, M., et al. 1975. The PSRO hospital review system. *Med. Care* 13 (suppl.) 18.

13. Nelson, A. R. 1976. Orphan data and the unclosed loop: a dilemma in PSRO and medical audit. *N. Engl. J. Med.* 295:617–619.

14. Payne, B. C. 1967. Continued evolution of a system of medical care appraisal. *J.A.M.A.* 201:536–540.

15. Payne, B. C., Lyons, T. F. 1972. *Method of evaluating and improving personal medical care quality: episode of illness study.* Ann Arbor, Mich.: University of Michigan Press.

16. Sanazaro, P. J. 1976. Medical audit, continuing medical education, and quality assurance. *West. J. Med.* 125:241–252.

17. American Medical Association Advisory Committee on PSRO. 1974. PSRO and norms of care. A report by the Task Force on Guidelines of Care. *J.A.M.A.* 229:166–171.

18. Welch, C. E. 1975. PSRO: guidelines for criteria of care. *J.A.M.A.* 232:47–50.

19. American Medical Association. June 1976. *Sample criteria for short-stay hospital review: screening criteria to assist PSROs in quality assurance.* Chicago: The Association.

31

Evaluation

Mildred A. Morehead

Unquestionably the "bottom line" for the future of the PSRO program will depend on the perception of the public and Congress, and to a lesser extent, the profession, of the impact that is made on the cost and quality of health services. Even to begin to address this issue will require accumulating a body of evidence that will show to the satisfaction of at least some of the players that the vast amounts of money, effort, and bureaucracy that have gone into this program are worthwhile. Furthermore, not only will extensive evaluation be necessary, but contrary to other such efforts, the results will, perforce, have to be positive, because data that fail to show any impact on the cost and quality of care will not be considered significant negative findings. If PSROs cannot show appreciable change or improvement in health care after their advent on the scene, it is probable that their days as a separate entity will be limited.

All of this places a heavy burden on those responsible for designing, accumulating, and analyzing data, and under the best of circumstances, answers will not be found in a short period of time. It is sad but true that our energetic country is geared to the "instant solution" and "quick answer," and when these are not forthcoming, patience is lost, funds diminish, and the public and Congress are off in search of another "innovative" or "definite" answer.

Quite aside from the problems created by pressures for instant success, there will be serious difficulties in identifying cause and effect among the various agencies and forces that are involved in the complex health scene. From the evaluator's standpoint, difficulties are also arising from unproved or newly developed methodologies available to measure effectiveness of PSRO efforts on the community, the providers, and patients.

Similar problems will also exist in efforts to examine the methodologies employed by the PSROs and the effectiveness of internal operations of individual programs.

I. OBJECTIVES OF THE PSROs

If the overall objectives of the PSRO program are considered, there are three major areas where evaluation efforts should concentrate.

1. Improved Quality of Care

In the past, reduction of mortality and morbidity have been equated to a considerable extent with the assumption that there has been improvement in health services. However, it has become increasingly apparent that many of the factors that led to longer life and a decrease in morbidity are not really a direct result of medical care per se. Improvements in economic and environmental status of many groups in the population as well as improved nutrition, education, and general living standards may well have contributed more to such health indices than the services offered by the health profession. Today, to examine questions related to improved quality of health care, more complex issues need to be faced: Is diagnosis being made at an earlier stage for those conditions where therapeutic intervention can reduce mortality and morbidity? Does greater access to preventive measures and maintenance care (such as prenatal or well-child care) reduce mortality and morbidity? With the increasing size of the therapeutic armamentarium, are we avoiding iatrogenic disease? Are appropriate medications prescribed and, more important, taken by the asymptomatic patient for conditions where their use is preventive, such as hypertension? Many of these issues are not yet being addressed by the majority of the PSROs, where concentration has been limited primarily to in-hospital utilization issues. But even in this more limited area, can we expect the inpatient review activities to have impact on the quality of care provided? Will definitive diagnoses be established earlier, and how can this acceleration be documented? How can unnecessary surgery be identified, or conversely, how can the necessity be demonstrated so that the arguments swirling about this issue can be stilled and action taken if indicated? Will consultants be brought into the care picture at a proper time in appropriate situations? Will there be fewer complications and less surgical mortality? Will patients at discharge understand their disease and the prescribed future regimen? These are not easy questions to answer, and again, the current methodologies are by no means able to address all of these issues in a clear-cut fashion.

2. Appropriate Use of Resources

Questions relating to the appropriate use of resources range from consideration of institutional beds (acute care, SNF, ICF, domiciliary, and so forth) to diagnostic modalities (CAT scanners) and treatment modalities (open heart surgery, organ transplants). Each of these will require specifically designed studies to answer the questions posed.

There will be a need to address the appropriate use of the increasing number of health professionals trained to provide care from subspecialties within the medical profession itself to midlevel practitioners in both medical and dental practice. The PSROs have yet to address in any depth the activities or the quality and cost implications of many of the professions that are allied to the physician-hospital axis (such as the optometrist, podiatrist, and mental health worker).

Ancillary services, including both programmatic components (ICUs, P.T.) as well as specific diagnostic and therapeutic modalities, will also need to be examined in relation to both quality and underutilization or overutilization. This area too is just beginning to emerge as an organized activity within a few PSROs.

3. Reduction of Health Care Costs

Not very subtly camouflaged behind the concern for the quality of health care lies a PSRO mandate to reduce health care costs. As governmental agencies at all levels and professional and consumer groups are aware, this, too, is a highly complex area. Patient demands, provider demands, and community demands are often at cross purposes: the public demands access to life-saving measures that are too expensive for the ordinary citizen to afford, and the profession demands access to the newest diagnostic modalities irrespective of questions of efficient utilization. Communities demand their "own" hospital and their "own" ambulance regardless of how much more sensible it would be if resources were designed and placed within a regional network rather than locally based.

Even if cost reductions are accomplished by PSRO efforts among providers and facilities in utilization and use of appropriate resources, it is clear that without close linkage with other agencies (particularly the Health Systems Agencies, which are able to bring about system changes), maximum benefits will not be obtained.

Although there can be anticipations that hospital care costs will be contained by PSRO efforts, the possibility exists that when unnecessary admissions and lengths of stay are decreased, the remaining patient days will be of higher cost because of the more serious nature of illnesses and the need for more of the expensive modalities available.

What cost reductions could occur in the ambulatory care field can only be speculative. Conceivably, inappropriate actions could be minimized, but could this in any manner counterbalance the expenditures required to see that all of the population has access to a high quality of preventive and maintenance care? It seems unlikely that this will be the case.

The complexities of the accounting systems of hospitals, outpatient departments, and emergency rooms have resulted in cost figures for these areas that appear to be totally unrealistic from the standpoint of the physicians, the patients, or the agencies involved in reimbursement. What conceivable effect the most active of PSROs could have on the cost of a single outpatient department visit is debatable in view of the current method of computing such costs.

Again, it must be stressed that primary responsibility for system changes, particularly in the areas of facilities and financing, rest elsewhere than

with the PSROs. Without such changes, it is unlikely that appreciable reductions in health care costs will be brought about solely by the PSROs.

II. MEASUREMENT TOOLS

Difficult and complex as the questions are that need to be asked to assess the impact of the PSRO program, they are equaled by the difficulties that exist in selecting the measurement tools to answer the questions. There are no universally accepted measurement tools for assessing the quality of care. The past decade has seen a proliferation of initials representing various approaches: PEP, QAP, MCAP CQAS, PACE, ASPERF, and so forth, all of which have vigorous proponents. Elaborate data systems have been set up in many of the government-funded programs (C&Y, CHS, FP) both to examine utilization and to obtain data that would permit inferences concerning the quality of services provided. None of these has been eminently successful, and all have been either gradually or abruptly discarded. As in other endeavors, the multiplicity of views indicates that definitive answers are lacking, that there is no universally accepted way of examining and reaching determinations of the quality of health care that would be acceptable to the majority of the spectators in the audience.

1. Structure, Process, and Outcome

Donebedian has classified the approach to quality measurement in three dimensions—structure, process, and outcome.[1] Within each area are numerous subcomponents and no universal agreement, not only about measurement tools, but about how to relate the three approaches.

Structural measurements have been utilized throughout the greater part of this century as almost the sole measurement of the adequacy of health care. Indeed, in the early part of the century and today in underdeveloped countries it is useless to inquire into the more sophisticated questions such as adequacy of the diagnosis or appropriate lengths of stay where facilities, personnel, or equipment are lacking or woefully incomplete. In this country, as medical knowledge, skills, and equipment have increased, as standards of living improved and the populace became willing (and even overanxious) to secure an adequate supply of the tangible aspects of medical practice, concern about strictly structural aspects of health care (the hospital beds, the number of nurses, the presence of ambulances, and so forth) has begun to shift to questions as to whether such resources were utilized effectively. Administrative policies and procedures, which create the matrix from which medical services stem, have increasingly important implications as to who receives care, how it is given, and what follow through occurs. At the moment evaluation of these factors has not been addressed by the majority of the PSROs, and problems in these areas surface only occasionally as they are encountered in the review process or the MCEs.

To examine the effectiveness of the care provided, the major efforts in the middle years of the century were devoted to what was done to the patient, the *process* by which care was provided. There have been a few recorded efforts to do this by observation, examining just what it is the physician does to and for the patient. Among these, the studies of Osler Peterson in the review of practices of randomly selected practitioners in North Carolina were most notable.[2] Although documentation is scarce, this is still probably the most widely used unofficial way to make determinations about the adequacy of physician performance. This method is in constant use in the teaching setting, where students, interns, residents, and attendings are observed and questioned. During the process, those in leadership positions come to conclusions, stated or unstated, as to the level of performance of the individuals within their environment. This process occurs even more unofficially outside of the teaching setting, where contact between colleagues, patient comments, and reactions slowly build over time to form an informal assessment of the quality of that "superb diagnostician," or "lousy doc." As a formal measurement tool, however, observation techniques are not generally in use. First, they are expensive, and the person hours required for sufficient observations are extensive. Although an immediate negative reaction to this approach is that the person or facility being observed would change practice patterns because of the presence of observers, in the North Carolina study as well as in other settings it was not difficult to identify less than optimal practice even in the presence of the observers. Ingrained practice patterns are hard to change, and over time the holder fails to be aware of "inappropriate" action. Another difficulty with the observation technique as applied to judgments about the care of a patient is that frequently the results of the examination or tests are not known, so that sequential actions over time (important in medical judgment) are not observed, and even more important, the follow-up of the patient is not known to the observer. One could make a case that the use of concurrent review in the hospitals by the PSROs is a process somewhat related to the observation techniques. However, concurrent review falls short of the earlier studies in this area, because only the record, not the patient or the provider, is observed, and at this time, major emphasis is given to utilization rather than quality issues.

Far more common as a quality review mechanism has been the retrospective examination of the medical record, the examination of the written word combined with reports from support services or other institutions, to assess whether or not what was done for the patient was adequate. The approach to such measurements has been generally through the use of criteria either implicit or explicit.

The use of *implicit criteria* depends on the judgment of the reviewer. The instruction to specialists in specialty areas in the Teamster studies[3] was, "We are asking you to judge the quality of medical care in line with your clinical judgment and experience. You will use as a yardstick, in relation to the quality of care rendered, whether you would have treated this particular patient in this particular fashion during this specific hospital admission." Judgments were then recorded in a pass/fail breakdown, "optimal" (excellent or good); "less than optimal" (fair or poor). Greater point determinations can be made, which tend to decrease the likelihood of agreement between reviewers.

The implicit review was by far the most flexible method by which to examine the total care provided to any individual patient, but it was questioned because of concerns about the subjective nature of the judgments made, the potential difficulties in reproducibility, and the amount of time required of expensive manpower, namely, the physician. To overcome these objections, increasing attention was given to *explicit review:* the development of criteria that could be applied to all similar cases, record abstracting by nonphysicians, and analysis as to what degree of adherence to the criteria existed. This approach could be performed and reproduced with relative ease. As the development of criteria and standards proliferated throughout the country, weaknesses in this approach also began to cause concern. Even though physician groups sat for long hours developing criteria for various conditions or health status examinations, the length of the lists proliferated,

until at one time the specialty academies of medicine and pediatrics had criteria extending into the hundreds of items to measure even the simplest of conditions. This increased not only the time involved in performing reviews but also increased the concern that such "laundry lists" would escalate the cost of health care unnecessarily without any solid evidence that many of the items were relevant to patient care.

In part to overcome these objections, methodologies that stressed examination of patient *outcome* came to the forefront. This was to be the most effective measure, because obviously the objective of health care was to improve the patients' and communities' health, and whether or not this occurred was really the only question that needed to be asked. Unfortunately, this simplistic approach has also rapidly proved not to be the panacea that was expected. There are too many conditions where medical science does not have the knowledge that permits successful intervention, where the natural history of the disease is not well understood and where the resilience of the human body can withstand medical intervention and can improve regardless of what is done. The eminent surgeon reviewer, Samuel Standard, had frequent occasion to refer to his maxim, "Folly that succeeds is still folly."

Although there are some conditions where the outcome approach is worthwhile and where adequate data exist to show that intervention will bring about improvement (for example, hypertension), a vast number of conditions remain where this is not the case, and to base judgments on outcome alone will not succeed in measuring either the effect of medical care or the role of the provider in delivering that care.

Observation of data relating to mortality, morbidity, and utilization over time is a time-honored measurement of change. Clearly, the most obvious way to show the impact of the PSROs is to examine such data before their operations began and to look again after they have been in operation. But like most simple questions, this will not give simple answers. There are indications that the lengths of hospital stays were falling in many areas before the advent of the PSROs, perhaps in part due to the emphasis placed on utilization review by the Medicare legislation, perhaps due to other factors, such as the decline in infectious disease incidence, so noticeable in the decrease in pediatric bed usage throughout the country. Although there are some PSROs where data are beginning to show decreases in both length of stay and in the number of admissions, data from which to make comparisons are not always readily available, are difficult to piece together from past records, and are subject to differences in interpretation when previous trends show a similar decline.

Another attractive approach would be to examine the effect of PSROs by comparing areas that do or do not have such programs in operation. This, too, will present problems, because the required matching of similar characteristics, ranging from diagnoses to characteristics of patients and providers, will be difficult.

2. PSRO Measurement Tools

The data system designed to examine the functioning of the PSRO programs is described elsewhere in this book. Considerable information is being accumulated at both the local and national levels about activities of physician advisors, the denial of patient days, the number of MCEs, and the like. Although this information will permit examination of activity levels and relationships to expended funds, of themselves they provide little or no information on the impact of the program activities on the delivery scene.

Data that contain information on individual hospital discharges are slowly beginning to ac-

cumulate also. In the future, considerable information from which to make comparisons among different PSRO areas in relation to diagnosis, length of stay, surgical procedures, mortality, and a few other basic demographic patient characteristics will be available. These data may well set the stage for future questions regarding medical practice in different areas, but the answers to these questions will in large part rest on further examinations at the local level.

The hospital data tapes will also contain extensive information about individual providers and their patterns of practice. These profiles have long been awaited by many of the PSROs as the first tool that will emerge that will enable intervention, be it educational or punitive. Here, too, the parameters will be somewhat limited: lengths of stay that are out of line, mortality that appears excessive, surgical procedures that do not appear to fit with the diagnosis. Again, these profiles will raise many questions, and the final answers will depend to a large extent on further explorative efforts to delineate the factors that caused the variations to determine whether the provider was indeed responsible or whether extenuating circumstances existed. Analysis of such data and, more important, subsequent action will depend primarily on the availability of local expertise to raise and answer the questions and on the willingness of the physician leadership to address issues that are going to be very difficult in view of the profession's longstanding reluctance to criticize peers or to undertake action that may impinge on a peer's freedom of action and professional judgment.

Current data from the reporting system relating to MCEs will not be helpful in examining the impact of these activities on care practices because of their simplistic nature (number of studies, hours, and so forth). It is exceedingly unlikely, for example, that the number of MCEs performed on cholecystectomy could be related in any meaningful overall fashion to reductions in mortality or complications.

On the local level, there will be a greater opportunity to examine in depth how specific diagnoses or problems are addressed, what the findings are, what action is taken, and what effect such studies have on patterns of care. Some of these may prove dramatic, as the marked increase in use of packed red blood cells for transfusion in the Washington, D.C. area reported by that PSRO or the increase in Pap smears noted by the Colorado PSRO. Others will be more difficult to document. Many of the observed deficiencies that are surfacing from the MCEs are related to problems of documentation, and even though there is almost universal agreement that the quality of recording improves after PSRO exposure, this, too, is difficult to document and, in many instances, difficult to relate to any actual improvements in the quality of care provided.

At this time, as previously mentioned, difficulties continue in the methodologies employed, so that, wisely, there has been no national push to assure that identical approaches are used throughout the nation. Even the PEP format, encouraged by the JCAH, is being seriously reviewed by that organization, because it is becoming clear that rigid adherence to that particular form is by no means the perfect answer to auditing. Although lack of uniformity will allow individual initiative and encourage further developmental efforts, it will not in the foreseeable future allow national comparisons of findings to be made so that conclusions could be drawn on the effectiveness and impact of this increasingly time-consuming and expensive activity.

Review of ancillary services for the hospitalized patient is just beginning to be addressed by a number of PSROs. This, too, will require accumulation of a considerable amount of data before inferences can be made as to whether or not concentration on this area has led to a reduction of unnecessary tests or procedures or to the increased use of such procedures where indicated. Again, data sets themselves in all likelihood will not provide the definitive solutions but merely will point the direction where further in-depth studies may provide the answers to the questions raised.

3. General Measurement Tools

The traditional measurements of an area's health status—mortality and morbidity data—will continue to remain tools to examine change. It is possible, for example, that concentration on obstetrical practices by an individual PSRO might result in lowering of perinatal mortality, prematurity, or other indices. Other improvements might be noted from changes made in the health care delivery system, be they by an individual provider or on an areawide basis. Here again, however, the difficulties in isolating the causative factors and attributing solely to the PSRO any changes observed will be difficult and are bound to be debated by other groups with different self-interests but similar motives to act as change agents.

The national health surveys, which illuminate many aspects of health care practices and patterns, have been a valuable tool in recent decades. These detailed studies permit analysis of not only what happens to recipients of care but also by inference the activities of health care providers.

The financial data available to the federal agencies involved with financing health care have not yet been examined in conjunction with PSRO activities to any extent. The recent merger of the PSRO program with the Title XVIII and XIX funding agencies should improve communication and facilitate linking cost data in a given area with the degree of the PSRO effort.

Many states also have resources to examine both cost and quality issues. States have already manifested uneasiness at having a physician-dominated agency responsible for the extent of their financial commitment and will be watching the cost issues closely. The few states that have contributed heavily to the Medicaid program are increasingly concerned with dollar expenditures, and cost is a far more burning issue among them than it is even at the national level. Concerns regarding quality appear to be even further down the list of priorities at the state level than they are at the national agency level. There are, however, exceptions to this. The Office of Health Systems Management of New York State has recently sponsored a major effort to develop a combined explicit-implicit method to examine the quality of both in-hospital and ambulatory care.[4]

The multitude of agencies already involved in gathering health statistics, from the American Hospital Association to voluntary agencies concerned with specific disease entities, will or should be examining in considerable detail the possible impact of PSRO activities on their special area of interest.

III. SPECIFIC AREAS REQUIRING EVALUATION

Overall answers to questions relating to the effectiveness of the PSRO effort undoubtedly will be based on a series of evaluations directed to the parts of the system where the major activities of the PSRO occur. As these activities are being phased in, it will take considerable time before answers for many questions are forthcoming. At the present time, the major program effort has been on the acute-care facilities, although a few PSROs are beginning to examine long-term care facilities and the ways that ambulatory care might be examined.

1. Acute-care Facilities

The questions relating to a decrease in the length of stay have already been mentioned; this is one area where the answers may be forthcoming in the relatively near future. In at least one PSRO area, however, questions already are being raised as to whether this reduction has led to a higher readmission rate, with the implication that perhaps the shortened stays occurred to the detriment of the patient's health. The issue of readmission rates should be part of the data sets being developed to analyze length-of-stay questions.

Determining the necessity for admission is also one of the prime objectives of the PSRO review system. Data acquired to date, however, show that very few (too few in the minds of many) admissions are being questioned and that some of the questions being asked will not enable clear answers to emerge. At this time, no serious effort is being made to assure confirmation of the diagnosis of the patient on admission. The present practices of not examining the patient and avoiding any questions relating to the necessity of surgery leave large gaps in the process of obtaining firm answers to the question of appropriateness of the admission.

Questions regarding costs of the hospitalized patient have already been mentioned. Will the diminution of unnecessary or inappropriate admissions and lengths of stays lead to a reduction of cost, and how much? If such reductions raise the cost level in specific institutions (such as tertiary care centers), will the total community cost be lessened by concomitant moves toward a reduction in beds? Do patterns of management of specific disease entities across institutions reflect different cost levels, and what can be said about efforts to equalize cost without at the same time impacting in a negative fashion on the quality of care provided? The same can be asked about the use of specific ancillary services on an areawide basis. Are there facilities where routine screening procedures of one type or another are provided without adequate medical indication and that merely escalate cost? Are there practices of specific providers that have cost and quality implications where intervention can bring improvements? One PSRO reported identifying a physician using extensive physical therapy modalities on patients with myocardial infarction; peers determined on further examination that such practice resulted not only in unnecessary costs but in detriment to the patients, and the practice was stopped. Much of the impact of the PSRO activities may occur in individualized practices in isolated settings, and presently there is no definite way to identify and compile information on such occurrences.

The concurrent review process itself should be more closely examined. This was introduced on a nationwide basis without a great deal of evidence to demonstrate its effectiveness. The lack of experimentation with review mechanisms has been commented on elsewhere,[5] and although the sense of urgency to have a uniform system in place is understandable, the opportunity is almost lost to examine whether other mechanisms might prove more effective.

2. Long-term Care Facilities

The weaknesses and lack of facilities to provide care to the patient who does not require acute hospital care but is not able to function independently in a home environment or does not have such an environment available are already beginning to surface as major problems causing inappropriate use of the acute facility and of skilled nursing home facilities. By ongoing evaluation studies of the use and impact of the use of such facilities, the PSROs may have data to support one of the most valuable contributions that can be made to the delivery system. In addition, continued patient studies that examine not only the quality of care but the level of patient function, both physical and psychologic, may lead to cost savings in the delivery system as well as improved quality of life for an untold number of the population.

Even more than acute hospital care, studies of the patients in long-term care facilities should be multidisciplinary in nature. Is physical function maximized by careful exposure to the physical therapy modalities? Is motivation encouraged, and are suitable recreational or work tasks available? Is nutritional status maintained? Do dentures provide proper occlusion? Have the surveillance efforts of the PSRO brought about improvement in these aspects of life? The slower entrance into the long-term care area will permit baseline studies that frequently were not conducted when the PSROs moved rapidly into the acute hospital field.

The movement of patients to appropriate facilities—skilled nursing homes, intermediate-care facilities, and domiciliary or protected environment—will provide opportunities to evaluate the cost to families and communities of the various levels of care, but inquiries should also be directed at the impact on patients and their families of the changes in patient ability to adapt, to improve or suffer from such relocations. Should studies of this nature indicate that there are adverse effects of relocation, particularly to the elderly, alternate types of payment, resources, and personnel might be employed to improve patient adjustment and to contain cost. As in other areas under the purview of the PSRO, documentation of the effectiveness and impact of the health delivery system will enable society to make more rational choices as to the level of funding and commitment that they are willing to place in health care.

3. Ambulatory Care

Some argue that if improvements were made in ambulatory care, not only would inappropriate use and the necessity of hospitalization be diminished, but the population's health status would also improve.[6] Just how much the cost of ambulatory care would be increased as a result of such efforts is speculative, because little has been done to document unmet ambulatory care needs that run the gamut of needs, from health assessments and immunizations to home care services and telephone support services (AA, drug abuse, suicide prevention, and so on). Evaluation efforts in ambulatory care must focus on the services provided as well as on those segments of the population who do not but should receive service.

Evaluation in the ambulatory sector will continue to be hampered in the foreseeable future by the lack of adequate data bases to examine the provider parameters of the questions in detail. Whether or not it will be justifiable or cost effective to introduce reporting systems for individual services remains an open question. Certainly, as previously mentioned, the federal efforts in detailed reporting systems not only to examine utilization but to glean inferences relating to quality (such as those used by the neighborhood health centers programs, the family planning programs, or the children and youth programs) were not conspicuous by their success, and after years of operation and large amounts of funds, the detailed approaches by now generally have been abandoned. Use of claims-based data is beginning to show some interesting findings,[6] and although these efforts are directed almost solely to gross deviations that come close to serving the purpose of identifying fraud and abuse rather than quality issues, perhaps this is a necessary first step.

The questions that need to be asked about the ambulatory sector are numerous. Obtaining the information will be time consuming, expensive, and as in other areas, not accomplished by any one specific approach. However, because this is by far the most frequent point of patient contact with the health delivery system, detailed evaluation studies of usage, quality, and cost are imperative. Among the issues that must be addressed are: What proportion of the population do receive health assessments? Of what do these consist? Do they indicate prudent use of resources, both manpower (nurse practitioners, physician assistants, and so forth) and technologic (tests and procedures)? Is the yield from the procedures employed such that they can be considered reasonably cost effective when employed on a communitywide basis? Are steps being taken to adjust the content and frequency of such examinations on an age-specific basis, related to occupational or environmental hazards and followed up to assure correction of identified abnormalities?

What is the content of the ambulatory care visit? Is it appropriate in terms of provider reaction to the presenting complaint, the underlying disease, the use of medications, or the charges for the service? Is there overscheduling of patients with no demonstrable need? Is there patient understanding of the frequently multiple types of medications dispensed? Do the patients understand their illnesses sufficiently so that less expensive types of contact might well be substituted for repeated physician contact?

What is the effect on quality and cost of the patient who "shops around" for medical care? What are the underlying reasons for this, and is this affected if quality is improved? Can patient perceptions of acceptability be improved with the use of more appropriate providers, for example, more social service exposure instead of physician placebo efforts?

What is the community pattern of referrals among the various specialties? Are the cost profiles for comparable types of conditions similar? Do certain patterns of referrals or practices correlate with hospitalization usage? Can the PSRO impact on both provider and patient knowledge and behavior to bring about change to meet goals adopted by local agencies?

In all probability, organized medical care settings, such as the outpatient departments and emergency rooms, will come under PSRO scrutiny before similar efforts are attempted in the private sector. Can the PSRO become an instrument of change in seeing that the increasing use of emergency rooms for nonurgent conditions is slowed or decreased? Are there changes in outpatient department organization and resources suggested by analysis of data relating to utilization, cost, and quality of services provided as well as by patient satisfaction with these services?

When the difficult issues of access to the solo practitioners' record are overcome, what will be necessary to assure that notations of varying brevity and legibility are adequate to provide justification for the payment of funds? Changing physicians' lifelong individualistic patterns of documentation will be extremely difficult and bitterly resisted.

4. PSRO Operations

Long before many of the answers about PSRO impact on the cost and quality of health care are available, questions will be raised about the activities of the PSROs themselves, their staffing levels, functions, efficiency of operations, soundness of purpose, integrity of the questions asked, the decisions made, and the actions recommended. Because of the difficulties in answering many of the basic questions relating to program impact, short-range questions will focus at both local and national levels on current expenditures and functions. Several levels of program evaluation are possible and currently are receiving attention.

Each PSRO itself should have in place an ongoing evaluation program of the institutions for which it is responsible (be they delegated or nondelegated) but should also examine its own operations as a coordinated whole on a periodic basis to ensure that maximum efficiency is being achieved. This type of *internal evaluation* (review by those involved in the effort) has both potential strengths and weaknesses. On the positive side, continual self-assessment is said to be the most effective manner to bring about change. Those who are in a position to change policy, to reallocate staff, and to effect modification in instruments are much more apt to do so when they are convinced of the need for change. On the other hand, the myopia of those involved frequently precludes objective assessment, and therefore the credibility of the effort, the conclusions reached, and the changes undertaken may be questioned by those observing the process.

External evaluations, assessments conducted by persons not directly involved with the specific program operation, present a special problem for the PSROs. At least at this time, a cadre of persons who are sufficiently knowledgeable about the details of legislation, regulations, or program directives who cannot be said themselves to have a somewhat vested interest in the program is not available. Whether those who review the program operations come from other PSROs, from various levels of PSRO agencies (support centers, state councils, AAPSRO) or from the national funding agency, questions can and will be raised about the objectivity of assessments, the concern that one peer might be reluctant to criticize another peer. This is particularly true in the early stages of such a massive undertaking when definitive answers on the efficacies of so many of the approaches in use are not available.

The past history of other governmental agencies in evaluating their own programs has not glittered with success. Quite aside from the protectiveness that is inherent in many such operations is the question of overdependence on adherence to agency regulations and requirements. Issues of compliance seem to dominate the bureaucratic mind, whether it be evaluating a PSRO or a community mental health center. And although it is acceptable for a funding agency to see that its regulations and mandates are followed, this often falls short of evaluating the effectiveness of the operation.

The PSROs are particularly difficult to evaluate by external review because of the large numbers of sites where actual program operations occur. The current external reviews have extensive questions built in regarding activities and documents of PSRO staff, but intensive review at the facility level, which is the cornerstone of the entire effort, is limited. To examine two or three hospitals out of 40 or 50, as current site visits do, is to glean a great deal of verbiage on what people say other people do without capturing even a representative sample of what occurs at the site where policy is turned into action. Ways to increase effectiveness, relevance, and validity of these evaluative efforts are needed.

There is another aspect of external evaluations that will have an as yet undetermined impact on the quality of the reviews, and that is the recent federal Freedom of Information Act. The intent of such legislation is understandable—the public does and should have the right to know what tax dollars are being spent for and what judgments are made as to efficiency and effectiveness of federally supported programs. Yet the fact that any one sentence may be taken out of context and utilized to the detriment of either the program, the reviewers, or both is bound to have an effect on the writers of any document that purports to present both the strengths and weaknesses of a given operation.

5. Community Impact

Quite aside from possible impact on patient health status, the public perception of the PSRO activities will have considerable effect on the ability of the PSRO, institutions, agencies, and professional bodies to bring about change. A citizenry aroused by examples of elderly near-indigent patients being harassed for payment of hospital bills because of PSRO denials, the change in patterns of "hospitalizations on demand" for certain individuals, nonpayment for long-accustomed injections of placebo medication or for certain provider visits may be vastly misunderstood by a number of per-

sons in any given community. Many of the changes needed to lessen the impact of such decisions, the availability of long-term care beds, home care programs, sheltered workshops or living accommodations, are far beyond the purview of the PSRO, yet their legitimate actions in denying access to inappropriate resources may cause a short-term (and possibly not too short) opposition by the population to an agency that is viewed as creating more impediments to care of patients.

Changes in institutional or provider practices that are perceived by patients as decreasing their satisfaction with the services, either in access or acceptability, will be a deterrent to PSRO growth, irrespective of how effective they might seem to professional eyes. It is difficult to imagine, for example, how the current activities in New Mexico that deny payment for unjustified use of the emergency room could possibly be transported to the heavily utilized emergency rooms in New York City.

There are areas where the PSRO operation alone will be expected to bring about change and improvement, but in the long run it is only in conjunction with a wide range of other agencies, both public and private, that the real impact of the program's operations can be judged. Has there been a decrease in the number of unnecessary acute-care beds? Is there a greater availability of alternate sources of care for the disabled, the feeble, or the disoriented older patient? Have the PSRO activities resulted in more appropriate use of health facilities, both institutional and ambulatory? Have other agencies, ranging from state Medicaid offices to professional societies of providers other than physicians, accepted and cooperated with the PSRO activities to bring about systemwide change? The American medical "system" or "nonsystem" has been famous for its resistance to change, for the failure of any one intervention effort, be it dollars (such as Title XIX) or programs (family planning or community mental health centers) to integrate with other resources. PSRO effectiveness in the long run will be measured by how the "system" responds, and many aspects of the change agents are beyond the influence of the PSRO.

6. Provider Impact

Again, aside from the impact on provider patterns of health care, the perceptions of the profession of the PSRO and its activities will be an important factor in the long-range effectiveness of the program. The initial response of organized medicine and many physician groups to the PSRO legislation was highly negative, and opposition was mounted in both printed documents and the courts of law. To a large extent this opposition has diminished at the present time. The reasons for this vary, and evaluation of the causes of the change may reveal much about the program direction. At one extreme, physician concern has been reduced by what has emerged in some PSROs at least as the reality of physician control. With this control has come a positive and professional approach to the medical issues of the day and a sense of ability to bring about change not hampered by lay interference. On the other hand, the acceptance of the PSRO entity by a number of physicians has come by virtue of their confirmed observations that there is no, or minimal, impingement on the traditional "freedom" of the physician to do as he or she chooses. The irritation caused by the untold number of review coordinators, who busily attach stickers to patients' charts and who ask questions that cause additional writing in some circumstances has been found to be completely controllable by virtue of the action (or nonaction) of a physician advisor. Often these physicians are close friends or colleagues and are irritated also by red tape and have no difficulty in using the physician advisor role consciously or subconsciously to subvert the purposes of the review process.

This is, indeed, one evaluation study whose results would be subject to vastly different interpretations should findings reveal that the once hostile medical profession is now wholeheartedly behind the effort of the PSROs to impact on the medical care system.

The increasing demands of the health professionals other than physicians for a meaningful role in the PSRO process is also one that evaluation efforts will need to address. Is there an impact on the practice of other health professionals? Are they having sufficient input into decisions that may affect not only their method of practice and income but also their perceived role in the health delivery system? Physicians have historically dominated the decision-making process in the health care industry, but their position is subject to continuing and increasing challenge not only by the public and lawmakers but by other professionals who are in a position to make significant contribution to the health care delivery scene.

The increasing number of professionals, lawmakers, and public citizens who are involved in making decisions regarding the health care system will have no difficulty coming to adverse decisions about the physician-dominated PSRO activities if indications of positive accomplishments are not demonstrated within the foreseeable future. Evaluation efforts, irrespective of the difficulties of methodologies and study design, need to be given high priority by all of those who continue to place faith in the medical profession's effort to effect change in the quality and cost of health care.

REFERENCES

1. Donabedian, A. 1978. A perspective on concepts of health care quality. Washington, D.C.: National Center for Health Services Research.

2. Peterson, O. 1966. Attributes of lifelong competence in medical practice. *JAMA.* 198(7):765–766.

3. Morehead, M.A., Donaldson, R., and Zanes, A. June 4–6, 1969. The Teamster comprehensive care program at Montefiore Hospital and Medical Center. *Proceedings, Nineteenth Annual Group Health Institute.*

4. Haggerty, R.J. (Project Director). 1975. Personal communication. Harvard School of Public Health, Albert Einstein College of Medicine, and New York Academy of Medicine.

5. Sanazaro, P.J. 1977. The PSRO program: Start of a new chapter? *N. Engl. J. Med.* 296(16):936–938.

6. Morehead, M.A. April 24–25, 1975. Ambulatory care review: A neglected priority. Presented at the 1975 Annual Health Conference of the New York Academy of Medicine, The Professional Responsibility for the Quality of Health Care.

Appendix A

Acronyms and Abbreviations

AAFMC	American Association of Foundations for Medical Care
AAPSRO	American Association of Professional Standards Review Organization
AC	Admission certification
ACAHC	Accreditation Council for Ambulatory Health Care
ACP	American College of Physicians
ACS	American College of Surgeons
AFDC	Aid to Families with Dependent Children
AGPA	American Group Practice Association
AHA	American Hospital Association
AIP	Annual implementation plan
ALOS	Average length of stay
AMA	American Medical Association
ART	Accredited Record Technician
ASIM	American Society of Internal Medicine
ASPERF	Assessment of performance
BC/BS	Blue Cross/Blue Shield
BHI	Bureau of Health Insurance
BHPRD	Bureau of Health Planning and Resource Development
BQA	Bureau of Quality Assurance
CAP	Colorado Admissions Program
CCS	Crippled Children's Service
CHAP	Certified Hospital Admission Program
CHDC	California Health Data Corporation

CHP	Comprehensive Health Planning
CHPA	Comprehensive Health Planning Association
CME	Continuing medical education
CON	Certificate of need
CONSERVE	Concurrent On-Site Evaluation and Review Effort
CPHA	Commission on Professional and Hospital Activities
CQA	Concurrent quality assurance
CQAS	Comprehensive Quality Assurance System
DHEW	Department of Health, Education, and Welfare
DME	Director of medical education
DOC	Days of care
ECF	Extended-care facility
ELOS	Expected length of stay
EMCRO	Experimental Medical Care Review Organization
EPAN	Evaluative profile analysis
ESRD	End-stage renal disease
FI	Fiscal intermediary
FMC	Foundation for Medical Care
GAO	General Accounting Office
GHAA	Group Health Association of America
HAP	Hospital Accreditation Program (JCAH)
HCFA	Health Care Financing Administration
HDS	Hospital Discharge Survey

HEW	Health, Education, and Welfare	OPEL	Office of Planning, Evaluation, and Legislation
HIAA	Health Insurance Association of America	OPSR	Office of Professional Standards Review
HICDA	Hospital-International Classification of Disease, Adapted	OSCHUR	On-Site Concurrent Hospital Utilization Review (Utah)
HIP	Health Insurance Plan (New York)	PA	Physician advisor
HMO	Health Maintenance Organization	PACE	Physician Ambulatory Care Evaluation (Utah)
HRA	Health Resources Administration		
HSA	Health Systems Agency	PAS	Professional Activities Study
HSP	Health systems plan	PAWG	Project Assessment Work Group
HSQB	Health Standards and Quality Bureau	PEP	Performance Evaluation Procedure (JCAH)
ICDA-8	International Classification of Diseases, Adapted for Use, 8th edition	PHDDS	PSRO Hospital Discharge Data Set
ICF	Intermediate care facility	PHS	Public Health Service
IOM	Institute of Medicine	PIPSRO	Private Initiative in PSRO
IPA	Individual Practice Association	PL 92–603	Social Security Amendments of 1972 (contains PSRO amendment)
IPS	Institute for Professional Standards		
JCAH	Joint Commission on Accreditation of Hospitals	PL 93–641	Health Planning and Resource Development Act
LOC	Level of care	PL 95–142	Medicare-Medicaid Fraud and Abuse Act
LOS	Length of stay		
LTC	Long-term care	PMIS	PSRO Management Information System
MAP	Medical audit program		
MCEs	Medical care evaluation studies	PRM	Program Review Manual
MCH	Maternal and Child Health	PPGP	Prepaid group practice
MGMA	Medical Group Management Association	PRN	Peer Review Network
		PSRO	Professional Standards Review Organization
MOU	Memorandum of understanding		
NABSP	National Association of Blue Shield Plans	QACE	Quality Assurance–Continuing Education
NAS	National Academy of Science	QAM	Quality assurance method
NAURC	National Association of Utilization Review Coordinators	QAP	Quality Assurance Program
		RC	Review coordinator
NCHS	National Center for Health Statistics	RMP	Regional Medical Programs
NCHSR&D	National Center for Health Services Research and Development	RRA	Registered record administrator
		RVS	Relative value scale
NHPRDA	National Health Planning and Resource Development Act	SHCC	Statewide Health Coordinating Council
NPSRC	National Professional Standards Review Council	SHPDA	Statewide Health Planning and Development Agency
OASH	Office of Assistant Secretary for Health	SMFP	Statewide medical facilities plan
OMB	Office of Management and Budget	SNF	Skilled nursing facility

SOSSUS	Study of Surgical Services in the United States	TAC	Technical Advisory Committee
		UHDDS	Uniform Hospital Discharge Data Set
SPAN	Supportive profile analysis	UPRO	Utah Professional Review Organization
SPSRC	Statewide Professional Standards Review Council		
SRS	Social and Rehabilitative Service	UR	Utilization review
SSA	Social Security Administration	URC	Utilization review committee

Appendix B
Methodology for EPAN Profile Development

The methodology for the development of EPAN profiles involves three steps: (1) formulating the objectives and goals of EPAN, (2) establishing a set of profiles in relationship to those objectives, and (3) generating a set of norms, standards, or criteria with which the profiles are analyzed. Although each step has been described in detail, a description of the type of data that should be used in a profile has been omitted for the mere reason that each PSRO has unique needs, health care patterns, and data. This fact, however, does not preclude giving examples of some possible profiles to clarify the extensive possibilities of EPAN.

This appendix contains four example profiles. All were developed according to the EPAN methodology in that they were designed to depict a specific component of the review system in terms of one of the many subobjectives of a PSRO. Each example profile contains a written description of the data elements to be profiled, the hypothesis about what the data elements may reflect, the criteria to be used in analyzing the profile, and, of course, the profile itself.

Although the data displayed in the profiles are imaginary, the information was developed with the intent of reflecting what would be realistically found in an active PSRO. The profiles were designed to depict the ten urban hospitals under the jurisdiction of a large PSRO and are conveniently labeled as hospitals A through J.

Example profile 1

Area for evaluation and monitoring: Health care providers

Area component: Administration

Profile subobjective: Appropriate utilization

Data elements: The percent of all hospital reviews along with the average number of days that are certified for each review where a reason code indicating "discharge planning delay" was used (Table B-1).

Hypothesis: Reason codes are used by the review coordinator during the concurrent review process to record certain aspects of a patient's acute-care stay. (The reason code indicating a "discharge planning delay" is used when the review coordinator feels that a patient's acute-care stay has been lengthened because of inadequate discharge planning.) It is hypothesized that when this particular reason code is used, it is an indication that there are acute-care days that are inappropriately utilized due to discharge planning problems.

Norms for the analysis of the profile: Realistically, there will always be a number of patients whose discharge is delayed for one reason or another. However, the number of times and number of days in which the reason code is used should be minimized. Using what occurs across the community as the supposedly normal extent of discharge planning delays, those hospitals above the eightieth percentile for either the average number of days that are certified or the number of times the reason code is used will be initially identified as having an excess of discharge planning delays. Additional investigation is then necessary to identify where those

384

TABLE B-1. Reason Code: Discharge Planning Delay

Hospital	1-3/76			4-6/76			7-9/76			10-12/76		
	No.	Percent	Average	No.	Percent	Average	No.	Percent	Average	No.	Percent	Average
A	20	0.47	3.60	49	1.37	10.70	20	0.44	2.91	45	1.04	2.00
B	14	0.30	3.60	5	0.07	3.10	46	1.10	4.17	30	0.72	3.68
C	44	2.48	3.03	50	2.69	3.34	31	1.72	3.47	21	1.04	3.04
D	5	0.20	2.10	9	0.92	1.90	18	2.64	1.60	7	0.49	1.77
E	12	0.81	2.47	7	0.47	2.10	17	1.28	6.87	14	1.14	4.00
F	37	0.84	6.74	24	0.55	4.35	68	1.65	4.77	25	0.54	5.00
G	15	1.01	3.01	19	1.60	3.10	25	1.83	4.20	7	0.35	3.10
H	16	0.43	3.50	26	2.48	2.55	17	1.37	3.25	36	3.25	3.32
I	17	0.21	3.60	4	0.04	2.10	13	0.37	2.88	15	0.46	2.92
J	20	0.33	3.66	16	0.27	2.68	6	0.09	3.10	16	0.31	3.85
Total PSRO	189	0.61	4.13	219	0.73	3.58	261	0.93	4.05	216	0.73	3.26

No. = The number of reviews for which the reason code was used.
Percent = The percent of the total reviews in which the reason code was used for each respective hospital.
Average = The average number of days that were certified when the reason code was used.
Those hospitals above the eightieth percentile are underlined (applied to both the percent of total certifications and the average days per certification).

discharge planning delays may lie. (There are ten hospitals in the PSRO area, therefore, the two hospitals with the highest values are those that are above the eightieth percentile.)

Example Profile 2

Area for evaluation and monitoring: Health care providers
Area component: Patient
Profile subobjective: Appropriate utilization
   Data elements: For those patients reviewed in each acute-care facility, the percentage distribution between the fiscal categories Medicare, Medicaid, and other (Table B-2).
   Hypothesis: It is hypothesized that different patient populations have unique health care utilization patterns. Although it is insufficient to identify different patient populations through the use of payment categories, if they are monitored in each acute-care facility, causes for different utilization patterns might be identified.

Norms for the analysis of the profile: This profile is one that describes the makeup of the patient population that is reviewed in each acute-care facility. Therefore, it is used as an aid in analyzing other profiles (particularly those profiles that are developed to evaluate utilization patterns), and no criteria are specified.

Example Profile 3

Area for evaluation and monitoring: PSRO
Area component: Review coordinators
Subobjective: Productivity
   Data elements: For each acute-care facility the average number of continued-stay certifications for each patient that is reviewed versus the average number of days certified for each continued-stay certification (Table B-3).
   Hypothesis: One of the main purposes for reviewing concurrently is that the review of the patient's acute-care stay takes place while the patient is hospitalized so that the review process has a greater

TABLE B-2.   Percentage Distribution by Payment Category

Hospital	1-3/76			4-6/76			7-9/76			10-12/76		
	MCR	MCD	Other	MCR	MCD	Other	MCR	MCD	Other	MCR	MCD	Other
A	61.7	24.7	13.6	61.2	26.5	13.3	58.2	26.9	14.9	61.0	25.5	13.5
B	75.1	24.9	0.0	76.6	22.7	0.7	74.9	25.0	0.1	74.1	24.3	1.6
C	74.0	8.7	17.3	74.2	7.8	18.0	74.6	8.7	16.7	73.7	10.0	16.3
D	74.5	9.7	15.8	75.9	10.1	14.0	75.1	13.7	11.2	75.8	11.7	12.5
E	64.5	35.5	0.0	68.3	32.4	0.3	68.5	30.0	1.5	61.5	36.6	1.9
F	42.8	48.4	8.8	39.1	48.7	12.2	42.8	45.7	12.5	43.4	43.1	13.5
G	72.7	11.5	15.8	71.7	16.3	13.0	69.9	16.4	13.7	73.0	17.1	9.9
H	97.0	1.0	2.0	95.4	4.6	0.0	93.9	6.1	0.0	96.0	2.0	2.0
I	64.5	17.8	17.7	64.4	14.9	20.7	61.8	15.9	22.4	63.9	14.9	21.2
J	60.6	4.4	35.0	83.5	8.9	7.6	60.2	7.9	31.9	75.5	8.2	16.3
Total PSRO	64.5	18.8	16.7	67.4	21.2	11.4	63.6	19.9	16.5	66.7	20.3	13.0

MCR = Medicare patients (percentage).
MCD = Medicaid patients (percentage).
Other = Those patients other than Medicare or Medicaid (percentage). (Private review).

immediate educational impact. Although in this PSRO the number of days that are certified on admission of the patient is statistically defined, the number of days for each continued-stay certification is up to the discretion of the review coordinator. The hypothesis for this profile is that there is a relationship between the average number of days that is certified per each continued-stay review and the number of continued-stay certifications per patient. The relationship between these two variables is that the longer the average days that are certified for each continued-stay review, the fewer average certifications per patient and vice versa. Although each hospital has its unique patient population and review procedures, extreme fluctuations between these two data elements may indicate that review resources are being allocated poorly.

Norms for the analysis of the profile: As the hypothesis implies, there is a reciprocal relationship between the average number of days assigned per continued-stay certification and the average number of continued-stay reviews per patient. Therefore,

the criteria for analysis assume that the total review community will set the proper relationship, and those hospitals that are above the eightieth percentile or below the twentieth percentile for either of the two data elements should be more closely analyzed for proper resource allocation.

Example Profile 4

Area for evaluation and monitoring: PSRO
Area component: Review coordinators
Subobjective: Productivity and efficiency
   Data elements: For each acute-care facility, the data elements include the average number of patients that are reviewed (average caseload) for each review coordinator in that facility as well as the ratio of that caseload to the average caseload for the total review community (Table B-4).
   Hypothesis: Although this is a rough indicator, it is hypothesized that the average caseload per review coordinator portrays the workload of that review coordinator. Although the number of patients that a

TABLE B-3.   Continued-stay Reviews

Hospital	1-3/76 Days	Ext.	4-6/76 Days	Ext.	7-9/76 Days	Ext.	10-12/76 Days	Ext.
A	4.19	1.25	4.74	1.16	4.08	1.12	3.76*	1.29
B	4.04	0.79*	4.07*	0.70*	3.95*	0.81*	4.06	0.76*
C	4.06	1.08	4.18	1.10	4.20	1.18	4.18	1.15
D	3.86	1.29	4.09	1.20	4.03	1.41	3.65*	1.24
E	3.78*	1.39	3.53*	1.18	3.75*	1.23	3.82	1.20
F	4.67	1.30	4.40	1.19	4.51	1.40	4.26	1.31
G	4.03	0.84	4.26	0.84	5.16	0.95	4.23	0.89
H	4.14	0.77*	4.45	0.66*	4.07	0.71*	4.20	0.82*
I	3.84*	1.16	4.60	0.93	4.05	0.91	3.86	1.03
J	4.21	1.16	4.15	1.13	4.38	1.07	4.30	1.07
Total PSRO	4.15	1.15	4.31	1.06	4.26	1.10	4.02	1.11

Days = The average number of days certified for each continued-stay review.
Ext. = The average number of continued-stay review per case.
* Those hospitals below the twentieth percentile.
Those hospitals above the eightieth percentile are underlined.

TABLE B-4.   Review Coordinator Caseload Analysis

Hospital	1-3/76 Average	Ratio	4-6/76 Average	Ratio	7-9/76 Average	Ratio	10-12/76 Average	Ratio
A	568	1.09	401*	0.78*	869	1.52	592	1.17
B	416	0.80	417	0.81	446	0.78	456*	0.90*
C	627	1.21	637	1.24	640	1.12	624	1.24
D	222*	0.43*	433	0.84	430*	0.75*	484	0.96
E	905	1.74	610	1.19	578	1.01	588	1.16
F	728	1.40	808	1.58	784	1.37	743	1.41
G	317*	0.61*	531	1.04	562	0.98	637	1.26
H	627	1.21	561	1.09	591	1.03	550	1.09
I	376	0.72	307*	0.60*	311*	0.54*	329*	0.65*
J	515	0.99	621	1.21	647	1.13	507	1.00
Total PSRO	519	—	513	—	573	—	505	—

Average = The average caseload per review coordinator (this is derived by dividing the total number of patients that are reviewed in each hospital by the number of review coordinators at that hospital).
Ratio = The ratio of the average caseload per review coordinator at each hospital to the average caseload per review coordinator for the total review community.
*Those hospitals whose average caseload is below the twentieth percentile.
Those hospitals whose average caseload is above the eightieth percentile.

review coordinator can review effectively fluctuates with review coordinator and hospital, there is a point beyond which the caseload is too great for effective review to be conducted. Similarly, extremely small caseloads may be an indicator that valuable review resources are being wasted. Therefore, the review coordinator caseload is one indicator of how review resources are being distributed across the community.

Norms for analysis of the profile: Based on the assumption that the average caseload for the total review community represents the appropriate caseload for review effectiveness, the criterion for analysis is that those acute-care facilities with the two highest average caseloads or the two lowest average caseloads require additional analysis to ensure that review resources are being properly allocated.

Appendix C
EPAN Hospital Profile

An EPAN hospital profile is one variation of the regular set of EPAN profiles that provides a comprehensive analysis of a hospital's review system and its health care patterns. Therefore, it follows that the EPAN hospital profile contains all EPAN profiles that are relevant to the particular hospital in question. A profile is determined to be relevant if it meets any one of the three following criteria:

    1. The profile is important in and of itself because of its descriptive aspects.
    2. The data for the particular hospital varies consistently from the standards or norms that were used in the evaluation of the profile.
    3. The profile helps to explain the data that are displayed in another profile.

The profiles that are chosen are combined into a document along with a brief summary analysis that is then used as part of the interaction process between the PSRO and the acute-care facility.

Based on the four profiles that were presented in Appendix B, an example of a hospital profile was developed for hospital F. The following is a brief summary analysis and the graphic displays that might be included in such a hospital profile.

Evaluative profile analysis: hospital profile
Hospital F—1976

This PSRO has developed a series of data profiles that were designed on a broad basis to identify and

monitor health care patterns as well as to serve as an aid in evaluating the concurrent review system. Four profiles appear to be particularly relevant to hospital F. These four profiles are displayed in Figures C-1 to C-4.

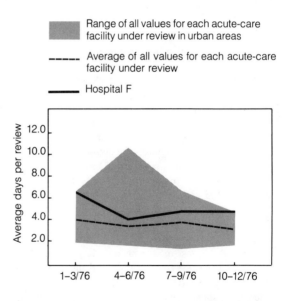

FIGURE C-1. Reason code: discharge planning delay. The average number of days that were assigned to each continued-stay review where a reason code indicating a "discharge planning delay" was used are consistently larger for Hospital F than what is observed as the average for the total review community.

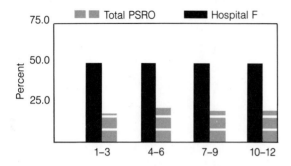

FIGURE C-2. Medicaid—percent of patients reviewed (1976). Of the three payment categories that are reviewed at Hospital F, approximately half of all patients reviewed are Medicaid. For all patients reviewed by the PSRO, 25% or less are Medicaid.

SUMMARY

Although the number of times the specific reason code indicating a "discharge planning delay" was used during the review process at hospital F is not high when compared with the average for the total PSRO, hospital F does tend to certify for a longer period of time. In the past, it has been suggested that discharge planning is more complicated at hospital F due to the unique problems that are continually presented to the discharge planning staff. These unique problems are due to the complexity of the patient population at this hospital. Hospital F is a large inner city hospital located in a neighborhood that is known for its high crime rates and also has the lowest median income in the city. These facts, along with the fact that hospital F, unlike any other hospital in the PSRO area, has the largest percentage of Medicaid patients, give some insight into the health, social, and economic problems of the patients at hospital F. Because of the length of the discharge planning delays at hospital F, this PSRO feels that investigation should be made into the possibility of adding staff or other resources to their discharge planning departments to better address the unique discharge problems of their patient population.

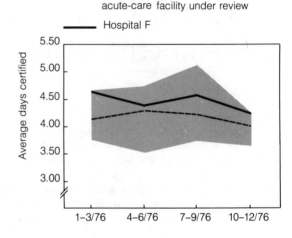

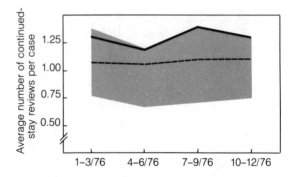

FIGURE C-3. Continued-stay reviews. Both the average number of days certified for each continued-stay review *(top)* and the average number of continued-stay reviews per case *(bottom)* at Hospital F are consistently higher than the same for all PSRO reviews.

Analysis of this PSRO's data has shown that there is a relationship between the average number of days that are certified for each continued-stay review, and the av-

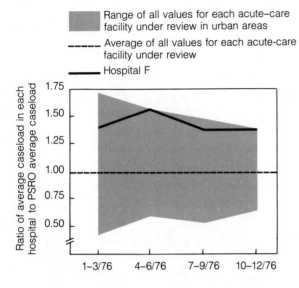

Range of all values for each acute–care facility under review in urban areas

Average of all values for each acute–care facility under review

Hospital F

FIGURE C-4.   Review coordinator caseload. The average caseload per review coordinator at Hospital F has been as much as approximately one and a half times the average caseload for the total PSRO.

erage number of continued-stay reviews per case. This relationship is such that the greater the average number of days that are certified for each continued-stay review, the fewer average certifications per case, and vice versa. How this relationship manifests itself depends on the individual hospital. Because of the complexity of the patient population at hospital F, it is felt that reviews for the continued stay of a patient should be conducted frequently. Therefore, the relationship between the average number of days assigned per continued-stay review and the average number of reviews per case at hospital F should be such that the average number of days that are certified are few, and the number of reviews per patient are high. The PSRO data reveal that the average number of days assigned per continued-stay review at hospital F are higher than that for the other nine hospitals in the PSRO area. When this information is reviewed along with the fact that the average caseload per review coordinator at hospital F is quite high, the conclusion becomes clear. The average caseload at hospital F is such that the review coordinators at hospital F do not have the resources or the energy to review as often as needed, the result being that to be able to review all patients, each continued-stay review is certified for a greater number of days than in actuality may be appropriate. This problem could easily be alleviated by increasing the review staff at hospital F so that effective concurrent review can take place.

Appendix D
Rural Tele-Audits: What Are They?

I would like to summarize our "rural hospital Tele-Audit project." The Health Care Review Center first became interested in the small hospital in early 1974 when it became obvious that a statewide program to meet the requirements of PSRO had to take into account the unique characteristics of rural hospitals. We held a 2-day conference to which we invited eight such hospitals to help identify and document those characteristics.

In the past fiscal year, while we have had a contract with the Washington/Alaska Regional Medical Program to develop a model for several rural hospitals in the central part of the state of Washington, we began looking for an alternative to the expensive multiple on-site visits required to develop the audit system in the rural hospitals. Furthermore, we needed a program that would recognize and deal with some of the unique characteristics of the rural hospitals as previously delineated. With the following objectives in mind, we decided to attempt to implement medical audit via telephone conference:

1. Combine continuing education at the beginning and during the development of criteria.

2. Help the hospital staff to develop valid and meaningful criteria for patient care in the isolated rural hospital.

3. Help the hospital staff interpret audit data to properly identify problems.

4. Help the hospital staff objectively select corrective action for identified problems.

5. Help the staff evaluate the results of its action.

6. Develop the multidisciplinary approach to review of patient care.

With these objectives in mind, the following procedure was developed for the rural hospital Tele-Audit:

1. The rural hospital audit committee selected a topic (a specific diagnosis, problem or procedure).
2. The Health Care Review Center, with the assistance of a physician specialist:
   a. Did a Medline search of the medical literature and selected two appropriate articles on the subject.
   b. Developed a list of ten key questions regarding the topic.
   c. Developed a proposed list of criteria based on the Health Care Review Center's experience at other hospitals and use of criteria sets available from various sources.

This material was mailed to the Health Care Review Coordinator at the rural hospital and distributed to the physicians and nurses who would participate in the Tele-Audit. The review of this material before the conference constituted the first element of continuing medical education.

3. The Tele-Audit conference:
Speaker phone sets had been installed in our Seattle office and the rural hospitals. The participants were as follows:
At the Health Care Review Center office:
The resource physician specialist

A moderator—a member of the Health Care Review Center staff

Other resource persons as needed, such as nurse and pharmacist

At the rural hospital:

One or more physicians

The director of nurses

Usually a nurse from one of the wards

The record room administrator

Depending on the subject, the pharmacist, a Medex, or other appropriate personnel would be invited to participate

Once the conference call is placed, the following procedure was followed after introducing the participants:

1. The topic was clearly identified and coded and a sample size agreed on.

2. The resource physician discussed the highlights of the topic for no more than 10 minutes (this is the second element of continuing medical education).

3. Using the criteria mailed to the rural hospital group, each category is discussed (criteria development). The physician specialist takes a very active part in settling controversial issues. (This is the third element of continuing medical education.) The rural hospital committee adopts its own criteria from the discussion.

This is the end of the first telephone conference, which usually takes from 1 to 1½ hours. A date for the second conference is set for 2 to 4 weeks hence. Between conferences the following activities take place:

1. The hospital record room person abstracts the data from the charts and displays them appropriately.

2. The local physician screens the data.

3. The data are mailed to the Health Care Review Center where they are studied.

The second telephone audit conference proceeds as follows:

1. Variations from agreed-upon criteria are discussed. The physician specialist is very helpful in deciding whether any of the variations are acceptable or not. (This is the fourth element of continuing medical education.)

2. Problems are identified.

3. Actions to solve the problems are agreed on.

These three areas of external support are keys to the success of the program since the isolated rural hospital often does not have the personnel or experience to properly identify the problems from the data or decide what is the best course of action. If the action decided on is an educational program for a staff meeting, the resource physician is an ideal person to go to the hospital and discuss the problems identified in the audit. This would be the final element of continuing education associated with the development of the criteria and identification of the problems. A re-audit of the topic would be planned for a year from the time the audit is completed to determine if the action taken corrected the problem. The time has not passed to take this final step.

Having completed eight audits now in nine rural hospitals, we can document the fact that the staff of each hospital has been enthusiastic about the procedure and wishes to continue the program. For the isolated rural hospital, the external support for internal decision-making supplied by the staff of the Health Care Review Center seems to be most meaningful. Combining it with the elements of continuing education seems logical and puts an entirely different flavor on a process which has often produced a negative feeling in the practicing physician.

Rural Hospital Program to Review Deaths

Purpose

1. To identify problems more effectively in the "quality of dying" as well as justifying death.

2. To provide documentation for Washington State PSRO or hospitals (or both) that deaths are systematically reviewed.

Management

Physician reviewer

Procedure	Responsibility
1. Pull "death charts" and attach check-off sheet.	Head nurse on ward

2. Review case using screening criteria.	Physician reviewer
3. Document comments and recommendations.	Physician reviewer
4. Written monthly report to executive committee.	Physician reviewer
5. Identify problems and action taken.	Executive committee

SCREENING QUESTIONS FOR MORTALITY REVIEW

_____ Chart No. _____

Questions	Comments
1. Was patient's condition on *admission* such that death was anticipated, for example, severe heart disease or failure, COPD with lung failure, renal failure, or advanced cancer?	
2. Did a complication related to treatment develop, and did it result in death, for example, hemorrhage secondary to use of antibiotics, drug reaction leading to renal shutdown, infection following surgery (peritonitis), death associated with anesthesia?	
3. Did the patient die during or within 48 hours after surgery?	
4. If patient was terminally ill on admission, was hospitalization justified?	
5. In your opinion, was treatment excessive, such as use of blood, antibiotics, cortisone, consultants for each body system?	
6. Was pain controlled? Did the physician order prn medication in a hopeless case with severe pain, or was medication given in anticipation of pain?	
7. Did the primary condition plus secondary diagnoses justify death?	
8. In your opinion, what was the factor(s) that caused death (may not be necessarily disease oriented)?	
9. Based on your evaluation, would you recommend further review of this death?	

Index